ANATOMY OF PSYCHIATRIC ADMINISTRATION

The Organization in Health and Disease

TOPICS IN SOCIAL PSYCHIATRY

Series Editor: Ellen L. Bassuk, M.D.

The Better Homes Foundation
Newton Centre, Massachusetts
and Harvard Medical School
Boston, Massachusetts

ANATOMY OF PSYCHIATRIC ADMINISTRATION
The Organization in Health and Disease
Milton Greenblatt, M.D., in collaboration with Paul Rodenhauser, M.D.

HOMELESSNESS
A National Perspective
Edited by Marjorie J. Robertson, Ph.D., and Milton Greenblatt, M.D.

RESPONDING TO THE HOMELESS
Policy and Practice
Russell K. Schutt, Ph.D., and Gerald R. Garrett, Ph.D.

A Continuation Order Plan is available for this series. A continuation order will bring delivery of each new volume immediately upon publication. Volumes are billed only upon actual shipment. For further information please contact the publisher.

ANATOMY OF PSYCHIATRIC ADMINISTRATION

The Organization in Health and Disease

Milton Greenblatt, M.D.

Olive View Medical Center—Los Angeles County
Sylmar, California
and University of California, Los Angeles
Los Angeles, California

In collaboration with

Paul Rodenhauser, M.D.

Tulane University School of Medicine
New Orleans, Louisiana

PLENUM PRESS • NEW YORK AND LONDON

Library of Congress Cataloging-in-Publication Data

Greenblatt, Milton.
    Anatomy of psychiatric administration : the organization in health
and disease / Milton Greenblatt, in collaboration with Paul
Rodenhauser.
        p.   cm. -- (Topics in social psychiatry)
    Includes bibliographical references and index.
    ISBN 0-306-44143-8
    1. Mental health services--Administration. 2. Psychiatric
hospitals--Administration.   I. Rodenhauser, Paul. II. Title.
III. Series.
    [DNLM: 1. Hospitals, Psychiatric--organization & administration.
WM 30 G798a]
RA790.5.G74   1992
362.2'068--dc20
DNLM/DLC
for Library of Congress   92-12133
                                                              CIP

ISBN 0-306-44143-8

© 1992 Plenum Press, New York
A Division of Plenum Publishing Corporation
233 Spring Street, New York, N.Y. 10013

Printed in the United States of America

To
LEW HARRIS,
1912–1991,
my wonderful brother

Preface

When the 13 founders of the American Psychiatric Association came together in 1844, hospitals were small, and the administrative aspects of a superintendent's job were relatively minor compared with their size and complexity today. Since the turn of the century, administration—the art and the science—has become a specialty of great importance, particularly in big business and government. Business recognizes fully that the success of organizational endeavors depends to a great extent on the talents and energies of top leaders. As a result, industry spends huge sums of money to train promising young executives and offers generous salaries and benefits to entice them. Anyone who wants to invest in a business first asks: "Who manages this organization, and is this management competitive in today's marketplace?"

Although health is today a great industry, emphasis on the executive role has lagged behind that in the general business field. In mental health circles, the strong emphasis on one-to-one therapy has delayed a full appreciation of the influence of organization per se on patient care and treatment. Yet there are now many signs of change. The popularization of behavioral science[1] and the rise of social and community psychiatry have brought organizational considerations forward. We are increasingly concerned with the human side of enterprise, with worker satisfaction, group dynamics, and organizational morale. Other flags have been unfurled. As a result of the growing influence of the Joint Commission on Accreditation of Healthcare Organizations and the multiplication of standard-setting and regulatory agencies, quality assurance has become an administrative subspecialty. Since 1954, the American Psychiatric Association has been conducting specialty examinations for psychiatric administrators.[2] Societies that recognize administration as an important specialty are growing in prominence. And administrative experience has become a requirement for the specialty diploma in psychiatry awarded by the American Board of Psychiatry and Neurology.[3]

More and more specialists in mental health fields—psychiatrists, nurses, social workers, psychologists, and rehabilitation experts, as well as people in community relations, marketing, development, research, planning, architecture, and psychopolitics—realize that mastery of at least the rudiments of good administration may spell the difference between success and failure. The twin administrative tasks of fostering high productivity and cultivating morale are only the beginning of the job. Even more important is the recognition that effective administration often holds the key to the very survival of an organization. In these endeavors the functions of the executive are crucial variables and bear the utmost scrutiny. The 1953 statement of the World Health Organization's Expert Committee[4] as to the influence of top leaders strikes a very responsive chord today:

> The most important single factor in the efficacy of the treatment given in a mental hospital appears to the committee to be an intangible element which can only be described as its atmosphere. . . . As in the community at large one of the characteristic aspects of the psychiatric hospital is the type of relationship between people that are to be found in it. The nature of the relationship between the medical director and his staff will be reflected in the relationship between the psychiatric staff and the nurses, and finally not only between the nurses and the patients, but between the patients themselves.

For anyone entertaining the thought of becoming an administrator, it is highly desirable that he* suffer no hesitations about assuming the role of a leader—that is, making critical judgments concerning the lives and welfare of many people and the programs and services of an entire institution. He should be attuned to the needs of workers, to the purposes of the institution, and to the changing times. At the same time this individual may be accountable to many agencies, must adapt to multiple limitations on his authority, and in all probability must also serve as cooperative subordinate in a larger organization. Thus, he is responsive to complex internal and external forces as well as to individuals and systems. The "social system clinician" view of the administrator's role, identified below, is an attempt to embrace both administrator and system in one theoretical perspective. The clinician role expresses the caretaking/treatment responsibilities of the administrator for a living system or organization that is subject to both health and disease.

My professional experience has brought a number of perspectives on administration into sharper focus: (a) The *systems view is the vital one* for the administrator. The leader of an organization must have information related to goals, resources, policies, and procedures necessary for the most effective functioning of the organization. He receives critical inputs from many

---

*The masculine singular pronouns are used throughout for the sake of convenience, with full acknowledgment of the bias inherent in the practice.

sources; then, using participatory management techniques, he integrates that information into a master plan, peculiarly adjusted to the realities of the times.[5,6] The process of decision making and the master planning associated with it involve many members of the organization at varying levels of responsibility.

(b) As indicated above, for leaders-to-be in the field of mental health, the primary and overarching role is that of *social system clinician,* a concept first advanced in 1957.[7] Briefly, the social system (the organization) is viewed as a living system, subject to health and disease. Borrowing from Claude Bernard,[8] we can see the system as subject to ups and downs—based on disturbances or dysfunctions—but with a decided tendency to reequilibrate or return to its former level of adjustment. The disturbances arise from either inner or outer stimuli, and their "pathological valence" is measured by the degree to which they inhibit the progress of the organization toward its avowed goals. Broadly speaking, these goals are to provide the best possible services to individuals and to a community.

The administrator is seen as playing the leading role in setting goals, recognizing as early as possible signs and symptoms of disturbance, planning appropriate interventions (treatments), and following through to restoration of organizational health. This formulation leans heavily on concepts borrowed from medicine, with its concern for the health of individuals and the effective functioning of systems of service delivery.

(c) Because pathology in a system manifests itself in the thinking, attitudes, and behaviors of the persons in it, I have emphasized in particular the analysis of *psychological and psychodynamic aspects of both workers' and administrators' behavior.* This of necessity includes an understanding of the myriad overt and covert ways in which individuals in a system display "neurotic residues," personality aberrations, and areas of emotional distress.[9] A system may be able to tolerate considerable immature behavior in some of its employees without serious disruption, but it may be very seriously affected by similar immaturities acted out by a top executive.

(d) To look at organizational disruptions, I have again introduced a *systems approach* that is familiar in this field. I discuss problems of executives entering the system (input), and then those happenings within systems that lead to disequilibrium and eventually to a new equilibrium (throughput). Problems and issues related to stresses and strains of executive careers and, finally, issues relating to the departure of the leader from the system (output) are considered. Economics of survival and the relations of the therapeutic system to the outer environment round out the presentation.

(e) A vital perspective used throughout the book is that *the social system itself is embedded in the matrix of the larger community.* Thus, the relationships of a hospital to the community network of agencies, services, and conditions—the political system, the media, professional organizations, educational institutions, regulating agencies, volunteers and citizen movements, surrounding clinics and facilities, labor, and the homeless—cannot be neglected. Since these outside influences have grown greatly in complexity and importance, the issues and problems they represent will be referred to often in the text.

(f) Finally, this volume is generously supplied with *case examples*—not examples of individual pathology, but examples of systems gone awry, of symptoms and dysfunctions that compromise the goals of the institution. Whereas casebooks in medicine have been popular since the time of Richard Cabot's famous *Differential Diagnosis*,[10] casebooks on system pathology in mental health organizations are notably lacking. I hope, to some extent, to correct that deficiency.

To whom is this book addressed? It is addressed principally to administrators of mental health facilities, meant to include psychiatrists who are or plan to become clinician-executives; also to trained professional administrators, as well as administrators from allied fields—nursing, social work, psychology, and so forth. Although the psychiatrist as system clinician is the main target, the numerous case examples and general principles expounded are relevant to all those who find themselves in leadership/executive roles. *Administrators of experience* appreciate the constant challenge of broadening their theoretical and practical perspective on organizations and the role of the leader; keeping up with the relevant literature is a formidable task. For them, the historical review of selected literature on scientific management (Chapter 2) and the conceptualization of their role as social system clinicians (Chapter 3) may be helpful. Entering and leaving the system (Chapter 4), a long-term special interest of mine, has not to my knowledge been dealt with extensively in other texts. The explorations of internal stresses and strains and human resource management (Chapters 5 and 6) may offer further insights into the administrator's everyday vicissitudes. The section on ethics of administration (Chapter 8) begins to do justice to the increasing importance of ethics to those in public life, particularly when resource strictures make critical decisions difficult. Economics (Chapter 7), the role of the administrator in education and research (Chapter 9), the relation of the organization to the outside world (Chapter 10), and executive careers (Chapter 12) are subjects worthy of special attention.

It is my hope that *young administrators* and students of administration will also profit from discussion of problems of entry, and the relationship of the administrator to governing bodies (Chapter 5); administrative stresses and strains and how they may be overcome (Chapter 12); vicissitudes in managing diminishing budgets (Chapter 7); power and decision making (Chapter 11); relation to the outside world (Chapter 10); and ethical dilemmas (Chapter 8). I also hope that the reader will gain a fuller appreciation of the extraordinary contribution a leader of an organization can make to his constituents, as simultaneously the shouldering of heavy responsibilities molds him into a more thoughtful and mature human being.

The reader is entitled to be informed about the author's background and experience. In my case, these include many years of administration in university, state, county, and Department of Veterans Affairs (VA) hospitals, and the planning and implementing of programs for the mentally ill at many levels. Specific positions include director of research and assistant superintendent at Harvard's Massachusetts Mental Health Center; superintendent of Boston State Hospital; commissioner of mental health in the commonwealth of Massachusetts; director of psychiatry at Sepulveda VA Medical Center (Los Angeles); chief of staff of Brentwood VA Medical Center (Los Angeles); director of hospital and clinics of the Neuropsychiatric Institute, UCLA; and chief of psychiatry for Los Angeles County–Olive View Medical Center. In the academic sphere, my appointments have been on the faculties of Harvard Medical School, Tufts School of Medicine, and Boston University School of Medicine; as assistant dean of the UCLA School of Medicine, and currently as professor and vice chairman of the UCLA Department of Psychiatry and Biobehavioral Sciences while serving as head of the psychiatry department at Olive View Medical Center. My experience spans more than 50 years. My colleagues have honored me with many local and national offices in professional organizations and associations. I have published over 300 articles and books, mostly in the fields of clinical psychiatry, organizational dynamics, administration, and psychopolitics.

ACKNOWLEDGMENTS

The exciting challenge in undertaking this book has been to try to fashion a *different*, if not entirely "new," book on administration. To the extent that we have been successful in this endeavor, my collaborator and I are indebted to our teachers and associates, our students, and the dedicated employees of the many organizations that have given us the privileges of studying and working with them. Above all, we appreciate the cooperation of our patients, who are the ultimate justification for all we do.

My genial and generous collaborator, Dr. Paul Rodenhauser, is currently director of medical student education in psychiatry at Tulane University School of Medicine and is the originator of a comprehensive course on administration that he has conducted for 10 years, and to which I was regularly invited as a contributor. His belief in what I might have to offer inspired the efforts that eventually resulted in this volume. He critiqued every chapter, offered valuable suggestions, and supplied specific material from his own experience. The three sabbatical months he spent with me in Los Angeles were vital to the completion of the manuscript.

Over many years, deans Sherman Mellinkoff, M.D., and Kenneth I. Shine, M.D., and associate dean Esther F. Hays, M.D., of the UCLA School of Medicine have been strongly supportive of all my endeavors, for which support I am eternally grateful.

Of the many people who have generously contributed to this effort, I mention specifically Louis Jolyon West, M.D., formerly director of the Neuropsychiatric Institute, UCLA; Douglas Bagley, director, Bruce Picken, M.D., medical director, and Marianne Z. Kainz, director of nursing, at Olive View Medical Center; and Milton H. Miller, M.D., chief of psychiatry at Harbor–UCLA Medical Center.

Individuals who carefully critiqued the manuscript or specific chapters in it, with considerable subsequent improvement in the quality of the book, include Ellen Bassuk, M.D.—who, in addition to serving as editorial liaison with our publishers, provided us with a penetrating analysis of the entire manuscript. Our debt to Gordon Strauss, M.D., who critically reviewed Chapters 1, 2, 3, 4, and 11, and in addition encouraged members of the UCLA Center for Group and Organizational Dynamics (of which he is director) to review other chapters, is very great. Members of the center who undertook serious editorial scrutiny of individual chapters include David Beck, M.D.; Vivian Gold, Ph.D.; James Lock, M.D., Ph.D.; John Lundgren, M.D.; Ronald M. Sharrin, Ph.D.; and Kathryn West, Ph.D. Charles J. Canales, chief of personnel at Olive View Medical Center, critically analyzed Chapter 6, resulting in significant improvement in that chapter. Other readers of individual chapters were Joan B. Barron, M.N., R.N., C.S.; Ching-piao Chien, M.D.; Frank A. DeLeon-Jones, M.D.; James Ketchum, M.D.; James Preis, J.D.; Mario Sewell, M.A., M.P.H.; and Pranav V. Shah, M.D. Raymond L. Eden, associate dean for administration at UCLA School of Medicine, was helpful with the chapter outlines.

In addition to the above generous contributors, Donald A. Schwartz, M.D., an expert in administration, examined Chapter 11 carefully, submitting many excellent suggestions; and Alan Steinberg, Ph.D., an expert in philosophy and ethics, gave much appreciated attention to Chapter 8. Jacqueline C. Bouhoutsos, Ph.D., an expert on the subject, gave critical advice on the section on therapist–patient sexual contact in Chapter 8.

Individuals who generously agreed to personal interviews include Douglas Bagley, Charles J. Canales, Howard Freeman, Oscar Grusky, Marianne Z. Kainz, Debrya J. Moore, William G. Ouchi, Carolyn Rhee, and Joel Yager.

In the course of my long career in many organizations, particular individuals stand out as having made a lasting impression on my life and work. I wish to express my deepest gratitude to Harvard professor and superintendent of Massachusetts Mental Health Center, Harry C. Solomon, M.D., my mentor and professional "father"; and also to Walter E. Barton, M.D.; J. Sanbourne Bockoven, M.D.; Wilfred Bloomberg, M.D.; Bertram S. Brown, M. D.; Esther Lucile Brown, Ph.D.; James W. Dykens, M.D.; Jack R. Ewalt, M.D.; Philip B. Hallen; Robert W. Hyde, M.D.; James G. Miller, M.D., Ph.D.; and Maida H. Solomon, M.S.W.

Representatives of Plenum Publishing Corporation were understanding and cooperative, making our collaboration most pleasant. We are especially indebted to Eliot Werner, Mariclaire Cloutier, and Christopher Dreyer.

REFERENCES

1. National Industrial Conference Board: The world of work and the behavioral sciences: A perspective and an overview, Chapter 1 in Behavioral Science: Concepts and Management Application. New York, The Conference Board, 1969, pp. 1–8
2. American Psychiatric Association, Committee on Administrative Psychiatry: Information Bulletin for Applicants, ed 9. Washington, DC, American Psychiatric Association, 1984
3. American Medical Association: Special requirements for residency training in psychiatry, in The 1988 Directory of Graduate Medical Education Programs. Chicago, American Medical Association, 1988, p 98
4. Expert Committee on Mental Health: Third Report. The Community Mental Hospital. Geneva, World Health Organization, Technical Series No. 73, 1953, pp 17–18
5. Rodenhauser P, Segal M: Performance appraisal and organizational issues in a mental health setting. Admin in Mental Health 10:181–194, 1983
6. McGregor D: The Human Side of Enterprise. New York, McGraw-Hill, 1960
7. Greenblatt M: The psychiatrist as social system clinician, in Greenblatt M, Levinson DJ, Williams RH (eds): The Patient and the Mental Hospital. Glencoe, Illinois, Free Press, 1957, pp 317–326
8. Virtanen R: Claude Bernard and His Place in the History of Ideas. Lincoln, Nebraska, University of Nebraska Press, 1960
9. Kets de Vries MFR (ed): The Irrational Executive: Psychoanalytic Studies in Management. New York, International Universities Press, 1984
10. Cabot RC: Differential Diagnosis. Philadelphia, Saunders, pp 1911–1915

Contents

List of Case Illustrations

Chapter 5

Chapter 6

Chapter 7

Chapter 8

Chapter 9

Chapter 10

Chapter 11

Chapter 12

1

Perspectives

Since 1900 there has been a virtual management explosion.* It is now universally recognized that the success of many enterprises depends largely on good administrators. Meeting today's intense competition puts a great premium upon the development of highly creative leaders, and effective management is ever more critical as organizations grow in size and complexity. The wealth of industry and of nations, government's ability to rule effectively, and indeed our place in the world affairs are all dependent on activities that are highly coordinated among many leaders possessing great skill and resourcefulness.

Big corporations have evolved *pari passu* with the emergence of extraordinarily talented administrators. General Motors, for example, enjoys revenues greater than most of the states in our country, and the 50 largest corporations in America have a larger gross income than all 50 states together.[1] The formation of conglomerates, the rise of arbitrageurism and business takeovers, and the emergence of multinational enterprises require managers who can direct organizations so vast that the comprehension of the details of any small section is far beyond the reach of the human mind.

The early management boom focused first on technical skills and competencies of managers. It was internally oriented and technocratic in its approach. But technical knowledge now is not enough. Leaders have learned to focus on worker motivations, public relations, and company reputation, as well as on outside economic and political trends. Even performance and profit are not enough, for executives are now searching for higher contribution and

*The literature in this field does not discriminate precisely between *manager, administrator,* and *executive.* The terms are often used interchangeably, and dictionaries tend to use one term to define the other.

achievement, even a new type of morality. Keenly aware of the mass of humanity that depends on them for sustenance and growth, administrators are thinking of the personal fulfillment of individuals in society, as well as the broader needs of society itself.

More and more, top management faces the daunting challenge of keeping up with changing demographic trends, political practices, and social policy. Drucker,[2] a prolific writer on management theory, estimates that top industrial executives spend four-fifths of their time in outside relationships. In Japan, top administrators classically relate to government, banks, other industries, and to the body politic. Their inside concerns are related primarily to training new leaders who will succeed them, and with plotting the very long-term course of their companies.

Drucker,[3,4,5] compares top management with a chamber ensemble. Players are equal, but one is the leader. In the future we will undoubtedly depend not on a single individual of great energy and talent, but on constellations of executives working together, it is hoped, in harmonious relationships.

The need for managerial talent is also very great in the field of health services. Here, too, increases in size and complexity of systems as well as rapid changes in technology and philosophy offer unending challenges.

As I view the history and present status of care systems in mental health from the vantage point of 50 years of experience, eight characteristics stand out above all others:

1. The enormous *diversity* of programs, facilities, and managerial perspectives
2. A great *turbulence* that characterizes the present scene
3. A national trend from *health policy* to *fiscal policy*
4. Changes in the *public attitude* toward the mentally ill (but still, see number 5)
5. Continuing *stigma* attached to mental and emotional disorders
6. *Competition* among health services organizations
7. Emergence of a *new trinity*—marketing, public relations, and development (i.e., fund-raising)
8. Changes in *patterns of care* of the mentally ill

DIVERSITY

The field of administration is very broad and its boundaries often vague. Within this field many *kinds* of institutions exist. They vary in size, in patient population, in governance, in the nature of their support, in community mission, and in treatment philosophy. Everyone would probably agree that a "typical" state hospital differs greatly from a "typical" university hospital. A Department of Veterans Affairs (VA) hospital differs greatly from a private institution. Since the 1960s, when the comprehensive community mental health center became the centerpiece of the deinstitutionalization movement, this model was added to the system of services dominated by the "old" state hospital. Yet, many of the "old" state hospitals underwent radical transformations during this period. The Boston State Hospital of the 1940s, for example, with 3,300 inpatients (mostly chronic) and a small outpatient service numbering around 200, was radically different from the Boston State Hospital of the 1960s, with its 1,400 inpatients; or the hospital of the 1970s, with less than 150 inpatients and an ambulatory population numbering in the thousands!

In governance, it makes a great deal of difference whether the hospital is ultimately governed by an administration a thousand miles away, as in the Department of Veterans Affairs, or by (in the case of a private institution) a selected and readily accessible group of citizens who meet regularly in a hospital building. The conceptions and goals that govern one institution among 172 similar institutions included within a grand VA national alliance are dramatically different from those ruling a for-profit hospital that is a member of a multihospital corporate chain.

As for administrators, they, too, vary greatly: in education, personal background, age, training, experience, and philosophy. The values, loyalties, conceptions, strategies, and general modes of thinking of administrators in one system may be vastly different from those in another.

Personality and style of administrators, too, are distributed along a very broad continuum—authoritarian versus egalitarian; "tight" versus "loose" style; outgoing versus reserved; entrepreneurial versus conservative, and so forth. Executive/administrative styles are probably as diverse and complex as personality itself. Executive style is also necessarily influenced by type of institution, background and philosophy, and current stage of development. Recently, in the book *The Irrational Executive*,[6] an attempt was made by a number of contributors to link executive style and its effect on systems to the personality and psychodynamics of the administrator—giving more weight than formerly to the influence of neurotic conflicts and behavior residues on their functioning. The assumption is made that relatively small immaturities or character deviations of individuals in powerful executive roles may have disproportionately large effects on the organizations they lead.

The staffs and patients of the various kinds of institutions also differ vastly from one another. The variations are determined by a host of factors, including sponsorship (private for-profit, private not-for-profit, university, state, county, or federal), services provided (acute, chronic, substance abuse, and/or child/adolescent/adult/geriatric programs), educational/research emphasis, and hierarchy of preferred or favored therapeutic approaches.

A gross example of staff differences is immediately apparent when comparing university personnel with personnel in a county hospital within one city in southern California. In the university system, professional staff members have the extraordinary privilege of time to think, discuss, study, and do research. In some county institutions, the burden of service to a superabundance of clients—with inadequate numbers of staff persons—gives personnel little time for creative reflection, research, or scholarly undertakings. Many staff persons of long tenure in such institutions look with envy, wonderment, and awe at those in the university system whose lives have been blessed with academic values and strivings.

Who, then, may be so bold as to present a book about administration in today's bewildering kaleidoscope of people, institutions, and missions? Indeed, the present author has hesitated long before embarking on such a hazardous task. However, it is because of the difficulties in comprehending a field of great diversity and vague boundaries and literally dozens of theoretical views (see Chapter 3) that a single perspective based on long practical experience may have value to the reader. Further, a theoretical position that I favor, outlined in Chapter 3, attempts to embrace and, it is hoped, simplify previous concepts related to the leader-organizational complex that we all strive to comprehend.

TURBULENT TIMES

The entire health industry has been facing turbulent times. In the 1960s and part of the 1970s, expansion and growth were the primary motifs. But in the 1980s the industry has been characterized by progressive restraints, stringent competition, and attempts at restructuring.

Survival has become an increasing preoccupation in organizational life. In one study,[7] 57% of CEOs stated that their hospital's survival was threatened. The smaller the hospital, the greater the perceived threat. Of the CEOs themselves, 28% thought their own survival in office was in doubt. More and more CEOs in corporations are asking for personal employment contracts with guarantees of at least three to five years of tenure.

As a result, much greater emphasis has been placed on strategic planning, enhancement of adaptive capacity, sales and marketing techniques, and broadening the health care mission, as well as the generation of new services (products). Stronger management teams and additional training for executives have been stressed. Closer cooperation between CEOs and staff and between CEOs and boards of directors is ever more critical. Staffs are learning to respect budget realities and to participate more in financial planning.

In a sense, the whole health care industry is under siege. Many hospitals have already folded; more are expected to follow. The old luxuries of long hospitalization and time to work with patients in dynamic psychotherapeutic relationships are essentially passé. The cherished professional ideal of the highest possible quality of care is being contaminated by practical budgetary considerations. Due partly to the increasingly complicated tasks facing management, medical leadership of health care organizations is yielding to professional management. Public access to care, particularly for the uninsured poor, is steadily being limited, as health care costs escalate and insurance coverage tightens. The organization of health care itself has become increasingly complicated, technologized, and difficult to administer.

THE NATIONAL TREND: FROM HEALTH POLICY
TO FISCAL POLICY[8]

Despite a formidable jump in health care expenditures for the nation, from $303.2 billion in 1980 to $438.9 billion in 1987, we are still far from the ideal of universal access to medical care. In fact, because of rising costs and reduced budgets, quantity and quality of services have suffered, and an actual phaseout of many "safety net" hospitals has occurred.

Rising costs of medical care have resulted from both social changes and great advances in medical science and technology. These include the aging of the population, inflation, expensive management information systems, costs of meeting regulatory and standard-setting agency requirements, the need to practice medicine defensively, and rapidly rising expenses of risk management. The growing sophistication of consumers asking for second and third opinions—in effect, functioning as a new body overseeing and monitoring patient care—adds further to the expense of medical services.

Quality Assurance

In recent decades, society has made considerable progress in the acceptance of the concept that health care systems must be subjected to careful monitoring, and that this monitoring must not be left to doctors alone. Since Medicare, Medicaid, and other third parties are paying the bills, these agencies want substantial returns on their dollars; therefore, they subject the institutions to additional accountability that adds greatly to their expenses. The proliferation of utilization review and quality assurance committees and the sudden emergence of quality monitoring as a new area of specialization attest to this phenomenon. Management information systems are expanded and refined to assist reporting required by monitoring agencies. It is a far cry from the days when Dr. Mesrop Tarumianz, supported by a grant from the DuPont Company of Delaware, conducted surveys of the mental hospitals of the 1930s and 1940s virtually alone and reported their deficiencies to the American Psychiatric Association.

Today, JCAHO (the Joint Commission on Accreditation of Healthcare Organizations) reigns supreme in the realm of accrediting agencies. Its triennial inspections are taken very seriously. No private or public hospital can afford to be put on probation, for the flow of governmental and insurance funds is often contingent on continued good standing with that body. An upcoming survey by JCAHO is a signal for broad-based mobilization of staff and departments. Memoranda fly, records are updated, and many directives are sent to individuals and hospital subunits for their compliance. Preparation for JCAHO reviews has become increasingly demanding of staff and administrative time—and increasingly costly (see "Regulation: Licensure and Accreditation" in Chapter 10).

Risk Management

In addition to the above drains on hospital finances, risk management has become a critical specialty in the effort to reduce unpredictable losses due to lawsuits charging negligence or faulty practice. Today the public is very alert. Mistakes made by the medical profession are sensationalized by the press. In a busy emergency room, the wrong leg may have been put in a cast, or a sponge left in the abdomen. A miscalculation in dosage may lead to complications, even death. The story of a confused attendant or nurse with peculiar notions as to when life supports may be turned off frightens the public. More lawyers specializing in malpractice are winning large awards; and large awards, in even a few cases, may threaten the fiscal stability of a medical center (see "Risk Management" in Chapter 7).

Government Involvement

Government was the big force in changing the shape of financial policy when in 1983 it shifted from reimbursing hospitals for costs incurred (and thus guaranteeing them a profit) to setting prices it would pay for nearly 500 different illnesses and treatments (i.e., prospective payments). Prices for so-called diagnostic related groups (DRGs) were based on national statistics and set at levels that would force the more costly hospitals down to a national average. Those hospitals that could not meet the standards were penalized by reimbursement cuts; those that did better than the national average would receive a financial reward. It was a new plan to control and reduce costs—but no sooner was the national average attained by a statistically outlying institution than the average was reset at a lower level. As the budget crunch got more severe, hospitals that earned a reward might find the reward reduced or even eliminated altogether. (Although DRG policy was relaxed for psychiatric hospitals, the trend established has been felt nationally.)

Medicare reviewers, over a period of years, looked critically over the shoulders of hospital physicians, warning that some medical procedures were overused or should be eliminated. Often reviewers ruled that hospital stays were too long and therefore reimbursements would have to be cut. Thus, many health care establishments ran into financial reversals; as a consequence, in many instances they cut back, sold out, or merged.

Ethical Questions

Extraordinary technological growth in the health sciences in the last decades has fostered a great interest in medical ethics. Many questions are being asked about the moral implications of the technology explosion. Callahan[9] of the Hastings Institute has formulated one aspect of the problem in his controversial book *Setting Limits: Medical Goals in an Aging Society.* He argues that as longevity increases and the incidence and prevalence of diseases in the elderly increases exponentially, many are kept alive through modern technology even though the *quality* of their lives has deteriorated enormously. As society's huge financial commitment to the elderly increases, too great a share of its resources is withdrawn from other sectors of the population, particularly children and young adults. Callahan recommends setting a limit beyond which society declares that there will be no further investment of scarce resources in particular individuals. How that limit is defined, or by whom it is decided or implemented, is not explicated. This concept, viewed by some as a "duty to die," has not gained instant acceptance. Yet, resources are in fact inadequate to take care of all our elderly persons with protracted illnesses. Limits are being set de facto, without adequate planning or resolution of the ethical issues involved.

The Response

Hospital managers responded with radical changes in practices and procedures. They reduced hospital stays and utilized less expensive services, such as outpatient treatment and home care (in surgery, in 1981, 19% of all procedures were carried out in outpatient departments; by 1986, it rose to 40%). Hospitals that were delivering substantial amounts of services to indigents took steps to change the mix of patients in favor of those who could pay. When insurance payments for patients were ultimately exhausted, financial imperatives forced hospitals to turn many patients away. Two public outcries were heard: that patients were being discharged prematurely; and that patients from financially stressed hospitals were being transferred, or "dumped," onto other hospitals.

As indicated above, many hospitals that were losing money had to close. The statistics are shattering. According to the American Hospital Association report of 1989,[10] 81 community hospitals in 28 states closed their doors in 1988, slightly increased from 79 hospitals in 1987. Since 1980, 445 community hospitals have closed. (Half of all urban hospitals, and 70% of rural hospitals, had lost money during the previous few years caring for patients with inadequate resources.) Of the 81 community hospitals that closed in 1988, 41 were not-for-profit facilities, 31 were for-profit facilities, and 9 were government owned. In addition, 21 specialty hospitals in 15 states closed in that same year. The principal reasons given were inadequate Medicare payments, loss of physicians, and assorted other economic problems. Where hospital beds became vacant, employees were laid off; perhaps a few were rehired when occupancy increased. To survive, hospitals paid more attention to marketing, public relations, and fund-raising (see "The New Trinity" later in this chapter).

Some say the health care industry as a whole is running toward bankruptcy. There is increasing clamor for governmental subsidies, especially for the safety-net hospitals serving the poor. People fortunate enough to afford health insurance find that copayments are larger, and that restrictions on coverage ceilings force them to pay a larger share of overall costs. All parties—government, insurance companies, and beneficiaries—are glad to turn to private industry asking for help. In some states, notably Massachusetts, legislation has been enacted requiring employers to finance minimal care for everyone. In 1988, the landmark Medicare Catastrophic Protection Act was passed to help the elderly avoid financial ruin. This was to be financed by a levy on both industry and the elderly. However, the plan was eventually overturned by a subsequent act of Congress, based on a determination that the tax was inequitable. Overall, during this period, as far as the consumer is concerned, critical ground has been lost, for the number of uninsured nationally has grown from 29 million in 1980 to 37 million in 1988.

To repeat: quality of care has suffered, the medical profession has lost much of its influence on health care, money has become an essential driver of health policy, and health care has become a product or commodity increasingly subject to measurement and manipulation. Many physicians also feel a loss of professional integrity and idealism. A strange uneasiness prevails that caregivers have become hired pawns in a chess game in which the dollar is king.

CHANGES IN PUBLIC ATTITUDES TOWARD THE MENTALLY ILL

Great shifts in attitudes toward the mentally ill have occurred in recent decades. In the years that I have worked in mental health, the following have been most impressive. Fifty years ago, institutions were almost exclusively governmentally endowed; relatively few private hospitals existed. Admissions were almost all involuntary, and medical decisions in the care and treatment of mentally ill patients reigned supreme. Regulations of psychiatric practice were few in number, widespread third-party coverage did not exist, research was at a low ebb, and medical student education in mental health (with Harvard a prime example) was given low priority. Treatment regimens consisted of a few drugs—barbiturates, bromides, and paraldehyde—together with some social and recreational activities, but very little psychotherapy, or family or group therapy. Seclusion, wet sheet packs, hydrotherapy, and physical and chemical restraints were regularly prescribed. The attitudes were custodial, and the patients regarded as dangerous. The profession of psychiatry had little esteem in the family of medical specialties, and the social stigma attached to mental diseases was pervasive.

We were at the beginning of a long climb toward greater understanding of the needs of patients, and reorganization of hospitals along egalitarian rather than authoritarian lines. The great postwar boom of interest in the mentally ill accelerated this trend. I have described elsewhere[11,12] the introduction of many new treatment modalities and the massive investment by the federal government and the states in research, education, and innovative clinical methods of care. Much of this boom became known as the "deinstitutionalization movement." Thousands of patients were discharged from hospitals to be managed in various ambulatory settings; the banner of social and community psychiatry was raised (see "the Deinstitutionalization Movement" in Chapter 7).

This whole movement peaked around the middle to late 1960s. In the late 1970s the pendulum swung back again to the negative side, and with its rapid acceleration many of the gains of 30 years were undermined. The liberal policies of more than a generation began to be replaced by regressive, reactionary trends that some have described as a movement toward "recriminalization" of mental patients. More and more admissions were involuntary, closed ward doors replaced open doors, patients were searched before admission for contraband, and many were prohibited from purchase and possession of firearms. The fear of violence in society found its counterpart in the fear of violence in the hospital—this despite great legal and judicial gains in patient rights in the last 25 years.

The deinstitutionalization movement gathered much strength during the 1960s and early 1970s, but adherents to social and community psychiatry then began to do battle with so-called hospital psychiatrists. I used to hear of community partisans who were "hospital busters," and hospital partisans who were "community busters." Further indicated in Chapter 7 is the fact that federal funds for community mental health centers began to decline after the Kennedy–Johnson influence abated. Critics within psychiatry bemoaned the lack of research that would permit evaluation of what the deinstitutionalization movement had accomplished. This falling off of interest and support for deinstitutionalization has at times been referred to as the "collapse of the community movement."

Nowhere was this reversal more striking than in California, which had formerly led the nation in its liberal policies. Voluntary hospitalization turned to involuntary detention for most acute and chronic cases. Hospitalization time was progressively shortened, personalized psychotherapeutic care and treatment almost vanished, drug treatment became more prominent, and admission policies based on clinical severity of illness often dominated selection of subjects for treatment. Many patients found that admission to a hospital might only be achieved by going through the penal route, for the department of corrections was given first priority in the admission of psychotic individuals.

The care and treatment of the mentally ill is a reflection of their economic, political, and humanitarian status in the body politic at any given time; relatively sudden, large pendulum swings can erase gains made over decades. Unlike the national economy, no regulatory agency like the Federal Reserve Board exists to iron out dangerous fluctuations. Unfortunately, the care of the mentally ill appears to be more susceptible to social, political, and economic shifts than other branches of medicine.

STIGMA ATTACHED TO MENTAL AND EMOTIONAL DISORDERS

Most will agree that the stigma attached to mental disease has decreased, especially where centers of education exist and many members of the intelligentsia have sought relief of emotional disturbance through consultation with mental health practitioners. Particularly after World War II, the popularity of psychoanalysis flourished in this country, and with it the utilization of dynamically oriented psychotherapy. Psychoanalytic training became the "in" thing among the growing population of psychiatric residents and practitioners. Practitioners from allied fields—psychology, social work, family practice—greatly expanded the number of patients receiving care for mental disorders. The advent of tranquilizers, anxiolytics, antidepressants, and antipsychotics gave hope to many that their illnesses could be alleviated or even cured. Many emotionally ill people were encouraged to seek help earlier in the course of their illness, when treatment results were more promising. Then, too, the increase in outpatient clinics greatly expanded the numbers of patients served. As the aggressive, violent behaviors of mentally ill cases were alleviated by medication, fear of the mentally ill decreased. Yet, the great, largely unconscious concern about "losing one's mind" and the published stories of violence attributed to the mentally ill continue to stoke the fires of fear. It is against such primeval dreads that psychiatry tries to make progress in its fight against prejudice.

In many general hospitals, discrimination is also felt. This is in relation not only to the mental patients but also to mental health service units or departments. Psychiatry often occupies a low place compared to other disciplines. When psychiatric services were gaining importance in patient care, and also in terms of financial returns, inpatient wards were established in many general hospitals—sometimes, to be sure, against considerable resistance. The concern was that disturbed patients would wander into medical and surgical wards and seriously disrupt treatment of other patients, or that they would act bizarrely, affronting staff and visitors. Hence, mental wards were often closed off from other parts of the general hospital.

How do we explain prejudice of this sort? In general hospitals, the concept of acute disease caused by defined etiology is still a familiar notion as well as an important assumption in medical education. In mental illness, etiology is more complex, including genetic, biological, psychological, and social factors entering into the patient's life in a complex, interrelated, developmental fashion. The treatment approaches are more fuzzy, the course of disease more chronic, and theoretical postulations more rampant and speculative. To hard scientists, psychiatry is a loose, less scientific field. Some medical students and even psychiatric residents find it hard to grasp the concept of the "therapeutic use of the self," or to employ this approach within the framework of subtly operating transference–countertransference mechanisms. Thus, a large gulf may separate the mental health department from more medically oriented departments in a general hospital.

The intensity of therapeutic activity on medical and surgical wards may give psychiatry a lower priority among administrators of general hospitals. Surgeons operate under tense conditions; their patients need a great deal of preoperative preparation and postoperative care. Surgical and medical personnel are occupied with intravenous fusions, lumbar punctures, gastric feedings, isolation precautions, cardiac monitoring, and respiratory care. The level of alertness is high, and emergencies are common. In contrast, patients on psychiatric wards walk around and wear street clothes. Their treatment consists of neuroleptic medication, psychotherapy, and group activities. Personnel *do* handle disruptions caused by aggressive or violent behavior, or by suicide attempts, but in general the pace of life is slower. Psychotherapy goes on behind closed doors, and recreational therapy is often outside the wards. Thus, medical and/or surgical personnel—and administrators, too—may view mental health workers as having an easier life. Administration responds quickly to the need for emergency equipment and nursing personnel to keep operating rooms functioning. Obstetrical patients may, therefore, get service before psychiatric patients receive attention.

To this may be added the fact that per diem costs for medicine, surgery, gynecology, and obstetrics are higher than psychiatry, and reimbursement for care and treatment proportionately greater. In many hospitals, departments other than psychiatry are much larger in size, both in beds and in numbers of personnel and patients; they, therefore, consume a greater share of the total budget.

Matters may be made even worse if two other factors exist: prejudice (conscious or unconscious) on the part of significant figures in the hospital chain of command, and ignorance in administrative circles as to how psychiatric patients should be treated or how a department of psychiatry should be run.

Case Illustration

What Can Happen When the "Security Motif" Takes Over

The following is an example of how reactionary concepts regarding the treatment of mental patients were incorporated into plans for a new hospital facility that opened in the 1980s. Custodialism and security were emphasized in many decisions pertaining to the mentally ill. All doors to psychiatric wards were locked; keys were issued only to "safe" persons. In fact, keys were denied to almost all therapeutic persons, but put into the possession of ward clerks. To obtain admission to the wards, doctors, psychologists, and social workers had to ring the door bell, then wait until the ward clerk opened the door! Normal traffic between therapeutic personnel and their patients was thus controlled by the ward clerk (who, it should be noted, was not always readily available). In this way, the relationships of treatment staff to patients were administratively obstructed—on the one hand by a heavy closed door, and on the other hand by the uncertain availability and possibly even the whims of a ward clerk. To cap it off, the department of psychiatry was not fully consulted as to this particular arrangement. This assumption that security was to be the main principle governing the care of the mentally ill—and the more security, the better—was obviously oblivious to major lessons or the past, namely, that in the name of "security" more hardships, injuries, confinements, restraints, restrictions, camisoles, and chains had been visited against the mentally ill than against any other group in history.

Thus, in ways subtle and not so subtle, discrimination is exercised against mental patients, even within hospitals supposedly dedicated to their health and welfare. Some of it undoubtedly arises from imbedded prejudices based on past unhappy experiences with the mentally ill. Some of it reflects lack of education concerning modern methods of care and treatment of the mentally ill.

Returning to the case illustration, the "key" fiasco was eventually resolved at the ardent insistence of the head of psychiatry that *all* therapeutic personnel be given easy access to the wards and their patients. Fears that keys might be lost and that the wards thus would be exposed to outside "evil" influences eventually yielded to the findings that risks were actually very low and that the staff was highly responsible in the use of keys.

COMPETITION AMONG HEALTH SERVICE ORGANIZATIONS

Competition among hospitals can be fierce, and indeed many hospitals have failed to thrive. To achieve a secure market share of paying clients, hospitals strive for diversity and richness in services and programs. In some communities, it may be impossible to survive without arteriography, cardiac bypass surgery, or advanced angioplasty. The capability for organ transplant surgery may make one institution stand out over another. The best house officers choose places for training that will best prepare them for future practice. Recruiting a specialist of renown to a hospital may make a critical difference in revenue enhancement and institutional fiscal health.

During the deinstitutionalization period, mental hospitals tended to be ranked according to their advancement toward goals set by national plans. If an institution lacked one or more of the five essential programs recommended by the federal government—namely, inpatient, outpatient, and transitional care, crisis management, and community education—it was difficult for an administrator to hold his head up, much less obtain federal funds. It was important then to serve a geographically defined population and to involve the community in both planning and implementation. Later it was necessary to develop programs to serve children and adolescents, geriatric individuals, and the chemically dependent. A flourishing day-care service was something one could brag about relative to fulfilling the requirement of a "transitional facility." Another mark of esteem was success in reducing the population of chronic patients by developing community alternatives for their care and treatment.

Competition between universities can also be fierce. It is in their natures to desire to be "number one"; if not overall, then at least in some sub-speciality. The appointment of a new dean in one university, for example, resulted in an 18-month master plan for the medical school's future, in which the planners averred that the medical center was to become the best in the nation within a specified period of time. This meant raising millions of dollars to support specialized research areas of promise (in this case, genetics and neuroscience). Some feared that this attempt to mobilize the creative talents of a mighty university towards a prescribed goal might constrain individual faculty members' natural curiosity or creative direction. Perhaps a freer exercise of talents might serve society and the university better in the long run.

How *does* one measure the relative worthy of academic institutions, and by what scales? Is it based on numbers of publications, their influence upon the thought and practice of the day, or on the number of "big names" attracted to the institution? Is it based on a reputation in teaching and research that makes students flock to its halls? Is it related to the impact of alumni on the community, the number of leadership roles they assume and their influence on society's future?

Within institutions, ideological differences may determine the areas in which special recognition is sought and where the money is spent. My experience in two university research and training institutions—one on the East Coast and one on the West Coast, both devoted to mental health and bio-behavioral sciences—highlights this difference.

The East Coast department, in its hierarchy of values, placed clinical care first, education second, and research third. Although that institution had considerable strength in all three areas, the director's creed was that "our first task is to achieve the highest possible level of care and treatment of our patients. Our greatest craft is to get them well."[13] Education, he felt, consisted in teaching professionals how this was done, mainly by progressively improving care and treatment, assuming personal responsibility for the minutiae of patient comfort, establishing warm and understanding therapist–patient relationships, prescribing with great wisdom, and artfully coaching the treatment team toward maximum use of its potentialities. Research, he said, was primarily in the interest of patient care. Although all kinds of research were encouraged, that which had the potential for early clinical application received most stress. He was a practical man, from a practitioner-oriented family, who himself had been a practitioner before becoming superintendent of the esteemed institution.

On the West Coast, the department of psychiatry was fashioned more along the lines of a Max Planck Institute. Research was held in highest esteem, education was next, and clinical care was last. Again, all three areas were heavily represented, but faculty valued above all their place in the academic ladder; ascension up that ladder was primarily through original research.

Both institutions held education of professionals, particularly psychiatric residents and medical students, in high esteem. A full panoply of ancillary professionals also received instruction—nurses, social workers, psychologists, rehabilitation counselors, and many others. In fact, both institutions functioned as small universities, with large numbers of undergraduates and graduates passing through their doors in the course of a year.

Which system is the better, the down-to-earth quality of the East Coast establishment and its emphasis on service, or the West Coast institute with its primary emphasis on research? Indeed, some of the professors in the western institute, illustrious in their fields, did not treat patients on the wards from one year to the next. One major professor stated that it would be unfair to patients for him to take on any duties of clinical care. He was too rusty!

THE NEW TRINITY

For many administrators, the "new trinity" is public relations, marketing, and development—the last of these being a euphemism for fund-raising. As has been mentioned, increasing competition for paying patients, diminished income from third parties, and escalating costs of new health technology have given this trinity of functions a new, survivalist meaning. Their functions are interrelated; their common purposes are to make the institution highly effective in treatment and, certainly, financially secure.

Here are some of the imperative goals of the trinity:

1. *Establish an image, both within the institution and in the community, of humane, individualized quality care and treatment for every patient—and concern for the feelings of the family.* If the hospital has developed a high level of care and concern for every patient in its charge, it is indeed fortunate, and word of mouth will eventually do well for its future. To achieve these ends requires careful selection of employees: kind and generous of heart, who enjoy caring for people, and who are themselves reasonably happy and satisfied with their lot in life. Equally important are kindness and caring attitudes in administration and other important norm-setting personnel, and good communication between top-level staff and lower echelons. There is no room for coolness, standoffishness, hostile criticism, impatience with patients and families—or for turning off employees, patients, or relatives when they hunger for a good word. Above all, morale within the institution must be maintained at a high level. A strike of hospital employees, for example, may tarnish the hospital's reputation for many months. However, rapid restoration of morale can be achieved after a strike, as the following example indicates.

Case Illustration

Morale Problems after a Strike

Morale among nurses was badly affected by a strike brought on by low pay, a shortage of nurses, poor working conditions, and the recognition that quality care of patients was suffering. Nurses faced the choice of joining the picket line, thus contributing to the dangers of thin staffing on wards with very sick patients, or staying on duty and looking after sick patients without the support of their striking colleagues. Administrative and training staffs of the nursing service pitched in, working together with those few nurses who remained "loyal." When the strike was over, some ward nurses were in tears because of exhaustion from overwork and the tension and anger directed against their coworkers for "deserting" them.

Severely troubled by such estrangements, nurse supervisors requested a group therapist to help restore morale among aggrieved personnel and to heal bitter wounds. A psychoanalytically trained psychiatrist of senior rank with considerable group experience took on the job. His kindness and objectivity in understanding the feelings of both sides, and his willingness to accept angry expressions as inevitable under the circumstances, quieted the turbulence in a few weeks, restored respect, and encouraged mutual forgiveness by the aggrieved parties. (When we speak of public relations, we often forget that there are two components to a public relations program—one is internal, the other is external. Internal public relations really is the process of cultivating the good will and efficiency [in Barnard's sense] of the employees; external public relations cultivates the goodwill of outside constituencies.)

Relying exclusively on word of mouth to spread awareness of the good work of the hospital, however, is not always enough. It may be a slow process, not sufficiently effective in the short run to meet the competition—because daily, in the media and many other ways, other institutions are also seeking clients based on *their* alleged high quality of care. Many public relations programs depend on the hiring of experienced professional public relations personnel who identify and promote a "theme" or "image" for the institution that is bolstered and supported by endorsements from patients and families, then repeated in best marketable forms.

2. *Relate the hospital and its program to specific target groups and to utilize the media to maximum advantage.* One key way to do this is to pay attention to the referring doctors and other referring professionals. That these individuals are worth their weight in gold is well-known in private institutions, but often neglected in public institutions. A small group of professionals with busy practices can be the heartbeat of the private hospital. They are cultivated by the following means, among others: (a) personal contact with staff as soon as their patients are scheduled for admission to the hospital or clinic, (b) discussion and sharing of treatment plans, (c) timely reports to update knowledge, (d) invitation to join the professional staff and to participate in the governance of the hospital, (e) invitation to participate in a clinical staff organization, (f)

dissemination of news about hospital life and times, and (g) invitation to social events designed to encourage interaction between referring professionals and staff members.

Another strategy is to target public relations toward selected societies, clubs, and uplift organizations in the community. An effective approach is to form a speakers' bureau, which assigns selected staff members to talk to outside groups on topics of the latter's choice. The requirement for this equation is to fit the appropriate staff member to the right club or selected group. Thus, a staff member who belongs to Kiwanis or Rotary may be a proper selection for one of these societies, provided that the individual is vivacious, enthusiastic about the institution, and capable of delivering an interesting speech. It should be noted that not all staff members are excited about forming bridges to community organizations; some resist on the basis that it is business, not medicine. They may be reminded that good community relations are an important element in patient care, let alone in the survival of the institution and, as such, the protection of their jobs. The reports of other speakers who have learned how much the community hungers for authentic health information and who have enjoyed their experiences may be even more convincing.

In addition to the above, spot announcements on radio, TV, or newspapers, often as fillers, may be accepted by the media without charge. Vignettes of public interest should be solicited from every department by the public information officer for release to the media. For example, the establishment of a new outpatient service, the acquisition of a major piece of equipment, an honor won by a staff worker, or the creation of a new clinic are all interesting to the citizens. The public relations expert educates the hospital staff to think in these terms.

It is not difficult to think of topics of great concern to the general public. Parents concerned about suicide or substance abuse in children want to hear about early manifestations of these disorders. Helpful information regarding the multiple crises of marital separation and divorce will appeal to almost everyone. Many will come to meetings to hear about management of the alcoholic person or the loved one with Alzheimer's disease. The hospital should become known for its experts who are willing to share knowledge that they are able to couch in terms understandable to laypersons.

Not all hospitals are equally interested in public relations, marketing, and fund-raising. Further, this interest is changing with the times. State and county institutions, for example, in the past have been almost totally dependent on governmental support; however, with the recent budget crunches, they, too, turn to third-party payers, and are interested in capturing a share of that market. State and county university-affiliated hospitals are particular examples of agencies that formerly received most of their funds from governmental sources, but as a result of escalating costs and restricted revenues have entered the competitive market for private support.

CHANGES IN PATTERNS OF CARE: INSIDE THE INSTITUTION

When the administrator, functioning as a social system clinician (see Chapter 3), looks at the organization, everywhere he sees movement, action, a system in dynamic change. A legion of questions come to mind. What kind of care and treatment is the patient really receiving? Is it the best that can be offered? Is it modern state of the art? And how shall we judge its efficacy?

Historically, treatment has varied greatly. In the time of the French Revolution, Pinel[14] propounded his philosophy of "moral treatment." It taught that mentally ill patients do not suffer from lesions of the brain or skull; they suffer instead from accumulated unhappy experiences of life, and all the chains and flogging that history has invented will not do for them what kindness and forbearance can do. During this period, enlightened understanding of the patient's psychological problems accomplished wonders under the guidance of men like the Tukes, Woodward, Todd, Butler, Ray, and Brigham.[15] Viewing this enlightened period of moral treatment in America, historians are struck by what moral treatment alone could accomplish without the modern trappings of neuroleptic drugs, individual and family therapy, social therapy, or psychoanalytic techniques.

In the 1930s and 1940s, somatic therapies prevailed, chiefly insulin coma and electrotherapy—the one soon discarded, the other highly popular until the advent of neuroleptic drugs. After World War I, penicillin proved to be *the* successful somatic weapon against neurosyphilis. However, somatic dominance was soon challenged by the rise of interest in social psychiatry. Biological treatments were complemented by social advances. In the 1950s, the age of psychopharmacotherapy came upon us—antidepressants, anxiolytics, and antipsychotics. And in the 1960s, deinstitutionalization became a national movement, supported by many of the professional associations in the nation and backed financially by both federal and local governments.

With all these historic changes, what seems to have endured through time is the importance of *kindness and forbearance* in interpersonal relationships as typified in the best moral-treatment hospitals of 150 years ago, and in the therapeutic climate of the best institutions of today.

This truism, accepted by many leaders, directs administrative attention to the quality of staff—not merely their technical expertness, but their humane characteristics. Everyone's morale, therefore, becomes part of the therapeutic climate, including that of the administrator.

What Helps the Patient?

In a therapeutic community, treatment of the individual patient is influenced by no less than the totality of all his relationships and experiences. The institution as a whole functions as a therapeutic milieu. It may be difficult, without careful study of all of the patient's contacts and activities, to decide where his greatest help comes from. Not infrequently, we discover, the patient's idea of what helped him differs from that of trained professionals.

> In a university teaching hospital with an open therapeutic community atmosphere, 60% of the patients were assigned to individual therapy on a once-a-week basis.
>
> When asked, "Who, of all the *people* around, helped you the most?" answers from a group of 120 patients, in order of frequency, were: doctor, 42; nurse, 26; other patients, 18; social worker, 5; occupational therapy personnel, 4; medical student, 4. (Some patients did not respond.)
>
> When the same group was asked, "What *things* that happened to you helped the most?" their answers were: doctors, 26; hospital in general, 16; somatic treatments, 13; other patients, 10; occupational therapy, 8; contact with people, 6; rest, 6; contact with community, 5.
>
> When asked, "If you had any troubles, whom would you go to talk to?" they answered: doctor, 67; nurse or attendant, 16; social worker, 9; other patients, 5; family, 5.[16]

In this example, patients pointed to a variety of influences that helped them; doctors appear to vary greatly in importance, depending on the form of the question. Patients and staff do not necessarily agree as to what was therapeutically effective. Sometimes, it was noted, an improvement that the clinical staff attributed mainly to electroconvulsive therapy was attributed by the patient to a kindly nurse or attendant. In some cases where the officially assigned therapist felt he or she was centrally significant to a patient, it turned out therapy was actually controlled by another person who had a greater hold on the patient's confidence. Finally, it is interesting that "other patients" are mentioned 18 and 5 times (in separate questions) as being of help, and that the "hospital in general" is mentioned as being of help to 16 different patients. Thus, it would appear that in an open community where natural affinities can be expressed, a patient may relate positively to many different individuals, or even to the institution as a whole, as if it were an organic entity. While it is possible that patients may be mistaken in identifying who or what truly helped them, it would also be shortsighted for management to neglect the patient's view of his therapeutic environment.

The Multiple Subcultures in the Mental Hospital

Each hospital is a small society with an ideology, values, beliefs, and behaviors that set it apart from other systems. In the 1940s and 1950s, social anthropologists and other social scientists published many studies showing how the hospital's social structure had an impact upon patient care and treatment. Their fascinating work led to many profound insights and some major reforms. They helped focus attention on the disgraceful living conditions existing in many of our large state hospitals, how these contributed to the patients' illness, and how neglect, rejection, and pessimism led many into chronicity. In this period several ardent students and some journalists were themselves admitted to mental hospitals as "patients" and exposed firsthand to what Albert Deutsch[17] described as *The Shame of the States.*

Case Illustrations

Researchers Admitted as Patients

As a "patient" admitted to the Yale Institute of Human Relations, social anthropologist Caudill[18] tells of eating lunch with other patients and explaining to them how he had become sick through a series of emotionally disturbing events. "Well," said one patient, "for someone so sick you sure have a good appetite." Whereupon Caudill suddenly lost some of his interest in food. This incident was used by Caudill to show how patient culture and expectations can shape the behavior of individuals in a system.

In another study, several "research" attendants (students from a nearby university) were allowed to work alongside regularly employed attendants in a large state hospital. From their reports it was learned that in order for new attendants to be admitted to good status among their fellows, it was sometimes necessary to beat patients or to steal. One of the attendants described how she gained entry into attendant culture:

> The general attitude went something like this: "There is no use trying to keep things nice on this ward. The patients tear up, mess up, or throw away every decent thing that is brought here. . . . I am poor and can't afford to buy all I need. Why shouldn't I take home one of these nice blankets. . . . This isn't on the same plane as stealing."[19]

The attendant was often urged to take things home and did steal a dozen eggs and a dress to demonstrate she was one of the gang and to incriminate herself with them. She helped others steal, for it was in poor taste to take things without the support of other attendants. It was a way of ensuring group cover-up in case of accusation by a supervisor.

Like a cancer growing on the body politic, this criminalization of attendants continued for a long time until it was discovered by a perspicacious administrator and finally rooted out. A system of protective corruption had been established (not unusual in the old mental hospital) that had allowed a steady rate of pilferage to drain the budget and cheat the patients of their due.

A last example concerns a group of college students who were "admitted" to a state hospital to learn firsthand what it was like to be a patient, and to report their experiences in the hope of effecting improvement in the patients' lives. The students spent several days and nights at the institution. What stands out in memory was the fear and revulsion, mixed with pity and compassion for the patients, felt by the students. They described fear of sleeping in the same dormitory with dozens of other patients who were disturbed, babbling, shrieking, and pacing restlessly about. Apprehensive that they might be attacked and pounded while they were asleep, they held a tense, wakeful vigil throughout the night; then, deprived of sleep, their mornings became a struggle against drowsiness as they attempted to carry on their work. Needless to say, the students' experiences gave the administration a deeper insight into the lives of patients, and incidentally had a powerful impact on the public when revealed by the press.

These examples point out that although each hospital has a character and image all its own, it contains within it many idiosyncratic subcultures. These cultural subgroups may be defined by functional divisions, as with those separating nurses, attendants, patients, and doctors. Others are totally informal and even hidden—for example, the patient cliques and friendships that form spontaneously, as illustrated in the case of Ruth (see "Commentary" on p 139), or the racial subgroups that spring up, as in the example of racism reported by a Pakistani doctor (see "Case Illustration: Racism in a Public Mental Hospital" in Chapter 5).

Administrators of any institution cannot afford to neglect these subsystems. Nurses and attendants, because of their close association with patients many hours each day, possess considerable knowledge of these relationships and are willing to teach us a great deal, if we will listen. Doctors who are in and out of the wards or administrators who periodically walk around do not acquire this information as easily. In one old-fashioned state hospital reported in the literature,[20] when the administrator made his rounds, the chief attendant (always interested in making a good impression on his chief and in keeping things quiet) was immediately notified by his wife, the telephone operator, who was positioned to know whenever the superintendent left his office. The superintendent going on rounds with the chief attendant then saw what he was programmed to see—namely, that all was well. In such a situation, the administrator may remain blind for a long time to what is truly going on in his own organization, a virtual captive of an unseen conspiracy.

SUMMARY AND COMMENTS

From the perspective of 50 years in the field, I identify eight characteristics of today's mental health scene that stand out above all others. First is the enormous *diversity* of programs, facilities, and managerial perspectives. Institutions vary in size, in staff and patient population, in governance, in the nature of their support, in the personality, philosophy, and style of administrators, and in their goals and missions.

A great *turbulence* also characterizes the present era. In the 1960s and part of the 1970s, expansion and growth were the primary motifs. The decade of the 1980s was characterized by progressive restraints, stringent competition, and attempts at restructuring. Survival has become an increasing preoccupation in organizational life. Many hospitals failed. Budgetary realities complicate professional ideals, and medical leadership of health care organizations is yielding to professional management.

Third, a national trend from *health policy* to *fiscal policy* has become dominant, with many changes resulting from the rising cost of medical care:

- *Quality assurance* has become a new specialty associated with the proliferation of utilization review and quality assurance committees, expanded management information systems, and the growing importance of regulatory and standard-setting agencies.
- *Risk management*, now a critical function, has developed specifically to
  reduce unpredictable losses related to lawsuits charging negligence or
  faulty practice.
- *Government involvement* has changed the shape of financial policy from
  reimbursement for costs incurred to prospective payments. Private insurers have followed suit. A variety of new insurance programs offers
  benefits of value to various classes of consumers. Governmental regulatory and standard-setting agencies have added their burdens to private-sector standard-setting agencies.
- *Ethical questions* have come to the fore, emphasizing principles and
  priorities in the *rationing* of care in a climate of austerity and reduced
  resources.
- All the above have given rise to new *patterns of coping responses* from
  administrators, providers, investors, and the government. Hospital
  managers reduce hospital stays, utilize less expensive services, and
  develop new, attractive revenue-enhancing programs. Merging of institutions, as well as phaseout of specific programs and even total
  organizations, has occurred. Marketing, public relations, and fund-
  raising have become the new trinity relied on to bail out embattled
  facilities.

Fourth, major changes in the *public attitude* toward the mentally ill have
occurred. Fifty years ago, most mental institutions were governmentally
owned; few private hospitals existed. Admissions were primarily involuntary.
Medical-psychiatric decisions reigned supreme. Regulations were fewer in
number and scope, and research was at a low ebb. In recent decades, many
gains in hospital management and treatment programs, as well as a great
movement toward community care, with emphasis on patient rights and
privileges have occurred. The deinstitutionalization movement accentuated
reduction in size or total elimination of state hospitals and their replacement
by comprehensive community mental health centers sited in populated areas.
Research and educational programs have enjoyed great expansion. Unfortunately, a recent serious retrenchment associated with economic hardships,
severe federal budgetary cutbacks, and a weakening of the thrust toward
community care has surfaced.

Fifth, the *stigma* attached to mental and emotional disorders is still prevalent, manifested as discrimination against mental patients both in the community and in some (especially general) hospitals. The low priority generally

assigned to social welfare programs for racial minorities and the poor is particularly noted during times of fiscal austerity.

Sixth, *competition* among health services organizations has become more acute as the number of such organizations has increased, as costs have escalated, and as resources have diminished. University hospitals are by no means immune, inasmuch as they compete for technological and scientific supremacy as well as for superiority in teaching and clinical care.

Seventh, the emergence of a *new trinity*—marketing, public relations, and development (fund-raising)—has been noted. The purpose of this trinity is to create a very positive image in the public mind so as to attract superior staff, loyal attending physicians, and a sufficiency of paying patients to render the organization financially secure. Thus, the media are heavily utilized, educational programs for both professionals and laity are emphasized, and new specialty service units are developed. Fund-raising from public and private sources may then be enhanced by the institution's improved reputation.

Finally, major changes in *patterns of care* have taken place. "Moral treatment" in the 19th century emphasized kindness, forbearance, attention to physical needs, recreation, and closer relationships between caregivers and patients in a climate of therapeutic optimism. Unfortunately, in the latter part of the century this gave way to overcrowding, custodialism, and therapeutic nihilism. The road back has been marked by great biological/pharmacological advances and major developments in social/community treatment. Major sociodynamic and psychodynamic insights into the patient's illness and recovery appear as staff–patient relationships become more central and meaningful in the treatment process.

In these rapidly changing times, executive jobs have become more complicated and challenging, and the need for effective administrators is greater than ever before.

REFERENCES

1. Jay A: Management and Machiavelli. New York, Holt, Rinehart & Winston, 1967
2. Drucker P: Conclusion: The challenge to management, in Drucker PF: Managing in Turbulent Times. New York, Harper & Row, 1980, pp 225–231
3. Drucker PF: Conclusion: Effectiveness must be learned, in Drucker PF: The Effective Executive. New York, Harper & Row, 1966, pp 166–174
4. Drucker PF: Conclusion: The legitimacy of management, in Drucker PF: Management: Tasks, Responsibilities, Practices. New York, Harper & Row, 1973, pp 805–811
5. Drucker PF: Conclusion: The challenge to management, in Drucker PF: Managing in Turbulent Times. New York, Harper & Row, 1980, pp 225–231
6. Kets de Vries, MFR (ed): The Irrational Executive. Psychoanalytic Studies in Management. New York, International Universities Press, 1984
7. Gifford RN, Davidson N: Gone tomorrow? CEO's speak out on institutional survival. Trustee 38:33–37, May 1985
8. Based in part on Malcolm AH: In health care policy, the latest word is fiscal: Living with the Reagan era's cost-consciousness. New York Times, Part E, p 3, Sunday, October 23, 1988
9. Callahan D: Setting Limits: Medical Goals in an Aging Society. New York, Simon & Schuster, 1987

10. [No byline]: 81 community hospitals closed in 1988: AHA. AHA News 25:3, January 23, 1989
11. Greenblatt M, York RH, Brown EL: From Custodial to Therapeutic Patient Care in Mental Hospitals. New York, Russell Sage Foundation, 1955
12. Greenblatt M: The evolution of models of mental health care and treatment, Chapter 7 in Greenblatt M: Psychopolitics. New York, Grune & Stratton, 1978, pp 99–109
13. Solomon HC: Personal communication
14. Pinel P: A Treatise on Insanity. Translated from the French by DD Davis. New York, Haffner, 1962
15. Bockoven JS: Moral Treatment in Community Psychiatry. New York, Springer, 1972
16. Greenblatt M: Formal and informal groups in a therapeutic community. Internatl J Group Psychotherapy XI:398–409, 1961
17. Deutsch A: The Shame of the States. New York, Harcourt, Brace, 1948
18. Caudill WA: The Psychiatric Hospital as a Small Society. Cambridge, Published for Commonwealth Fund by Harvard University Press, 1958
19. Wells FL, Greenblatt M, Hyde RW: As the Psychiatric Aide Sees His Work and Problems. Genetic Psychology Monographs 53:3–73, 1956
20. Cumming J, Cumming E: The Locus of Power in the Large Mental Hospital. Psychiatry 19:77–85, 1956

Toward Scientific Management

The science and art of management have developed with staggering speed over the last 50 years, although leadership itself has been important ever since people have come together in groups, divided a task in achieving some objective or goal, manufactured a commodity, or lived under some system of government. The recent rapid growth in the size of organizations, however, has been a decisive factor in bringing the managerial role into prominence, for any system that expends huge resources sooner or later must come under scrutiny for the good of all.

It should be noted that students attracted to medicine and psychiatry are selected primarily because of their interest in individual human service, not for their interest in systems. Courses in management are not taught in medical school. Only recently have professional organizations been formed in the field of psychiatry to advance the art and science of management. However, the prestige of administrative positions is growing, although salaries are still low, and many hospital administrative positions formerly filled by M.D.s are being taken over by nonphysicians.

As management has come into focus, more and more emphasis has been given to the development of a *science of management*.[1] This has occurred *pari passu* with the development of the field of "behavioral science."

WAYS OF LOOKING AT HUMAN SYSTEMS

Executives in charge of human organizations often remark upon the difficulty in comprehending their organization in all its complexities and details. In a sense, one can say that the first task of a top executive is to make peace with his limitations; an obsessive leader who must know everything and control everything is bound for disaster. The second task is to realize that the organization must be run through others to whom authority is delegated. Once carefully selected and tested, they must be willingly endowed with the appointing officer's trust.

Many thinkers have grappled with the problem of comprehending human organizations, but although many interesting concepts have been advanced, it is probably fair to say that no one concept or theory has won the day. The dilemma has some analogies with efforts at understanding human beings in health and disease at the one-to-one level. Freud gave us new ways of looking at human thinking, feeling, and emotion, and new ways of intervening for therapeutic purposes. But even here we have counterposing theories—witness Jung, Adler, Horney, Kohut, the psychobiologists, and the social psychiatrists.

Greiner's "Recent History of Organizational Behavior"[2] starts with the caveat that all ideas about management are "in process," each insight representing a small step in the evolution of thought. I could not agree more. The view of history presented below borrows heavily from Greiner's perspective.

Max Weber

Max Weber (1864–1920) introduced the word *bureaucracy,* together with a theory of formal organization.[3] Tasks and authority in organizations were central to his interests. Authority was divided into three types: legitimate, charismatic, and traditional. *Legitimate* authority is granted by the organization or by law. It is rational and legal and subject to defined limits. *Charismatic* authority arises from the personality of the leader who evokes strong emotion and personal devotion from his followers. Through some "divine grace," he is able to reach the deep needs of people and lead them towards goals consistent with his personal ideology. *Traditional* authority rests on belief in the sacredness of a social order, based largely on historical precedent. Thus, the Pope's authority, although formally bestowed by election of the cardinals, is exercised in the name of God; his pronouncements are considered sacred and are not readily challenged by the laity.

Weber's concept of bureaucracy did not have the negative connotations ascribed to bureaucracy today. It was a rational, legal system in which competent persons occupied positions in a hierarchy, and in which rules, regulations, and policies were specified. Managers, who were *not* owners, were held administratively responsible for the proper functioning of the organization.

Labor was divided into horizontal and vertical levels. Horizontal levels were represented by programs and departments; vertical levels by a hierarchy of supervision over defined tasks. The organization was further characterized by clear lines of authority and communication, formal rules and regulations, and a staff of administrators and clerks.

Criticisms of Weber focus around his assumption of a perfect "fit" between labor and the goals of management, and the further assumption of rational motivations of the several involved parties. Today we pay greater attention to motivational discordances and the irrational behaviors of both management and labor.[4]

Frederick W. Taylor and Henri Fayol

The founding father of the principles of scientific management is commonly recognized to be the engineer Frederick W. Taylor, who in his *Principles of Scientific Management* (1911)[5] emphasized work measurement, standards, and a pay formula that rewarded workers' efforts. He stressed the role of the foreman as a planner rather than a task worker or a disciplinarian. The French engineer, Henri Fayol[6,7] (1916) followed with emphasis on planning, coordination, and control. He espoused the importance of unity of command, division of work, equity, and orders for carrying out these functions.

In the early part of this century, the science of "industrial psychology" was born. It emphasized the motivational needs of employees and their integration with the organization.[8] Psychological testing was employed to fit the abilities of the individual to the demands of his job, but since these tests did not prove to be accurate predictors of work success, attention shifted to employee training, merit rating, and promotion policies. Welfare benefits and better working conditions were also emphasized, with attention to worker recognition and satisfaction. This humane "warming trend" received further elaboration in the work of Follett, Mayo, and Roethlisberger.

Chester I. Barnard

Chester I. Barnard's book *The Functions of the Executive*[9] (1938) has been an enduring source of enlightenment for generations of executives and a standard textbook in many schools. He pictured the organization as a complex system in which the executive maintains equilibrium in an environment of physical, biological, and social forces.

Barnard conceived of organizations as made up of individuals who cooperate together to achieve a purpose not achievable alone because of their physical and biological limitations. Cooperation is essential to the survival of the organization and the achievement of its purpose. There must also be sufficient "inducements" to encourage communication and working together. Barnard visualized the organization as a social system—indeed, a *living* system—in which both *effectiveness* and *efficiency* play important parts. "When the purpose of a system of cooperation is attained we say that the cooperation was effective; if not attained, ineffective."[10] "Efficiency relates to the satisfaction of individual motives, and is personal in character. . . . The test of efficiency is the eliciting of sufficient individual wills to cooperate."[11]

Barnard also distinguished carefully between formal and informal aspects of organizations. "Formal organization is that kind of cooperation that is conscious, deliberate, purposeful."[12] "The functions of the executive . . . are those of control, management, supervision, and administration in formal organizations . . . exercised not merely by high officials in such organizations but by all those who are in positions of control of whatever degree."[13]

Barnard defined informal organization as "the aggregate of personal contacts and interactions and . . . associated groupings of people."[14] Informal interactions may be accidental or incidental to organized activities or purposes, either friendly or hostile. ("Informal association . . . is a condition which necessarily precedes formal organizations."[15]) An important and indispensable part of an organization is its informal aspects, which unfortunately are often not fully appreciated by officials. Communication and maintenance of cohesiveness and of a feeling of integrity are the main functions of the informal organization. It is "a means of maintaining the personality against certain effects of formal organizations which tend to disintegrate the personality."[16]

Barnard's analysis of authority was profound for its time, and is valid still for our own. Authority does not arise from above but depends on the acquiescence and cooperation of individuals at the lower level (see Chapter 11). For example, whether or not an order is obeyed lies with the person to whom it is addressed and not with the person who issues the order.

> A person can and will accept a communication as authoritative only when four conditions simultaneously obtain: (a) he can and does understand the communication; (b) *at the time of his decision* he believes it is not inconsistent with the purpose of the organization; (c) *at the time of his decision*, he believes it to be compatible with his personal interest as a whole; [and] (d) he is able mentally and physically to comply with it.[17]

Since purpose is the unifying principle of cooperative systems, the efficiency of the organization arises from the perception that the organization's purpose is proper and important. The executive, in Barnard's view, has the moral obligation to rationalize the organization's goals in an insightful and responsible way. "This creative function . . . is the essence of leadership."[18]

Wallace S. Sayre

Sayre (1956)[19,20] suggested four ways that administrators may look at human organizations: (a) as technological systems, (b) as systems for policy formation, (c) as social process systems, and (d) as systems of responsibility and accountability. This helpful fourfold perspective is directed only at a better comprehension of the human organization; it does not examine the role of the executive in relation to the system.

Technological System

This view, most often emphasized in the business world, stresses efficiency and work performance at the least cost. Because hospitals and other mental health facilities may be loosely integrated (with many semi-autonomous units staffed by persons with loyalties to both the institution and the professions that nurtured them), cooperation tends to be based to a large degree on mutual agreement. The tight pyramidal authority implied in a technological approach is more characteristic of business organizations. Cost-effectiveness, however, has become a prominent theme in psychiatric care. Executives in the public sector of mental health, particularly during times of austerity, strive to evaluate the effectiveness of programs and account for expenditure of all funds. Sophisticated budgeting, accounting, and evaluation procedures and automated information-processing systems are part and parcel of successful operations.

System for Policy Formulation and Decision Making

Here the primary questions are: How is policy developed, and how are decisions made? Who participates? Alternatives and choices are constantly placed before decision makers for analysis, argument, and persuasion. If many minds are at work in policy development and decision making, the process may be regarded as having a proper base of participation. A broad base of participation usually contributes significantly to the morale of patients and staff and to the health of the organization.

Social Process

This perspective, insofar as it emphasizes a human interactive point of view and respects the individuality of persons working together, is likely to be especially appealing to psychiatric administrators. This view also assumes that individuals, more than technology, shape organizations—thus, participation, cooperation, morale, and consensus are all important. Leadership is regarded as the skill necessary to evoke maximum expression and cooperation within a climate of healthy, nondestructive competition.

System of Responsibility and Accountability

The emphasis here is on accountability both within and outside the organization. Trustees and constitutional authorities must be informed and their approval requested. Evaluation, criticism, and reporting are the major themes. In recent years, the psychiatric administrator has assumed responsibility for integrating the work of his organization with third-party payers, as well as with outside standard setters such as the JCAHO, professional societies, labor unions, and citizen groups with special interests.

Ludwig von Bertalanffy, James G. Miller, and Jessie L. Miller

Bertalanffy's[21,22] general system theory (1955) views organizations as open systems, exchanging information, goods, and services across boundaries with the outside world. Their functions are categorized under three headings: input, throughput and output. Feedback of information allows adjustment of the organism to a changing environment. James G. Miller[23] and Jessie L. Miller[24] have enormously expanded and developed systems theory, especially in the classic book *Living Systems* (1978). They identify eight levels of systems (cell, organ, organism, groups, organizations, communities, societies, and supranational systems) and show how the movement of matter/energy and information into, through, and out of each system is controlled by 20 distinct functions.

System theorists focus their attention on the organization, and elaborate primarily on similarities across organizations; they are not primarily focused on administrative roles or tasks, or on the relationship between leadership and system functions.

E. J. Miller and A. K. Rice

Miller and Rice (1967),[25] with others at the Tavistock Institute, use open system theory together with concepts of *primary* task and *sociotechnical* systems as tools for the analysis of different enterprises. They find that two systems, one geared to task performance (task systems) and the other to relationships (sentient systems), rarely have common boundaries. Usually a three-part organization is required: (a) for controlling performance, (b) for ensuring interest of members in enterprise objectives, and (c) for regulating relations between task and sentient systems. They emphasize the importance of boundary management as a means of control within the enterprise, and between the enterprise and the environment.

Elton Mayo; Douglas McGregor and Theory X and Theory Y

Elton Mayo[26] and his colleagues, who studied human relations in the Hawthorne Plant of Western Electric between 1927 and 1932, were prime initiators of a new trend. Their classic work (1927) demonstrated that people in factories formed a group with common purposes, psychological awareness of each other, interdependent roles and relationships, and shared norms and values. Productivity was influenced by intensely personal factors—personal needs, cooperation, cohesion, and gratification. A variety of changes in their working situation could enhance productivity, as long as workers felt that changes were carried out for their benefit and were experienced as benign.

Work satisfaction, said Mayo, was dependent on the *informal* social pattern of the group. Many problems in work–management relations were the result of emotionally based attitudes. Therefore, one of the tasks of management is to discover how spontaneous cooperation could be achieved. Through these highly important studies a much fuller realization of the importance of the human factor, of group affiliation, and of the values and norms of the group came forth. In effect, a "human relations" movement was started and "industrial sociology" was born.[27] These studies laid the foundation for further interest in research on groups by organizational psychologists, a field pioneered by Kurt Lewin.[28,29]

The Hawthorne studies, therefore, stood in opposition to the work of Frederick W. Taylor and others, who emphasized primarily time and motion studies of worker efficiency. Mayo and associates, on the other hand, focused on friendly relations between management and workers as the key to greater productivity—thus setting the background for McGregor's[30] Theory X and Theory Y.

In his *Human Side of Enterprise* (1960), McGregor identified these two opposite conceptual positions. Theory X holds that (a) the average human being has an inherent dislike for work and will avoid it if he can; (b) he must be coerced, controlled, directed, or threatened with punishment in order to achieve organizational objectives; and (c) he prefers to be directed, wishes to avoid responsibility, has little ambition, and wants security above all. Tight control and close supervision are the natural consequences of this point of view.

Theory Y, in contrast, holds that (a) the expenditure of physical and mental energy in work is as natural as play or rest; (b) people will exercise self-direction and control to achieve objects to which they are committed; (c) commitment to objectives is a function of rewards associated with their achievement (i.e., esteem and self-actualization); (d) the average person learns under proper conditions not only to accept but also to seek responsibility; (e) most people are capable of a high degree of imagination, ingenuity, and creativity in solving organizational problems; and (e) under conditions of contemporary industrial life, the average person's intellectual potentialities are utilized only partially.

Thus, McGregor argues that a worker's motivations to a great extent are in response to management's view of his potentialities. Under X, control is externally imposed; under Y, control is internally introjected. McGregor did not argue for consensus management or abandonment of authority. His was not a black-and-white choice; he merely assembled management attitudes into two conceptually polar extremes for purposes of elucidating the general field.

William G. Ouchi: Theory Z

Theory Z applies to organizational patterns prevailing in Japanese culture. Much attention has been drawn recently to Japanese industrial organizations because of their great successes competitively in capturing American markets. Ouchi[31,32,33] is an outstanding student and theoretician of this model.

Ouchi points out that since World War II, productivity in Japan has increased two to three times faster than in the United States; and recently productivity in Japan has grown at a faster rate each year, whereas in the

United States productivity barely increases and even declines in some quarters.

In Japan, the whole system of employment is intimately bound to social and cultural patterns. In a typical Japanese industry, a most important element is lifetime employment in one company where the managers take responsibility for the health, welfare, security, and morale of each employee. Promotions are almost entirely from within; once hired, the new employee is retained until mandatory retirement at age 55. Each year a large share of the employee's salary is provided in the form of a bonus (which may add up to as much as five to six months of total income) that is contingent on company as well as individual performance. Thus, the risks of business are shifted not so much to stockholders (as in this country), but to employees—who consequently have a very large stake in the company's future. They ally themselves with managers in organizational vicissitudes, in good times and bad.

The Japanese believe that the relationship between a foreman and his workers is best when it has the positive ingredients of intimacy, subtlety, and complexity. Indeed, they see the relationship as a highly sensitive one in which, through long association and mutual trust, employees learn how best to work with each other.

> A foreman who knows his workers well can pinpoint personalities, decide who works well with whom, and thus put together work teams of maximum effectiveness. These subtleties can never be captured explicitly, and any bureaucratic rule will do violence to them. If the foreman is forced . . . to assign work teams . . . on the basis of seniority, then that subtlety is lost and productivity declines.[34]

Japanese firms have available to them a large group of temporary employees—women. This arrangement allows for flexibility in hiring to meet the ups and downs of business fortunes; at the same time it increases income for families who may need it. The firms also manifest flexibility in accommodating women who have children. Another feature is that every employee is simultaneously a member of 8 to 12 work groups, through which experiences employees learn more about the business, appreciate their workmates' tasks and problems, and open up possibilities of role interchangeability. Such common experiences form a base upon which trust and confidence between management and the workers, and among the workers themselves, can be developed. The common culture, thus shared, facilitates planning and decision making. Indeed, decision making in Japan is shared with a very large number of people, much more so than in this country. Teams of employees assume responsibility not only for setting tasks but also for decision making.

By integrating the economic with the social life of the individual, Japanese companies have been able to reduce turnover rates greatly as compared with American firms. They have also reduced resignations and layoffs, and minimized costs of training new people. The stability of organizational personnel extends to the executive as well as the worker level. "We believe that the typical United States rates of twenty-six percent annual turnover and of eight percent average absenteeism are an irreducible minimum, but annual turnover among European firms average twelve percent and among Japanese firms six percent, with lower absenteeism rates as well."[35]

Ouchi's fascinating book came out in 1981 and immediately made its way onto the best-seller list. We interviewed Ouchi eight years later to obtain his personal reflections on the impact of eight years of Theory Z-type industrial models on American companies. Having followed national trends closely, he believes that the impact on U.S. industry has been great, forced by increasing dominance of Japanese products in American markets. The concept is being accepted in the United States that an organization can reach its fullest potential only by delegating decisions to its employees as to how best to do their own work. To delegate more such freedom, management must be assured that the goals of the employees are compatible with those of stakeholders.

More and more, U.S. companies are discovering the practices and techniques of Japanese companies.[36] In the auto industry, for example, United Auto Worker agreements now include profit sharing toward lifetime employment security. Further, U.S. companies must develop more techniques to stabilize human capital. In America, education takes place in the university; in Japan, more of the employee's education takes place in the firm. American universities, by and large, do not hire their own Ph.D.'s. In Japan, they do.

Ouchi sees no countertrend in Japan toward using American models. However, he believes American cars are now catching up to Japanese cars in quality and durability.

Recently, James R. Lincoln[37] has cast additional light on the debate as to whether Japanese productivity successes are due to management styles that can be transplanted to America, or instead are dependent on nontransplantable cultural factors. The widely used seniority system in Japan and the participatory style fostered particularly by their quality circles breed greater worker loyalty, strong social bonds, and more positive work attitudes. In addition, employee services, company-sponsored sports, recreational outings, and company ceremonies contribute to better morale. The same conditions, it is claimed, can produce similar results in American plants.

Rensis Likert: The Likert System

Likert (1967, 1969)[38,39] puts the group at the center of his system. He sees departmental managers as the linking pins between several groups, facilitating the flow of information horizontally, upward to higher echelons, and downward as disseminator of policies and practices and as interpreters of change. Open lines of communication, development of trust, group goal setting, consensus decision making, and shared responsibility are to be encouraged.

In Likert's view, which is consistent with Barnard's, the manager's authority is dependent on how much authority his subordinates *allow* him to have. In turn, the influence he asserts over his subordinates depends on how much he allows himself to be influenced by them. The extent to which he considers their opinions determines in large measure their commitment in carrying out decisions effectively. Mutually supportive relations are essential to individual motivation and identification with the goals and objectives of the group. He believes the participative-group style is the most creative and effective.

In his book on *The Human Organization*,[40] Likert expounds a theory of *human asset accounting* as a means of measuring return on investment with respect to the people who make up the organization. He uses two criteria of employees' value at any time: productive capacity and customer goodwill. If able, well-trained people leave a company, the worth of the human organization is reduced. If well-trained people join the company, its human assets are increased. Irreconcilable conflicts reduce human assets, but cooperative teamwork and the capacity to use differences constructively increase human assets.

This concept will ring true to those who strive to upgrade quality of personnel and to boost morale. It certainly deserves much research attention, including efforts to quantitate the variable involved.

Chris Argyris: Integrating the Individual and the Organization

One of the major themes underlying Argyris's writings (1969)[41] is the dichotomy of individual needs and organizational needs. This is immediately reminiscent of the theories propounded by Miller and Rice. The organization, insofar as it frustrates the social and egoistic needs of the individual, may be the source and cause of human problems. With its pyramidal structure, formally designated roles, division of labor, lines of authority, rigid communication channels, tight job descriptions, hierarchical reporting, budget limitations, and so forth, the organization fails to recognize human needs and thus thwarts the worker. His personal value and self-esteem, sense of contribution to the group, and need for recognition and independence are unfulfilled. His psychological energies are then directed away from the organization's needs to his personal needs. If organizational aims are thus subverted, the organization, viewed as a living system, is then regarded as "unhealthy" or "sick."

Fundamentally, says Argyris, the problem is to effect a better accommodation between organizational and individual needs. He recommends face-to-face group laboratories to develop a more optimal organization. These work groups, directed toward encouraging honesty, candor, cohesiveness, and mutual support, should in many cases cut across formal organizational barriers, bringing together the most appropriate and able people necessary to define the job. As interpersonal competence develops, group work improves.

Another Argyris theme is "job enlargement," or expansion of job content to include a wider range of tasks and to broaden the worker's control over his tasks. He recommends that workers can set their own pace and assume discretion in the methods of performing their tasks and in performing their own quality control checks. Interchangeability of tasks broadens knowledge of how the organization functions, and increases the workers' appreciation of other workers' roles. Argyris's view of the organization as a living system, manifesting "health" or "sickness" and dependent on direction of workers' energies, correlates well with views expressed in Chapter 3 ("Toward Better Theory and Practice").

Abraham Maslow

Abraham Maslow's[42] theories assume that human needs may be ranked along a continuum. His work, supported by Herzberg (see below), has been widely adopted as useful in understanding management–worker relationships.

Maslow's hierarchy of needs starts with the most primitive and archaic needs and moves up: (a) physiological needs, (b) safety needs, (c) the need for belonging and love, (d) the need for esteem, and (e) the need for self-actualization. The idea is that once a lower-level need is satisfied, the individual is no longer motivated by rewards at that level but seeks satisfaction at increasingly higher levels. Self-actualization, which refers to activities that enhance the expression of the real self, is the only one of the needs that is essentially unlimited; the individual at this level enjoys a sense of freedom, spontaneity, and creativity and gains satisfactions in the realization of his innate capabilities.

The aesthetic and artistic professions, by nature, indulge this self-actualizing need; but self-actualization possibilities can be found in many other jobs and professions, provided the individual's life and work can be arranged to gratify his innate drives. In this sense, management may regard most, if not all, individuals as motivated, and must seek the proper conditions for release of their energies into healthy organizational channels.

Frederick Herzberg

Herzberg's[43] theories complement Maslow's. He studied factors he called "satisfiers" and "dissatisfiers," as reported by 200 engineers and accountants. Good feelings about the job were related to so-called *content* factors such as achievement, recognition, growth, advancement, responsibility (satisfiers). Bad feelings about the job were related to *context* factors such as company policy and administration, supervision, interpersonal relations, salary, status, and working conditions (dissatisfiers).

In analyzing his findings, Herzberg discovered that factors associated with job satisfaction were those stemming from people's need to realize their human potential. On the other hand, factors associated with job dissatisfaction arose from the individual's need to avoid physical and social deprivation. The latter were basically concerned with the job *environment*, extrinsic to the job itself; hence, he refers to them as "job hygiene" or "maintenance" factors. Their lack will cause dissatisfaction. It is the set of factors intrinsic to the job, concerned with motivation and growth and development, that cause satisfaction—and their absence will lead to lack of satisfaction, but not dissatisfaction. Thus, satisfiers and dissatisfiers are not opposites, but represent two relatively different levels of human needs.

Herzberg's findings direct managers to focus on job enrichment, opportunities for growth and learning, increased individual accountability, additional authority and freedom on the job, and allowing a person a complete natural unit of work. Recognition is a strong factor leading to job satisfaction, increased motivation, and productivity. Herzberg's research, which supports both Maslow's and McGregor's theories, has been validated in a number of practical demonstrations.

How psychological energies may be revivified, released, organized, and directed is one of the major tasks of management. The organization, like the individual, may be healthy or sick, depending on how its energies are utilized. If pathologically directed, that energy spends itself in desultory, undirected activities, with much of it diverted into factional strife and destructive behaviors. If properly directed, energy flows into imaginative and creative channels that spark morale and affirm the organization's purpose.

Sociological Views of Mental Health Organizations

The Multitiered System

In America we have not one psychiatry, but many psychiatries. We have believers in somatic therapy, drug therapy, psychotherapy and psychoanalytic therapies, and social therapy—and also eclectics who mix these up in proportions that suit themselves. Likewise (as pointed out in Chapter 1), our hospitals vary greatly, not only in the values attributed to various forms of therapy—the therapeutic hierarchy, so to speak—but also in general service missions and goals. They also vary in size, complexity, type of university affiliation, research and training emphasis, public versus private sponsorship, religious affiliation, and in relative dominance of the various professional groups with their varying strengths of loyalty to their professional societies.

Despite America's apparent commitment to equal opportunities for all, we still have in his country several tiers of mental health care, with a general level of quality attached to each tier.

The *university hospital* usually is characterized by much involvement in research and training, with intensive patient care and treatment and high staff-to-patient ratios forming a background to the teaching and research mission. Admissions policies are usually selective, catering to "interesting teaching cases" or "tertiary cases" useful in research. Whereas special endowments may make it possible to carry indigent cases of unique teaching and research value, university hospitals require a substantial base of paying clientele for financial stability.

The *private hospital* is characterized usually by affluent surroundings and well-appointed interiors, good staff-to-patient ratios (but usually not as high as in the university), and essentially a middle- or upper-class clientele either well insured or otherwise able to pay their bills. There is heavy emphasis on client and family satisfaction, and on cultivating excellent relationships with referring physicians and other outside referring sources. Although fiscal soundness and good profit margins are major criteria of success, the best places know that high-quality care and treatment are also a royal road to success. In recent years, the rapid development of many private psychiatric hospitals and their takeover by large for-profit chains have introduced highly competitive elements into the picture. Heavy emphasis on advertising and marketing by these chains, as they seek to enroll additional clients and to market new or improved techniques of care and treatment in specially targeted areas of need, is an increasingly prominent feature of the market place.

The *Veterans Affairs* hospitals are units of the largest health system in the world, catering to those "who have borne the brunt of battle."[44] The major emphasis is on service to veterans with service-connected disabilities, although many non-service-connected veterans are still receiving care and treatment in these institutions or their ambulatory divisions.

Only about 10% of the population (veterans) receives care in veterans' hospitals—usually free, for means tests have as yet not been systematically applied. Quality of care, and per diem expenditures, are generally less than in university or private hospitals. Since World War II, the Department of Veterans Affairs has managed to develop academic affiliations with university medical schools, and thus has vastly upgraded its quality of care, teaching, and research.

This vast system is dominated by an administrative hierarchy in Washington, D.C., which in turn receives guidance and financing from the Congress, with final responsibility and decision in the hands of the president. The president, in turn, appoints a cabinet secretary who is invested with large powers to run the organization. As a result, local initiative in the numerous hospital units may be limited. In times of austerity, the hospitals in the field are forced to lower the quality of care. This elicits aggressive counterlobbying efforts by a large built-in constituency, the various veterans' organizations in the community.

The history of *state and county hospitals* has been a sorry one. When moral treatment collapsed after the Industrial Revolution of the middle and late 19th century, these hospitals started to slide; indeed, they reached very low levels of service. Overcrowding, inadequate staffing, impoverished environments, chronicity, and custodialism were rampant. Physical plants were often allowed to deteriorate. The term *total institution* has been applied by Goffman[45] to describe the total control over the lives of patients exerted by many of these hospitals. For years, however, the state and county hospitals were practically the only refuges for the seriously disabled mentally ill. After World War II, national, state, and local efforts were mounted to improve these hospitals, but today, the underfunded state and county hospitals are still the major treatment facilities for the poor, the dispossessed, and the multiply handicapped. Despite efforts to upgrade them, these hospitals remain at the bottom of the ladder in terms of quality of care and treatment.

Finally, there are millions of Americans today who are seriously neglected or who receive no treatment although they may have severe disabling diseases (see "Homelessness: The New Epidemic" in Chapter 10). These include the homeless, cast aside as a result of withdrawal of billions of dollars of federal support, or a lack of low-cost housing, or economic turmoil and loss of employment. Many are psychiatric casualties of the deinstitutionalization movement; many others are chronic alcoholics or drug-dependent people, and many are chronically mentally ill derelicts who refuse treatment. Still others are neglected mentally ill persons who cannot afford health insurance or are not covered by insurance after the death of a breadwinner. Thus, it is fair to say that a fifth tier exists—a large group of needy people for whom the absence of care for their mental illness is the most striking characteristic.

Sociological Characteristics of Mental Institutions

Because of the great diversity in levels of care and types of therapeutic organizations, sociological analysis presents a major theoretical challenge. Yet it appears that mental health organizations in general may be differentiated in several ways from other public service organizations, or from industrial institutions. The following is distilled from Blau's[46] sociological analysis of mental institutions, modified by personal reflections.

1. The tasks of mental institutions are different from many other enterprises in that mental institutions are dedicated to *transforming people* rather than *manufacturing tangible products.* They try to help people move from lower to higher levels of adaptability, to improve their self-image and sense of self-worth, to reduce or eliminate symptomatology, and to enhance their capacity to relate to other people. Restoration to society, self-sufficiency, and productivity in the workaday world are ultimate goals to be achieved after symptoms are alleviated, and insight and self-confidence are restored.

Work that transforms people is much less susceptible to standardization and precise evaluation than work that produces a commodity like a toy or an automobile. This greater uncertainty, which permits differences in philosophy, opinion, and role concepts, may be translated into conflict. Additionally, diagnosis is not an exact science, and where diagnoses are uncertain treatment patterns vary. Boundaries between the several professionals working in the same arena, and on the same patients, are not sharp. Overlapping activities and diverse training backgrounds further complicate the scene.

2. *Diversity and specialization of occupations* bring the patient under the treatment of a team rather than a given individual. The tendency for different teams in the same institution to handle outpatients as opposed to inpatients may create a high degree of fractionation, as well as discontinuity in patient

care. The patient has the added task of adjusting not only to the different therapeutic settings but also to different therapists, perhaps with different concepts or techniques. Discontinuity of caregivers is increased in institutions with heavy psychiatric training commitments, which require that trainees change sites in order to provide them with an appropriately rich set of experiences. For this reason, generalists have become an important element in case management. They bear various names—"ombudsman," "case manager," "case administrator," or "treatment coordinator"; their role is to integrate the efforts of the various caregivers working with a given patient.

The high degree of occupational diversity must nevertheless be respected, or staff morale will suffer. Each occupational group not only has strong loyalty ties to its own profession and pride in its area of expertise, but also strives to ascend the ladder of professionalism in terms of gaining added educational and training credits—symbols of achievement—and progressive refinement of its knowledge base. A further complicating element is that over time the roles of the various professionals tend to change, usually toward more supervisory or teaching roles rather than front-line care. Psychiatrists, in recent decades, have tended to leave administration to others, and in many new mental health centers they function primarily as prescribers of medication, case consultants, group leaders, and in-service teachers and trainers of other professionals. As noted in Chapter 12, "Executive Careers", in many hospitals the role of administrator has been taken over altogether by nonmedical people trained as professional hospital administrators.

3. The balance of *centralization versus decentralization* is a major variable affecting both hospital organizations and patient care. Small organizations favor a simple structure and coordination via collegial relations, whereas large hospitals are coordinated mainly through administrative communications. Small organizations give more opportunities for direct egalitarian contacts with patients; large organizations are more custodial and hierarchically controlled. The American Association of Superintendents of Asylums for the Insane, when first formed, wisely prescribed that the treatment of the mentally ill was best carried out in hospitals with less than 250 patients. Some believe that no hospital should be larger than the number of patients the superintendent himself can know and relate to. In large hospitals, much of the care and treatment is relegated to individuals at the bottom of the hierarchy with little training. They take direction from nursing, occupational, or recreational departments or from other attendants—while the superintendent himself loses touch.

There is evidence that decentralization is associated with belief in milieu treatment, whereas centralization is associated with drug treatment. Many believe that decentralization of decision making is associated with greater autonomy of staff, improved morale, and better quality of care.

4. The *matrix structure* characterizes many institutions. In this structure, individual caregivers have multiple relationships and status positions within an organization, which is thought to improve morale as well as patient care. A

given staff person is linked to many groups engaged in a variety of functions. In some groups he or she is an expert, in others a learner or observer. This enlarges the network of communications, tends to break down barriers, broadens the base of involvement in organizational goals, and increases respect and tolerance of others' opinions and values. (Matrix structure is an important element in Theory Z Japanese institutions.[47])

5. Administrators of mental hospitals suffer from both *role conflicts and role ambiguities*. Boundaries between their clinical and administrative functions are often vague and/or strained. Administrative functions are often managed best by centralization, clinical functions by decentralization. Administrative functions emphasize quantity, control and efficiency, while clinical functions emphasize high standards and quality of care. Hodgson's[48] research emphasizes the need to divide and share among different executives the many functions needed to run a hospital. In the small university-connected hospital he studied, the functions of administration, teaching, and research were each headed by different individuals who, in their cooperative family-type interactions, provided role complementarity that worked effectively. Hodgson argues that a constellation of role functions is necessary to administer any large psychiatric organization, however those functions may be divided among individuals.[49] (See "The Executive Constellation" later in this chapter.)

6. In mental hospitals, *forces outside the organization are very influential*. Consumer interest in health care has increased, and so has the number of standard-setting and monitoring agencies that play an all-important role in quality assurance. In addition to rules and regulations stemming from controlling legislative bodies, there now exists a large body of judicial decisions from litigation related to patient rights. Among the regulating and monitoring agencies are JCAHO and agencies monitoring safety, food preparation, fire protection, rights of patients, Medicare and Medicaid, laboratories, and vivaria.

In governmental hospitals, special investigations are launched frequently where complaints of patient abuse, or administrative mismanagement, are involved. These investigations may be used unwisely or even abusively when they serve political purposes rather than the goals of effective patient care.

Citizen bodies play a significant role in influencing policy and use of resources. They affect institutional functions through advisory boards, volunteer organizations, and service organizations (see "Volunteerism and Citizen Involvement" in Chapter 10).

Professional organizations exert a constant influence on health organizations, inasmuch as they represent professional identifications of their members, formulate standards of practice, and uphold professional ideals (see "Professional Organizations and Boards" in Chapter 10). They also promote public recognition of the profession, and may function like labor unions, pressing for better wages and conditions of work. The professional employed in a hospital has loyalties to his professional group or society as well as to the institution that employs him. These divided loyalties tend to become exaggerated when budgetary curtailments occur, when shortages of professionals dominate the marketplace, or when strikes occur (see "Labor Unrest and the Strike" in Chapter 10.)

Indeed, the interpenetration of the health organization with powerful professional organizations is one of the most distinguishing hallmarks of the health system. Professional societies are to a surprising extent self-governing; membership requires training that involves years of hard study and field experiences. They are also influenced by codes of ethics, and by periodic technical and ethical reviews of their status. Having met the requirements of accreditation and licensure, professionals cherish independence and do not lend themselves to easy control by others. Although today (as seen in "Psychiatrists in Leadership Positions" in Chapter 12) medical directorial powers have been largely superseded by lay managers, medical professionals—by virtue of technical knowledge and the ability to bring patients and funds into the hospital—still remain a corps with great influence, rewarded with relatively higher incomes.

In the multiplicity of supervising and monitoring agencies, and in the numerous influential lay bodies that press upon the executive, the job of administrator of a mental hospital is unique today, and the role of administrator one of the most complex and sensitive in the whole sphere of public or private service.

Psychodynamic Views

An important publication by Spiro[50] on psychodynamic theories points out that insights from psychodynamics may be applied to organizations in two ways: to identify and elucidate the character problems and neurotic elements of individual administrators, policymakers, and policy implementers; and to elucidate how psychodynamic insights may be applied to *organizations*. In the first instance we are on more solid ground than in the second, for the application of psychodynamic insights (derived mainly from work with individuals) to large groups is fraught with peril. In this field, Spiro outlines several ways the unwary thinker may be trapped: poor data collection, "wild" interpretation, or inappropriate emphasis.

Freud pointed out that civilizations are possible only when gratification of dependency needs, acceptance of interdependencies, and curbing of unbridled narcissism permit the development of ego-dominated reality-based relationships. Thus, inhibition makes civilization possible.[51] In the expression of instinctual impulses, however, the individual almost always has someone in mind as a model, an object, or an opponent. Libidinal ties may be formed to leaders or to the organization itself. These then involve mechanisms of introjection, identification, and idealization. When group members bind themselves strongly to the leader, a setting materializes for the emergence of charismatic leadership.

Freud wrote about mythology and taboos surrounding leaders. Followers tend to be suspicious and to fear enslavement. They attribute dangerous magical powers to the leader. In tribal life, the primal father may be murdered by rebellious sons,[52] who then take over organizational power. The modern leader whose management style is excessively authoritarian may stimulate similar archaic hatreds and incite staff rebellion.

Shortcomings in the leader's personality (such as those discussed in Chapter 5) aggravate latent hostilities and promote regressive behavior in subordinates. Particularly important are aggressive–masochistic trends; sexist needs to dominate, demean, or possess; and excessive narcissism that hungers for praise and affection and demands centrality in everything. Self-understanding in a leader implies not only a balanced nature and sensitivity to one's own feelings, but also sensitivity to the feelings of others; for in relation to his position of power and authority, his workers often manifest anger, fear, and rebelliousness—or, to the contrary, the need for approval and love, all of which may affect their attitude toward their jobs (see Kernberg[53] and others in *The Irrational Executive*[54]).

Another important phenomenon, "organizational regression"[55] (i.e., deterioration in organizational morale and performance), is often attributable to personality aberrations of the leader, as Kernberg points out. However, "the very nature of the task carried out in psychiatric institutions, particularly in settings where severely regressed patients are treated, also exerts a powerful [regressive] influence."[56] Serious distortions may also arise when "political objectives replace task oriented or functional ones." In institutions where disturbed characters possessing huge drives for power may dominate, there can be a virtual affective dictatorship of groups as well as of individuals, leading to organizational regression. Excessive monitoring from outside agencies saps the strength of the organization and stifles creativity. Excessive use of consultants who foster dependency, or budget cuts severe enough to make people angry, anxious, and frustrated may impair competence or exacerbate rivalries among individuals and factions, and may also lead to organizational regression.

In his work on organizational functioning, Bion[57] described three types of regression that take place in group processes. In a *dependency group* the leader is seen as omnipotent and omniscient; the members of the group see themselves as inadequate, immature, and incompetent. The idealization of the leader is matched by efforts to extract knowledge and power from him. The group is united by a common sense of helplessness and fear of the outside world. Personal growth toward independence and self-reliance is therefore retarded. In a *fight–flight group,* the members fear external enemies and expect the leader to protect them not only from their enemies but also from their own infighting. In a *pairing situation,* the group focuses upon a pair who through some magical reproductive experience, they believe, will resolve anxieties, preserve the group, and guarantee its survival as if larger group and system issues were not a problem.

In these psychoanalytic views, as also in the work of Schwartz[58] on the paranoid and depressive positions, "the overarching concept is that there is a direct and continuous relationship between basic assumption states and the kinds and capacities of leadership which arise therefrom. Each state creates a different kind of leadership. Here is one place where the intersection between individual personality and system can be located."[59]

The psychoanalytic views above are fascinating; however, the "regressive pull" theory of Kernberg needs further validation and refinement through acute observation and research in different institutional settings. As for Bion's views, it remains to be seen how his theories, derived from small groups, may apply to large system operations, as well as how their "regressive" influence is exerted and how regressive effects can be prevented or mitigated.

Developmental View of Organization

Extrapolating from constructs derived from observations of small groups, Kaplan[60] posits a theoretic model of phases of organizational development. During the 1960s and early 1970s, when a large number of comprehensive community mental health centers, supported by federal grants, came into being, I had occasion to observe the genesis of several centers. My personal observations support the propositions advanced by Kaplan.

At its *beginnings* (the first phase), one finds looseness of organizational rules and regulations, strong commitment from a few men and women, optimism, excitement in creating something from nothing, and the joy of sharing inspirations sanctioned by sponsoring agencies with enough power to bring dreams to life. Organizational issues and problems then exist mainly in the abstract, to be solved by intellectual discussion and compromise. Intense leader dependency and loyalty may characterize this stage.

During the next stage, that of *expansion*, staff members representing various disciplines and programs are recruited. They, too, share the idealism, sense of purpose, and dreams of the pioneers. Competency of staff and availability of resources now tend to define limits to the rate of expansion. Often resources expected and resources provided are at variance. A burgeoning economy that spawned the idea of new buildings and programs may fade into a climate of austerity. Needless to say, sudden introduction of reality disappoints people and cools their ardor. Disappointments are more likely if the time from planning to construction and program development is great. In state and county systems, 5 to 10 years may pass, whereas in private systems, 12 to 14 months is often enough to start active operations. A 5- to 10-year lag, in a changing field, may mean that priorities of many programs may have to be restructured. Increasing complexity in the period of accelerated growth requires a flexible organizational structure. Limited resources may thrust the new organization into unexpected competitions or into political activism.

Phase three, *consolidation and efficiency,* is characterized by quality considerations, promulgation of rules and procedures, negotiations with outside agencies for accreditations, and creation of training and research programs. Gradually, more and more subgroups develop, each adding to its power base as the number of personnel increases and their expertise grows. Power, formerly concentrated primarily in one individual, is now subdivided and differentiated. As time passes, seniors become differentiated from juniors, the "old guard" from "young Turks." Enthusiasm and flexibility merge into practical functionalism contained by fiscal realities. By this time, a core of middle managers has inserted itself between upper authority and clinical workers. Program tracking and feedback systems emphasize the growing need for control consistent with larger size and complexity.

Kaplan[61] holds that leader mystique changes as the organization changes. In the early phases, the leader is very prominent and often seen as charismatic. The leader mystique appears to be proportional to the lack of definition of organizational goals and lack of clarity about rules, competence, and resources. In the next phase, the leader changes from "omnipotent one" to "plenipotentiary ambassador." Charisma of person is changed to "charisma of office." As structure and function are progressively clarified, and subdivisions are unequally developed, rewards may be unequal and rivalries emerge, creating a climate for disruptive internal events.

The Life Cycle of the Organization

The stages of development noted above occur in the early years of the life cycle of organizations. Although some organizations, once established, may endure in perpetuity, a great many are destined after a period of time to decline and demise. The deinstitutionalization period ushered in many new small mental health centers, but it also ushered in dramatic phasedowns of large institutions and the total phaseout of many.[62] In Massachusetts, as commissioner of mental health I was empowered to phase out totally Grafton State Hospital, housing 750 mostly chronic, elderly mentally ill. Between 1970 and 1973, in the country at large a total of 15 state hospitals were reported as having been phased out completely. Since that time, many more have ended operations or have been converted to other types of facilities. (Altogether, the adult mentally ill population of state hospitals in our country, through one means or another, has declined from more than 600,000 to approximately 130,000 since the deinstitutionalization movement began.[63])

I have learned that the closing of hospitals is not a quiet affair proceeding smoothly according to a well-defined plan, but that it can be an upheaval of major proportions. Not a gradual slipping into oblivion, but often more a terminal convulsion.[64] Patients, manifesting varying degrees of reluctance to move, are transferred to other facilities, or to a variety of community programs, or to nursing homes. Mortality rates may increase, especially among those with existing poor health or mental confusion.[65,66,67] On the other hand, follow-up of Grafton patients[68] after closure of that hospital in Massachusetts revealed that 40% of chronic geriatric patients were successfully placed in various community settings, of whom 42% were placed in nursing homes. In general, Grafton patients reacted positively to their new environments. However, many of the patients still lead isolated lives, and local citizen resistance to state-hospital patients discharged to the community has been vocal and vigorous.

Effects of closures on staff have been studied.[69,70] Morale falls when jobs are in peril; personnel must either move to a new location, undergo "retread" training, or retire. Ties are broken with other staff members, the community, and patients with whom they have formed meaningful relationships. Families with children may take the disruption badly.

Where the hospital has been a major employer in a rural community, the financial impact becomes a matter for labor unions, local politicians, and community organizers. There is concern that patients and employees may become dependent on welfare, and that the local economy may crash. Thus, there have been many efforts to slow the tide of depopulation and delay the demise of mental hospitals.

Those who have experienced such trauma, or have dealt personally at the planning and implementation phase, write passionately of the demoralization, sadness, and tension accompanying these closures.[71] The life-cycle view of hospitals can be expected to come into greater prominence if the closing of health facilities throughout the country continues at its present rate.

The Executive Constellation in Organizational Leadership

Turning rather abruptly from analysis of total social organizations, their growth and development and their life cycles, I bring to the reader's attention a seminal study of leadership groupings that I believe has not received sufficient attention in the literature. Yet, with the increase in size and complexity of organizations to which I have referred again and again as perhaps the most striking phenomenon of organizations in modern times, leadership at the top has become more diffuse, power more divided, and communications more intimate and collegial than hierarchically related.

Based on intensive study of three top leaders in a prestigious research/training mental hospital, Hodgson, Levinson, and Zaleznik[72] developed their concepts of the *executive role constellation*. Their theories move the management focus away from the single man, the final decision maker who confers on occasion with subordinates, to a multiperson system that—whatever the formal titles of its members—carries out a number of irreducibly important functions for the organization. They go behind the formal facade to what happens informally in a system. This is an early (1965) example of the applications of dynamic insights to executive-organizational functioning. The assumptions in this work are that the

> top executives in any organization—except one that is being pulled apart—form a close-knit group that is of key importance in all aspects of that organization's operations. Such executive groups, we think, usually

consist of two or three (rarely more) central individuals, although some others may be peripherally involved. . . . We use the term "constellation" rather than group to emphasize the significance of the personal relations among members, the emotional climate of the group, and the psychological properties of the interactions that define the group.[73]

Constellations involve three elements: "(1) role specialization of executive members, (2) differentiation among individual roles, and (3) complementary relations among them."[74] Without specialization there would be little differentiation of vital executive functions, and without trust and ability to work together, complementarity could hardly exist. This does not suggest that there is no disagreement, competition, conflict, or tension among members of the constellation, but these factors must be kept in check if effective management is to be forthcoming.

In the hospital studied, Hodgson et al. identified three role types acted out by upper management: the paternal–assertive, the maternal–nurturant, and the fraternal–permissive. The paternal–assertive was largely assumed by the superintendent; the fraternal–permissive role by the assistant superintendent, who was also head of research; and the maternal–nurturant role by the clinical director, who was also the director of residency training. "The functional similarity of this executive role constellation and the familistic triad of mother, father, and uncle was . . . unmistakable."[75]

The authors speculate that not only are these roles common in organizations, they are also based on common early experience with these roles in family life. The subordinates in an organization project these basic familial roles upon superordinate figures as the superordinates, characteristically and to an extent unconsciously, assume the roles. The superordinates' assumption of these roles stems both from internal drives as well as from external assignment by subordinates.

Types of constellations may vary from a *single person* attempting to introject all three roles, as in Freud's concept of the dominant father and the primal horde, to dyads, triads, and larger aggregates. Each model has its pros and cons in terms of institutional efficiency, built-in conflict tendencies, stability, and succession. For example, the single great executive may do well in the early developmental stages of a small organization, but may suffer as his powers wane with age and the "primal horde" becomes eager to take over.

The *dyad* incorporates the roles in father–mother, sibling, or parent–child relationships. One of the pair may look after boundary relationships (inside–outside), and the other internal dynamics. The *triad* constellation is viewed as intrinsically unstable. A constant pressure is asserted for the third person to remove himself from the constellation. Indeed, in the hospital studied by Hodgson et al., the third person (the assistant superintendent) eventually removed himself by taking a job as superintendent in another hospital.

Returning again to the three roles studied, the authors hypothesize strengths and weaknesses in each role. The paternal–assertive role may attract those who are dependent and need strong leadership, but repel those who disdain subservience to an omniscient father figure. The maternal–nurturant appeals to those who need warmth and affection, but unfortunately, aggression tends to arise in the group of subordinates competing for that warmth and affection. The fraternal–permissive builds on camaraderie, but contains within it the threat of erotic (homosexual) transference.

In summary, the executive role constellation construct greatly expands theories of management by groups, which more and more typify large organizations. However, this particular study is based on one triad in one specialized hospital. How well it applies to other systems of different size and goals, and to what extent other constellatory models function successfully, remains to be determined by future experience and research.

Fairness and the Span of Discretion[76,77,78]

Elliott Jaques, a psychoanalyst and social analyst, is responsible for fascinating insights into the basic laws governing business organizations. Jaques led a study of worker and management activities in the Glacier Metal Company, an engineering factory in London, that "may well come to bear comparison with the Hawthorne studies for their impact on management thinking."[79] Jaques's method involved the "working through" of problems by groups of investigators and employees together, which related to management–worker differences and their ramifications in terms of wages, job satisfaction, and "felt fairness."

In addressing the workers' continuing dissatisfaction with wages and salaries, attention focused on what was the right pay for a given level of job. From this the concept of *time span of discretion* as the main criterion by which a job should be evaluated was developed.

> Time span of discretion is defined as the maximum time during which an employee continues to exercise discretion without the results being reviewed.[80] . . .
>
> The essence of time-span measurement is that it is based not on vague general statements about "responsibilities" but on specific and concrete statements of real tasks that a real manager expects his real subordinates to carry out.[81] . . .
>
> Every concrete task that someone is required to do has a target completion time. . . .
>
> The higher a person goes in an executive system, the longer is the time framework within which he or she works. . . . The time span at which successive levels emerge in all managerial hierarchies is remarkably consistent. New levels emerge at . . . 1 year, 2 years, 5 years, 10 years and longer. For each time-span level there is a corresponding level of pay that people at that level feel to be fair.[82]

In effect, Jaques holds that if a payment system is based on discretion differences between jobs, it will generally be seen as equitable. The significance of this to the administrator is that many employees may justly feel that their pay is *not* fair; this is communicated outward as low morale, absenteeism, lowered productivity, grievance agitation, or (at times) strikes. What employees want, as Jaques points out eloquently, is fair pay, a share in the determination of policy, the right to appeal, and the right to work at the level appropriate to their capacity. In this day and age, 80% to 90% of workers in democratic industrial nations gain their livelihood by working for wages or salaries. They may spend more time in the manager–subordinate relationship than they do with their spouses. In this dependent relationship, adequate compensation and gratifying work determine to a great extent their status in society, their ability to educate their children, and the overall quality of their lives and the lives of their loved ones.

SUMMARY AND COMMENTS

Throughout history, analysis of organizations and the roles of management has received higher and higher priority as organizations have grown in size and complexity and have come increasingly under scrutiny of organizational psychologists, standard-setting groups, the legislature, and the judiciary.

I have selected 18 examples of contributions to the literature from the time of Max Weber onward to illustrate the remarkable diversity and originality of views on organizations and administration. This is not an exhaustive list. It is a selection of contributors who over the years have become significant to students of the field.

It is a formidable task to analyze and integrate the thinking of so many significant individuals. Consider the diversity of ideas and emphases: Weber looked at organization, workers, and managers and provided us with a general framework that has endured. Taylor and others, tackling employee productivity as their major variable, were the first to attempt to introduce objective data and analysis of work processes with a view toward reducing and simplifying those processes and helping the employee carry out his task in the shortest period of time.

Barnard's *The Functions of the Executive* remains a theoretical tour de force by a person with a long career in administration, heading up a variety of national organizations. It integrates the functions of organizations, employees, and executives in a brilliant way.

Sayre's fourfold perspective on organizations is a favorite piece repeatedly consulted by students. However, it does not attempt to delineate specifically the role of the executive. Bertalanffy and J.G. Miller have added penetrating insights on similarities of apparently different systems. J.G. Miller's *Living Systems* is a remarkably detailed study of 20 functions in eight different systems. Although much is said about the "decider" function, the main thrust of the work is on the system per se.

Miller and Rice of the Tavistock group, expanding greatly on Weber's approach, turn to organizational tasks, the needs of the people involved, and the necessity to integrate the two, based on intensive study of group and organizational processes. They have gained many followers on both sides of the Atlantic.

McGregor's Theory X and Theory Y are historical nuggets, organizing concepts related to worker potentialities into two polar philosophies that summarize a great deal of the thinking up to that time. Theory Z of Ouchi, based on intensive analysis of the Japanese industrial model, further strengthens McGregor's contention that Theory Y is the preferred way to deal with workers' productivity.

Likert emphasizes the centrality of groups, the important of linking pins, and the concept of human asset accounting. Argyris calls attention to the fact that the system tends to depress and thwart the worker, reminiscent of Barnard, Mayo, McGregor, Ouchi, Likert, and others. He recommends job enlargement, worker discretion in pace and performance of task, and use of the group laboratory to promote worker morale and involvement.

Returning to a consideration of the worker per se, Maslow and Herzberg are two whose insights into workers' needs and drives have been incorporated into management's thinking. Finally, from the more strictly sociological perspective, the characteristics of mental health systems are analyzed, and a national view of therapeutic organizations is considered that identifies the several levels of care and treatment given to our mentally ill citizens, and the ways in which mental health organizations may differ from other institutions in our culture.

But that is not all. With the development of psychodynamic theory and practice since the turn of the century, it is inevitable that psychodynamic theory should be applied to an understanding of organizations. Here Kernberg, in particular, offers a special point of view with his examination of leader and organizational regression and the multiple causes thereof. The developmental view and the life-cycle view of organizations contribute further to a broadening of perspective on organizations and how they function over time.

Particularly intriguing is still another study, by Hodgson, Levinson, and Zaleznik on the executive role constellation, which directs our attention to the multiple functions of management teams, how those functions are divided, and how the several managers must relate to each other. The panorama of theoretical and scientific attempts to comprehend our systems ends with Jaques and his unique contribution to the employee's concept of fairness and how the time span of discretion relates to the type of work performed, the supervision required, and the compensation assigned to the particular job.

So much for diversity. What about similarity of findings and theoretical constructs? Overlapping themes in this area are indeed numerous. Worker morale and worker participation and identification with the goals and purposes of the organization are increasingly stressed. Ever since the Hawthorne studies, "humanization" of the worker has become a prominent theme. Indeed, Japanese successes suggest that in America the humanizing trend has not gone far enough. Group methods of encouraging greater worker experience, cohesion, and dedication are mentioned more and more prominently in the literature. The worker as shareholder or stakeholder in the organization is upheld by many as an ideal. Should a greater part of the worker's educational, social, and cultural life be centered about his place in the organization? Should workers be made more secure about their long-term future?

Another theme has do with the functions of the executive—his multiple responsibilities and roles, the necessity for distributing executive tasks among several interrelated individuals (the executive role constellation), and the stresses and strains on executives, especially from increases in competition during austere times. Steadily growing is the realization that executive rationality may be hampered by character quirks and aberrations arising from unresolved conditioning in early life. In this connection, executive-renewal retreats and seminars to stimulate greater self-awareness and self-understanding are encouraged.

Implicit in the study of organizational development and organizational life cycles is the growing assumption that executive styles must be adapted to the historical stage of development of an organization, its changing purpose and community mission.

Impressive also is the view of writers that organizations dependent on human energy and skills are living systems. This is implicit in almost all the contributions mentioned above, but is overtly stated by Barnard, the system scientists, McGregor, Argyris, and others. Although the living system approach seems to be increasingly useful in studying and analyzing systems, a widely acceptable comprehensive theoretical perspective that includes worker, administrator, and organization together still lies ahead. One senses that most of the writers mentioned in the above review are striving for such a touchstone, but no single perspective has been adopted by the large majority of scholars.

A final point of interest. In reviewing the literature, the question arises: How much is offered that is science in the classical sense, as opposed to distillation of practical experience, or the development of "theoretical postulates?" The field is, indeed, rich in theoretical speculations, founded on the scholarly research and the experience of persons responsible for managing organizations. They delineate the *art* of administration, which is now, and perhaps will always be, a necessary talent of leaders in this field. It should be noted, however, that many who have made outstanding contributions to knowledge and theory have leaned toward a social-anthropologist type of approach, absorbing impressions and information through participant and nonparticipant observation, not by using the more formal, structured methodologies of the natural sciences.

REFERENCES

1. Boettinger HM: Is management really an art? Harvard Business Review 53:54–74, Jan.–Feb. 1975
2. Greiner L: A recent history of organizational behavior, in Kerr S (ed): Organizational Behavior. Columbus, Ohio, Grid Publishing, 1979, pp 7–11
3. Kraft AM: Behavioral and organizational theories, Chapter 9 in Talbott JA, Kaplan SR (eds): Psychiatric Administration. New York, Grune & Stratton, 1983, pp 123–133
4. Kraft AM: Behavioral and organizational theories, Chapter 9 in Talbott JA, Kaplan SR (eds): Psychiatric Administration. New York, Grune & Stratton, 1983, pp 123–133
5. Taylor FW: Scientific Management. New York, Harper & Brothers, 1911, 1939, 1947
6. Fayol H: Administration, Industriale et Génerale. Bulletin of the Société de l'Industrie Minerale, 1916
7. Fayol H (revised by Gray I): General and Industrial Administration. Published under the sponsorship of the IEEE Engineering Management Society. New York, IEEE Press, 1984
8. Greiner L: A recent history of organizational behavior, in Kerr S (ed): Organizational Behavior. Columbus, Ohio, Grid Publishing, 1979, pp 7–11
9. Barnard CI: The Functions of the Executive. Cambridge, Harvard University Press, 1938
10. Barnard CI: The Functions of the Executive. Cambridge, Harvard University Press, 1938, p 43
11. Barnard CI: The Functions of the Executive. Cambridge, Harvard University Press, 1938, p 60
12. Barnard CI: The Functions of the Executive. Cambridge, Harvard University Press, 1938, p 4
13. Barnard CI: The Functions of the Executive. Cambridge, Harvard University Press, 1938, p 6
14. Barnard CI: The Functions of the Executive. Cambridge, Harvard University Press, 1938, p 115
15. Barnard CI: The Functions of the Executive. Cambridge, Harvard University Press, 1938, p 116
16. Barnard CI: The Functions of the Executive. Cambridge, Harvard University Press, 1938, p 122
17. Barnard CI: The Functions of the Executive. Cambridge, Harvard University Press, 1938, p 116
18. Barnard CI: The Functions of the Executive. Cambridge, Harvard University Press, 1938, p 281
19. Sayre WS: Principles of administration—1. Hospitals, J.A.H.A. 30:34, 35, 92, 1956
20. Sayre WS: Principles of administration—2. Hospitals, J.A.H.A. 30:50–52, 1956
21. Bertalanffy, L: General system theory. General Systems 1:1–10, 1956. Reprinted from Main Currents in Modern Thought 71:75, 1955
22. Bertalanffy, L: General System Theory: Foundations, Development, Applications. New York, Braziller, 1968
23. Miller JG: Living Systems. New York, McGraw-Hill, 1978
24. Miller JL: The timer: A newly recognized subsystem at eight levels of living systems. Behavioral Science 35:157–196, 1990
25. Miller EJ, Rice AK: Systems of Organization. The Control of Tasks and Sentient Boundaries. London, Tavistock, 1967
26. Mayo E: The First Inquiry, in Merrill HF (ed): Classics in Management. New York, American Management Association, 1960, pp 407–416. Reprinted from Chapter 3 in Mayo E: The Social Problems of an Industrial Civilization. Boston, Division of Research, Graduate School of Business Administration, Harvard University, 1945, pp 59–67
27. Pugh DS, Hickson DJ: Elton Mayo and the Hawthorne investigations, in Pugh DS, Hickson DJ: Writers on Organization. Newbury Park, California, Sage Publications, 1989, pp 172–176
28. Lewin K: Field Theory in Social Science. Selected Theoretical Papers. D. Cartwright (ed). Westport, Connecticut, Greenwood Press, 1975
29. Lewin K: Resolving Social Conflicts: Selected Papers on Group Dynamics. New York, Harper & Row, 1948
30. McGregor D: The Human Side of Enterprise. New York, McGraw-Hill, 1960
31. Ouchi WG: Theory Z: How American Business Can Meet the Japanese Challenge. Reading, Mass., Addison-Wesley, 1981
32. Ouchi WG: Organizational paradigms: A commentary on Japanese management and Theory Z organizations. Organizational Dynamics 9:36–43, Spring 1981

33. Ouchi WG: Organizational culture. Annual Review of Sociology 11:457–483, 1985
34. Ouchi WG: Theory Z: How American Business Can Meet the Japanese Challenge. Reading, Mass., Addison-Wesley, 1981, p 7
35. Ouchi WG: Theory Z: How American Business Can Meet the Japanese Challenge. Reading, Mass., Addison-Wesley, 1981 pp 220–221
36. Ouchi WG: Theory Z: How American Business Can Meet the Japanese Challenge. Reading, Mass., Addison-Wesley, 1981
37. Lincoln JR, Kalleberg AL, with the collaboration of Hanada M, McBride K: Culture, Control, and Commitment: A Study of Work Organization and Work Attitudes in the United States and Japan. Cambridge, England, Cambridge University Press, 1990
38. Likert R: The Human Organization: Its Management and Value. New York, McGraw-Hill, 1967
39. Rush HMF: A science-based management: Rensis Likert, in Behavioral scientists: Their theories and their work, Chapter 2 in Behavioral Science: Concepts and Management Application. Studies in Personnel Policy, No. 216. New York, National Industrial Conference Board, 1969, pp 31–40
40. Likert R: The Human Organization: Its Management and Value. New York, McGraw-Hill, 1967
41. Rush HMF: Integrating the individual and the organization: Chris Argyris, Chapter 2 in Behavioral Science: Concepts and Management Application. Studies in Personnel Policy, No. 216. New York, National Industrial Conference Board, 1969, pp 26–30
42. Maslow A: Self-Actualizing People: A Study of Psychological Health. New York, Grune & Stratton, 1950
43. Herzberg F: Work and the Nature of Man. Cleveland, World Publishing, 1966
44. Lincoln A: Second inaugural address, March 4, 1864
45. Goffman E: Asylums: Essays on the Social Situation of Mental Patients and Other Inmates. Garden City, New York, Anchor Books, 1961
46. Blau JR: Sociological theories. Chapter 10 in Talbott JA, Kaplan SR (eds): Psychiatric Administration. New York, Grune & Stratton, 1983, pp 135–146
47. Ouchi WG: Theory Z: How American Business Can Meet the Japanese Challenge. Reading, Mass., Addison-Wesley, 1981
48. Hodgson RC, Levinson DJ, Zaleznik A: The Executive Role Constellation. Cambridge, Harvard University, Division of Research, Graduate School of Business Administration, 1965
49. Hodgson RC, Levinson DJ, Zaleznik A: The Executive Role Constellation. Cambridge, Harvard University, Division of Research, Graduate School of Business Administration, 1965
50. Spiro HR: Psychodynamic theories. Chapter 11 in Talbott JA, Kaplan SR (eds): Psychiatric Administration. New York, Grune & Stratton, 1983, pp 147–165
51. Spiro HR: Psychodynamic theories. Chapter 11 in Talbott JA, Kaplan SR (eds): Psychiatric Administration. New York, Grune & Stratton, 1983, p 155
52. Spiro HR: Psychodynamic theories. Chapter 11 in Talbott JA, Kaplan SR (eds): Psychiatric Administration. New York, Grune & Stratton, 1983, p 154
53. Kernberg OF: Regression in organizational leadership, Chapter 2 in Kets de Vries MFR (ed): The Irrational Executive: Psychoanalytic Explorations in Management. New York, International Universities Press, 1984, pp 38–66
54. Kets de Vries MFR (ed): The Irrational Executive: Psychoanalytic Explorations in Management. New York, International Universities Press, 1984
55. Kernberg OF: Regression in organizational leadership, Chapter 2 in Kets de Vries MFR (ed): The Irrational Executive: Psychoanalytic Explorations in Management. New York, International Universities Press, 1984, pp 38–66
56. Kernberg OF: Regression in organizational leadership, Chapter 2 in Kets de Vries MFR (ed): The Irrational Executive: Psychoanalytic Explorations in Management. New York, International Universities Press, 1984, pp 38–66
57. Bion WR: Experiences in Groups, and Other Papers. New York, Basic Books, 1961
58. Schwartz DA: A précis of administration. Community Mental Health Journal 25:229–244, 1989
59. Sharrin RM: Personal communication, 1991
60. Kaplan SR: Phases in development in psychiatric organization. Chapter 12 in Talbott JA, Kaplan SR (eds): Psychiatric Administration. New York, Grune & Stratton, 1983, pp 167–175
61. Kaplan SR: Phases in development in psychiatric organization. Chapter 12 in Talbott JA, Kaplan SR (eds): Psychiatric Administration. New York, Grune & Stratton, 1983, pp 167–175

62. Greenblatt M: The closing of state mental hospitals. Chapter 11 in Greenblatt M: Psycho-politics. New York, Grune & Stratton, 1978, pp 157–180
63. Greenblatt M, Norman M: Deinstitutionalization: Health consequences for the mentally ill. Annual Review of Public Health 4:131–154, 1983
64. Greenblatt M: Historical forces affecting the closing of state mental hospitals, in Plog Research, Inc., Stanford Research Institute (preparers): "Where Is My Home?" Proceedings of a Conference on the Closing of State Mental Hospitals. Menlo Park, California, Plog Research, Inc., and Stanford Research Institute, April 1974, pp 3–17
65. Aldrich CK, Mendkoff E: Relocation of the aged and disabled. A mortality study. J Amer Geriatr Soc 11:185–194, 1963
66. Markson EW, Cumming JH: The Post-Transfer Fate of Relocated Patients in New York. Mental Health Unit Research Monograph. New York State Department of Mental Hygiene, 1974
67. Marlowe R: The Modesto Relocation Project: The Social Psychological Consequences of Relocation of Geriatric State Hospital Cases. Project 1-60 (MOD), Bureau of Research, Department of Mental Hygiene, State of California, 1972
68. Khan NA, Kaplan RM: Phase-Out of Grafton State Hospital. Interim Report to Department of Mental Health, Commonwealth of Massachusetts, 1974
69. Weiner S, Place D, Ahmed P: A report on the closing of a state hospital. Admin Mental Health, Summer 1974, pp 13–20
70. Glover R (Ohio State Department of Mental Hygiene): Personal communication, 1975
71. Stotland E, Kobler AL: Life and Death of a Mental Hospital. Seattle, University of Washington Press, 1965
72. Hodgson RC, Levinson DJ, Zaleznik A: The Executive Role Constellation. Cambridge, Harvard University, Division of Research, Graduate School of Business Administration, 1965
73. Hodgson RC, Levinson DJ, Zaleznik A: The Executive Role Constellation. Cambridge, Harvard University, Division of Research, Graduate School of Business Administration, 1965, p 284
74. Hodgson RC, Levinson DJ, Zaleznik A: The Executive Role Constellation. Cambridge, Harvard University, Division of Research, Graduate School of Business Administration, 1965, p 284
75. Hodgson RC, Levinson DJ, Zaleznik A: The Executive Role Constellation. Cambridge, Harvard University, Division of Research, Graduate School of Business Administration, 1965, p 482
76. Jaques E: Taking time seriously in evaluating jobs. Harvard Business Review, 57:124–132, Sept.-Oct. 1979
77. Dowling WF (interviewer): Conversation with Elliott Jaques. Organizational Dynamics 5:24–43, Spring 1977
78. Jaques E: A General Theory of Bureaucracy. New York, Halsted Press, 1976
79. Pugh DS, Hickson DJ: Elliott Jaques and the Glacier investigations, in Pugh DS, Hickson DJ: Writers on Organization. Newbury Park, California, Sage Publications, 1989, pp 31–36
80. Jaques E: Taking time seriously in evaluating jobs. Harvard Business Review, 57:124–132, Sept.-Oct. 1979
81. Jaques E: Taking time seriously in evaluating jobs. Harvard Business Review, 57:124–132, Sept.-Oct. 1979, p 126
82. Jaques E: Taking time seriously in evaluating jobs. Harvard Business Review, 57:124–132, Sept.-Oct. 1979, pp 126, 127, 128

Toward Better Theory and Practice

THE SOCIAL SYSTEM CLINICIAN VIEW

The Need for a General Approach to Leader–Organizational Dynamics

In discussing the origins of general system theory, Ludwig von Bertalanffy[1] stated in 1956, "Today, our main problem is that of organized complexity. . . . General Systems Theory is in principle capable of giving exact definitions for such concepts and, in suitable cases, of putting them to quantitative analysis." Similar thoughts about "organized complexities" inspired the writings of Mary Parker Follett,[2] who in the 1930s examined complex industrial systems not merely to enlighten how they pursued the two objectives of producing commodities valued by the public and maximizing profits, but also because of her larger concern that unless organizations learn how to operate effectively in serving the individual, we are on the road to chaos. Her idea was that although the individual's welfare is greatly dependent on the ability of business organizations to solve the problems of producing goods and services, clearly it is also dependent on governmental organizations to maintain equality among people in rights and privileges, as well as to provide protection and safety for them. In addition to the business organizations she studied, organizations and institutions dedicated to law, education, and justice, as well as health and welfare, are also vital to the safety and welfare of the individual citizen.

Many attempts to elucidate the phenomena of leader–organizational dynamics in complex systems stress either the leader or the organization, without necessarily joining the two. The dynamic balance sought herein would take into account (a) the leader's characteristics, talents, and operational style; (b) the organization's goals, regulatory mechanisms, disturbances of homeostasis, institutional pathology, and interventions necessary to restore equilibrium; and (c) relationships between these two groups of factors.

Much of the literature describes characteristics for successful leadership, stressing such desiderata as intelligence, resilience, common sense, creativity, persistence, and so forth, often without reference to organizational context. Undesirable characteristics are also discussed, particularly in the book *The Irrational Executive*,[3] which stresses the harm that can be done by leaders who are overly narcissistic, obsessive, anxious, or guilty. However, lacking organizational specifics, we are often afloat on a sea of vagaries, not knowing how these traits operate in real life in a given context. Further, terms such as *narcissism, obsessiveness,* and *anxiety* are broad concepts. In nature these traits rarely exist in pure form; they are mixed with other traits, expressed with varying intensities, in varying relationships, and evoked by special, often unique situations.

On the other hand, structural/functional analyses that are focused primarily on organizations also can fall short if they neglect goals, pathological deviations, cybernetical mechanisms, or interventive strategies. They are even more lacking in meaning if they neglect the system role of the leader—his plans and dreams for the organization. The two together, leader and system, represent a dynamic, interacting complexity, the understanding of which presents a major challenge to all of us.

The Systems Clinician Model: An Embracing Concept of the Administrator's Role?

Bearing in mind the above, I have found it useful to view the organization as one would look at an *organism,* subject in the course of its career to changes and disturbances that bear on its health and welfare. In this perspective, the administrator becomes the *social system clinician*[4] (a term coined in 1957), looking after the organization as it goes through a series of disturbances of varying severities and durations, but with a strong tendency to return to its preexisting level. The reader will note that this concept of reequilibration (borrowed from Claude Bernard,[5] the great French physiologist) can apply equally as well to organizations as to individuals. The principle, using W.B. Cannon's term, is that of "homeostasis"—that is, the tendency of the organism to maintain constancy of its *milieu interieur* in the face of disturbances of equilibrium.

The principle of disturbance of equilibrium and the principle of homeostasis exist side by side, two aspects of life, inevitably intertwined. For example, if we consider the physiology of the human organism, a rise of blood pressure (for whatever cause) sets off a homeostatic mechanism that restores blood pressure to normal. What is remarkable is that throughout each day, although the blood pressure rises and falls many times, each time the homeostatic mechanism is equal to the task of reequilibration. The same applies to a great many other functions: control of blood sugar, cardiac rate, blood volume, and so on. Organizations, too, are subject to frequent alterations in their equilibrium, but mechanisms exist to set the organization right again and again.

Claude Bernard's concept of reequilibration was derived mainly from studies of acute, short-term changes in physiology of the organism. However, some of these changes, repeated often or with great exaggeration over a longer period of time, may result in permanent pathological deviations. Thus, blood pressure elevated to high levels too often and over a long period may lead to arteriosclerosis, which then becomes established and permanent. The organism is able to go on—apparently, in the early stages, functionally unimpaired—but in the long run, stenosis of arteries affects vital organs such as heart, kidneys, or brain.

Although the mechanisms for homeostasis operate in the short run with great efficiency, nevertheless a third principle of organismic change manifested over the long run must be introduced. The human organism, and in an analogous manner the human organization, changes inevitably with time. Thus, three principles—acute disturbances, homeostatic reequilibration, and *change in basic structural/functional status* must be accepted together as fundamental to living systems. Constancy in the short run, change in the long run; both relate to the deviations produced by stress.

Primary Requirements of Effective Top Management

Before going further with this theoretic model, I must point out that management, however we define it—whether as the functions of a single individual, an executive constellation, or a management–board interacting system—is responsible for the *functioning of the total system*. Under normal conditions, management receives more vital information about the functioning of the system as a whole than any other individuals or groups within it. The information as far as possible is confirmed for reliability and accuracy and should be purified of gossip, conjecture, or guesswork. Reliable information, whether it concerns "hard" items like the budget or "soft" items such as morale, intradepartmental friction, or community image, is a precious commodity in the business of management. It is also assumed that the system is managed by trustworthy individuals—worthy by virtue of training, experience, intelligence, wisdom, judgment, resilience, and personal maturity. If the leaders do not excel in their grasp of the total organization, then some other party or parties will, informally at least, gain greater influence in directing the organization.

An important implication here is that not only must top management be well endowed and equipped to lead, it must *work* assiduously at the task, for the challenge of comprehending the system never lessens. A system, however much it defies total understanding, nevertheless is better led the more management knows about it. Since the organization always changes, the need for understanding of both acute and long-term changes is ever present. Taken together, mastery of short- and long-term events also changes management: It diminishes their errors, sharpens judgment, and improves predictive ability.

At this point two common myths about administrators may be interjected. One is that administrators have an easy job: "They simply think up orders that everyone else has to follow." "They are out of town a lot, take frequent vacations, and receive high salaries." "They are masters of their own time, have a lot of assistants, and can do as they like." Such thoughts, often unspoken, nevertheless may be exchanged in the privacy of the informal organization. For those workers tied to front-line jobs such as the eternal processing of mentally ill admissions, with the inescapable burden of responsibilities, paperwork, and technical details, an administrator's job may look like paradise. Closer contacts between administrators and staff, together with shared information about each other's jobs, participatory planning, and cultivation of mutual respect, may go a long way toward ameliorating such attitudes.

The second myth applies to a considerable extent, but by no means exclusively, to middle managers—many of whom aspire to become top managers eventually. This particular fallacy is that once one becomes top manager, the heavy load of managerial details can be shifted to others, and one's life can suddenly become more relaxed. Then, at last, one can think, create, plan, even teach and do research. This fantasy also appears repeatedly among middle-level academic personnel in universities and medical schools, where education and research are foremost values. What is often not understood is that although delegation of work to others is a necessary factor in the organization of information and control systems, *delegation does not diminish the administrator's authority and responsibility for work done.* Each employee to whom work is delegated must be carefully selected, trained, and monitored, thus enlarging the top executive's sphere of responsibility. If too much is delegated, or if vital information is neglected, the leader's grasp of his organizational responsibilities weakens. For this reason, ensuring adequate input of vital information, particularly at critical times, can be a near-obsessive preoccupation of a conscientious administrator. He can diminish his value and even threaten his very existence in office if he neglects too many details.

The Nature of the System

What is the nature of the system in which both management and all the workers in it are involved? It is a *living social system,* as described comprehensively by J.G. Miller in his remarkable book *Living Systems.*[6]

Living systems are "open" systems that admit persons, matter, energy, and information through semipermeable boundaries into the interior, where these elements interact and may be transformed. The output from the living system is again people, matter, energy and information, but in modified form. The system is self-maintaining and can be self-reproducing—reproducing "organisms" similar to itself, or reproducing one or more of its many subsystems. Maintaining an organization in a relatively steady state requires feedback (cybernetical) mechanisms that correct its deviations in accordance with the theory of homeostasis (originated by Claude Bernard[7]). The larger system is divided into subsystems that serve special purposes. The processes and interactions that effect the transformations should be made consistent with the goals and purposes of the organization. An overall, intelligent "decider" mechanism governs the integration of subsystems, the transformations, the timing of events, the storage of matter and information, and the expenditures of work and energy (i.e., the "costs"). A self-critical function of the organization evaluates the efficiency and effectiveness of the system and directs the cybernetical (self-correcting) mechanisms.

This is but the merest summary of Miller's work. The many functions, subsystems, interactive processes, and transformations controlled by the decider mechanism need a further word of explanation. In the model presented here, the system clinician is the decider. His work is not limited simply to the interactions of the human elements, but includes all other elements: food, medical and surgical supplies, the communications network, information systems, transportation apparatus, and so on. In this maze, it is true, human elements claim the majority of "nonsentient" resources; but without both human and nonhuman elements the system cannot function properly.

The Social System in Health and Disease

The most important aspect of the systems clinician theoretical model is that the deciders view the system not only as a living organism, but also as an organism subject to *health and disease*. The first task, then, is to make a *diagnosis* of the social system. H. Levinson's[8] case study of the Kansas Power & Light Company is an early contribution in this regard. The study was undertaken to develop a diagnostic instrument that would eventually enable researchers to relate work organizations to mental health. The work organization—like any other living system, Levinson says—has a history, experiences crises, and adapts. His concept of a diagnostic outline is borrowed from psychoanalytic theory, clinical practice, and organizational theory, and he uses open system theory to expose three manifest tasks: maintenance of equilibrium (a) among subsystems, (b) between the system and other similar systems, and (c) between the given system and the larger system of which it is a part.

Organisms (including organizations) suffer insult and injury from their environment. An organizational diagnosis is therefore necessary to understand its identity, image, values, morale, tasks, goals and purposes, necessary interventions, and plans for the future. A diagnostic method would be a basis for training students and executives and for assessing organizational change as well as the results of managerial efforts.

The task, then, in the social system clinician model is to identify healthy and unhealthy trends in the system, determine if there are indications for intervention, and intervene at the proper time and with the proper corrective actions. Follow-up evaluation and a review of lessons learned from each significant system event complete the picture. A case file or casebook of system disturbances then becomes a valuable reference resource in teaching the art and science of administration.

Euphoristic Events

We commonly concern ourselves with disruptive happenings, and they do indeed take most of our time. But many system events are "euphoristic" or morale building, and they, too, deserve discussion.

Euphoria can be stimulated by internal or external events. When the organization or any part of it receives recognition in the media, most employees and administrators share pride in its accomplishments. When JCAHO confers full accreditation after a vigorous attempt by all hands to meet criteria, this event is marked by mutual congratulations and special acknowledgments to those who have participated in the success.

Internal events that have a positive effect on morale and productivity are classically illustrated by the Hawthorne studies alluded to in Chapter 2. Manifestations of personal interest by important supervisory figures affect worker productivity. As Herzberg has also shown (Chapter 2), achievement, recognition, advancement, and responsibility are internal "content" factors that give workers a good feeling about their job.

The personality and style of the leader are also very important in setting the morale and tone of an organization. Who does not wish to work for the benign, caring, protective father figure? On the other hand, who wants to work with a mean-spirited, irritable boss? Such qualities are quickly perceived by workers, who are often remarkably sensitive to the leader's personality, behavior, and operative style.

The euphoristic effects of the compassionate behavior of a benign leader are very welcome. Even a pat on the back and a word of encouragement are often more meaningful than a tangible reward. Interest in a worker's family, his recent promotion, recognition by his friends, or a reward given by his community can go a long way toward improving morale. What makes this kind of knowledge possible is an information-input mechanism sensitive to what really counts in human life. Since the executive cannot get around to everyone personally, memos and letters to individual employees and groups remind them he is always interested in their welfare.

Beyond these informal touches are the more formal recognitions: the employee-of-the-month award, a mention in the institution's newsletter, a bonus for an innovative suggestion for greater productivity, and the annual banquet or staff retreat to broaden the base of interaction between workers and supervisors.

Harry Solomon, professor at Harvard and superintendent of Massachusetts Mental Health Center (1943–1958), taught that his greatest concern was staff morale. When he made his unscheduled walks through the center, he often sat down to pass time with a member of his staff. His presence attracted others; together they talked and joked unhurriedly about anything and everything. His unprepossessing style had a "euphorogenic" effect on hospital morale. It increased the "smile index"—something he was fond of noting as he cruised through the halls.

Pathological Events

Unhealthy or pathological disturbances, too, can be the result of internal or external events. An example of a primarily *internal* event is disruption consequent to loss of a significant member of the organization (through promotion, transfer, firing, or death). An example of a primarily *external* event is disturbance that arises from budget cuts imposed from without (as a result, say, of a legislative mandate). In both cases, the internal reverberations can be widespread.

Disturbances may affect the organization as a whole, or be more or less confined to a limited segment. They also vary in severity, duration, and kind. Some are mild and of short duration; others may be severe, crippling, and extended in time, as when severe budget cuts threaten quality of care, professional integrity, and/or security of employment. How seriously these changes impact upon morale as well as on institutional goals and purposes may be used as a measure of their effect. When the organization reacts negatively, we may refer to such disturbance as *institutional pathology.*

This formulation, borrowed heavily from medicine, assumes that management, in fact, functions in the role of diagnostician as well as therapist of the organization. It is the job of the leader to be aware of—and anticipate, where possible—system disruptions that may be inimical to organizational health, and to effect those critical interventions that restore it as far as possible to health. If total restoration is not possible, then certainly the aim is to minimize damage and to help workers accept the new realities with the fewest scars upon morale and organizational functioning. *In short, the system clinician (leader) is concerned with the causes (etiology) and manifestations (signs and symptoms) of system disturbance, the varieties of euphoristic or disruptive changes created, the application of interventions (treatments), and the possible consequences or outcomes (prognosis).*

It is well to point out at this juncture that the administrator and the organization are intimately involved together in this health-and-illness model. Unlike the mechanic who fixes the vehicle after it has broken down, or the doctor who waits for patients with established disease to come to his office, the interactions of leader and group are intensive and ongoing—thus making it possible, after sufficient experience, to anticipate many institutional crises. At times the administrator himself actually contributes to the disturbances, not only because he is committed to a master plan for change, but also because his personal stresses and strains may interfere with organizational imperatives.

Examples of disturbances that are produced by leaders in the act of advancing institutional goals may include (a) a redistribution of resources between various divisions of the organization; (b) introduction of a new goal for the enterprise, necessitating changes in tasks and relationships; or (c) recruitment of a new person to head up an existing section or to become a coordinating agent among several sections. These changes may be part of a plan consistent with institutional goals in which the leader's actions are appropriate and wise. On the other hand, examples of leader-produced disturbances that are negative may include the promulgation of bad decisions, expression of inappropriate anger or bitterness, or playing favorites among his personnel. Institutional pathology derived from personal inadequacies of the leader is likely to be given more attention in the future than it has been in the past.[9]

Pathological disturbances limited to one part of the organization may include tensions and hostilities arising among personnel who work within the boundaries of a given subdivision. However, it should be borne in mind that because of the intimate interrelationship among the parts of a living system, a disturbance in one area tends to reverberate or network into other areas.

To classify the common types of pathology manifested in a system, the types of intervention practiced, and the efficacy of efforts to restore order and health will require objective research by individuals trained in field observation. Such research would yield much of value to the art and science of administration. It will help students make sense out of the maze of events going on in organizations, and it will provide more scientific underpinning to a field that is now an unruly mixture of art and science.

The Myth of the Uninvolved Leader

The social system clinician model has been criticized as ascribing to the leader a role similar to that of an all-knowing, wise physician who is coolly detached from the feelings of his patient. This tends to place the administrator exterior to his organization, immune to the processes he is attempting to ameliorate.

If some such image occurs to the reader, I hasten to point out that this is not the usual state of affairs for either the therapist–client relationship or the administrator–organization relationship. On the contrary, a dynamic partnership tends to be built up, for this partnership in fact establishes the best conditions for achieving the much-desired state of health and well-being of the respective organisms. I have never known a physician who is not sorely troubled when his patient suffers or presents a suicidal or homicidal risk, or when treatment is not going well. Indeed, in some cases empathic identification may be so acute that judgment is impaired and the clinician is drawn into the patient's pathological system (a specific example being therapist–patient sexual contact; see Chapter 8).

Whatever the shortcomings of the social system clinician model, there is no intent to paint a picture of an easy, relaxed, detached job as the administrator's lot. He is always a vital, interacting part of the culture of the organization he has helped to create—a culture that, in turn, molds both his character and his leadership style (see "Stresses and Strains of Administration" and "Rewards" in Chapter 12).

Inherent Stresses within Organizations

At all times, stresses or potential stresses are identifiable in every organization; I will recapitulate some of these stresses and strains here. In Chapter 5, examples are given of how stresses and strains occur between administrative and clinical divisions, between doctors and nurses, among members of a treatment team, or as a result of the emotional problems of workers or executives. Further problems are inherent in the relationships between staff and patients as a result of discrimination, favoritism, racial barriers, and the emotional baggage that people bring to the therapeutic environment.

There are also built-in stresses incidental to the division of labor among workers, the separation of organizational functions by departments or bureaus, and the differences that may arise among various hierarchical levels of command.[10] In Barnard's view, workers' contributions depend on inducements, but inducements do not necessarily elicit the desired contributions.[11] In another view, as Miller and Rice[12] have pointed out, the needs of the people ("sentient system"), and of the organization ("task-centered activities") do not always jibe.

Or, using Sayre's[13] fourfold approach to human organizations, difficulties may arise in or among any of the elements he identifies—the technological system, the system for policy formulation and decision making, the system of social processes, or the system of responsibility and accountability. The organization model presented by J.G. Miller, in which 20 functions related to input, throughput, and output are delicately balanced, again provides a matrix in which incompatibilities and malfunctions may arise.

Social scientists tell us that because of the diversity of occupations in the mental hospital, role ambiguities and conflicts may readily occur. Powerful forces outside the organization may be at odds with each other or clash with the organization's avowed direction.

Psychodynamicists see the organization as a microcosm of civilization and its discontents. Power and authority problems are ubiquitous, and the desire to displace the leader exerts a constant regressive pull. Those concerned with the life cycles of organizations call attention to stresses associated with early developmental stages as well as late phases of deterioration and demise.

Hodgson et al.[14] remind us that leadership today is often associated with a special "executive constellation" rather than with the prerogatives of one man, and that members of the constellation may evoke hostile reactions from staff or develop bitter rivalries among themselves.

Finally, Jaques points out that if the workers' feelings about fair pay, participation in management decision, access to appeal mechanisms, and the need to work at their appropriate capacity are repeatedly violated, labor–management struggles may be exacerbated.

Thus, we may conclude that none of the prevailing perspectives envision utopian harmony in the functioning of human systems. On the contrary, organizations are rich breeding grounds for pathological disturbances as instinctive needs, drives, and fantasies are acted out. It therefore becomes the administrator's task to modulate these drives within the bounds of organizational goals and imperatives.

Summary and Comments

Attempts to elucidate leader–organizational dynamics must take into account (a) the leader's characteristics, talents, and operational style; (b) the organization's goals, disturbances, regulatory (homeostatic) mechanisms, manifestations of pathology, and the interventions necessary to restore equilibrium; and (c) relationships between these two groups of factors. Much of the literature centers either on characteristics and problems inherent in the leadership role or on the structural/functional elements of an organization. This chapter is an effort to link the two together in a unifying theory.

I take the view that the social system clinician concept best epitomizes, in the fewest words, the unity of the administrator role in relation to goals and functions of the organization. The organization is seen as a living, open system, with inputs, throughputs, and outputs, capable of maintaining itself through its several functions (which include feedback mechanisms, timing mechanisms, and overall "decider" activities). Normally these functions maintain the organization in a steady state (homeostasis) despite perpetual disturbances in its equilibrium. Over time, however, the organization itself changes in a more fundamental sense as a result of repeated impact from inner and outer sources.

The changes an organization undergoes may be euphoristic (healthy) or dysfunctional (pathological—i.e., unhealthy) in response to stimuli (inner or outer). The system as a whole, or any of its parts, may be affected. As viewed from the perspective of basic goals and purposes, its disturbances may be regarded as major or minor.

The system clinician (leader/administrator) is concerned with the causes (etiology) and manifestations (signs and symptoms) of system disturbance, the euphoristic (healthy) or disruptive (pathological) changes produced, the application of interventions (treatments), and the consequences or outcomes (prognosis). This structure, borrowed heavily from medicine, can be applied to human organizations as well as to individual human beings.

It should be noted that in his role as leader, the administrator himself initiates and encourages changes in the system as part of his responsibility to serve his constituents and to maintain the health of the organization. In turn, the administrator is affected by such changes and undergoes both personal development and modification of his style of management.

At all times there are stresses within the organization, for the needs of the individuals and the goals and purposes of the system do not always jibe. Indeed, none of the prevailing organizational perspectives envision utopian harmony in the functioning of human systems.

INSTITUTIONAL CHANGE

It is not sufficient to comprehend how our health systems work and how it may be possible to restore balance quickly by specific interventions when institutional equilibrium is acutely upset. Beyond these are changes of the system over time, many of which depend upon the views of the citizens in the organization as to the *missions* of the organization and the steps to achieve these missions.[15] Some of these changes may occur without consciously directed influence from administration, but many involve active input of ideas, energy, and force from management.

In the 1930s and 1940s, social scientists studying mental institutions pointed out that to change some of the stagnant, custodial, entrenched, authoritarian hospitals of that day, the most important factor necessary to jar them out of their rut was change itself—almost any kind of change.

Aims and Goals

The aims and goals of an operation are expressed originally in formal documents created at the founding of the organization. They are then modified to conform with the needs of the times. Goals are usually translated into aims, identified as specific targets of accomplishment, with assignments as to who will be responsible within a given time frame. Resources needed are then tied to objectives in what is popularly known as management by objective (MBO).[16]

At IBM, goals and objectives are spelled out for seven years ahead, and revised annually for the next seven years. Each department draws up schedules of objectives and needs that are then integrated into a final program by management. In many places the general aims are first drawn up by management, then translated by individual departments as guidelines for their units. A broad base of participation is encouraged through departmental meetings and organizationwide retreats where all units are represented.

In industry, goals are relatively easy to define. Profit is the primary motif, and the relationship between the commodity (or service) offered the public and profitability is a central consideration. Industry asks: Will a particular investment in a new plant pay off in terms of supplying the market with a more saleable product? Will a greater investment in research be required? Will the introduction of a management information system facilitate data acquisition vital to planning, and at the same time generate savings in personnel? Or, more subtly: Will a rearrangement of foreman–worker relationships or the introduction of incentives yield a higher quality product and reduce product errors?

In the mental health systems, the variables are more subtle, and planning for institutional progress is more closely affected by the human equation. The "commodity" is an improved human being—more fit to adapt to current society, more capable of looking after himself, and (it is hoped) happier and more content with his lot in life. We ask: Have his hallucinations abated? Is his reality sense improved? Is his self-esteem restored? Are his relationships with family, friends, and workmates happier, less tense, less dominated by projections or distortions? Or, more subtly: Who, in our multidisciplinary staff, is most suited to form a productive relationship with this drug-dependent young adolescent, maltreated by his father after his mother's death? Or: Can we make explicit the determinants of a good therapeutic match?

The goals of an organization may be implicit or explicit. An implicit goal in industry is exemplified by the assumption that a good profit year means greater worker security of employment, and perhaps a bonus at Christmas time. For mental health institutions, just as at IBM, explicit goals may be set in writing, distributed to all departments, and made the subject of lectures and demonstrations. Before explicit goals are hardened, contributions come from all departments. The individual units are invited to become involved. The final version is hammered out by an expert committee whose recommendations are adopted, often with modifications, by management. In the process of contributing to the final product, implicit goals and assumptions are aired. Problems of morale, rights and responsibilities, and grievances may be addressed.

In the mental health system, an example of goals for the year as expressed by one mental health chief of a governmental agency were as follows:

1. Correct revenue deficiency by (a) increasing bed occupancy, (b) changing the mix of patients by admitting more patients with third-party coverage, and (c) maximizing revenue from "covered" patients by more careful financial analysis.
2. Open a new service for adolescent patients.
3. "Academicize" the department further by (a) increasing the quality of teaching in every division, and (b) stimulating greater interest in research and scholarship.

Goal Slippage

It is not enough to enunciate goals, and/or to assume that somehow the institution will move toward those goals. The possibilities of "goal slippage" begin at the point of enunciation. To avoid slippage, plans for attainment of these goals must be carefully developed. Each step of implementation is worked out in detail, and methods for measuring progress toward the goals are defined. Considerable energy and effort must be forthcoming from the administrator's office and from many other levels to make the goals come true.

1. The first possibilities for slippage arise from *inadequate, unrealistic framing of the goals.* They should be stated in clear, simple language that is understandable to all echelons. Goals expressed in vague, abstract terms are an invitation to failure; the average worker wants something he can sink his teeth into. They should be formulated so as to ensure the broadest possible base of involvement. Thus, a goal such as "the employment of three new clerks in the division of revenue enhancement" is hardly likely to guarantee mass cooperation.

2. The goals should be communicated so as to evoke *personal interest.* Workers should be made aware that accomplishment of goals will impact not only on the way they do their jobs, but also the way their performance will be evaluated. This will require repetition of targets throughout the year, and feedback of information to workers.

3. The goals must be *accepted* by a sufficient number of workers to make achievement possible. Acceptance starts with rationalization, involvement, and participation. Where serious resistances (either overt or covert) occur, attention is directed to establish a process of working through the resistance. This is a fundamental mechanism in resolving institutional resistance to change, used with patience, understanding, and effectiveness by good administrators. The following quote from H.C. Solomon is an example:

> We want continuing change, not by ukase, but by discussion and argument, perhaps continuing for months; with respect for the opinions of all. Issues can be decided by logical debate rather than direct orders. The "High Moguls" should be willing to justify themselves to the "Low Moguls." This will lead to a feeling among staff that they are not being pushed around. Let personnel and patients, rather than doctors only, use their imagination in developing enterprises.[17]

4. The *means of measuring progress* should be at hand. Thus, the goals mentioned above (" 'Academicize' the department . . . by increasing the quality of teaching . . . and stimulating greater interest in research and scholarship") may be meaningless unless some ways of measuring progress can be defined. For those involved with academic organizations, it is sufficient to remind them that in fact the means *are* at hand to measure many subtle variables. Quality of teaching can be measured by the satisfaction of students

with their instructors' performance; thus, student rating sheets are important. Annually, psychiatric residents—for another example—take the PRITE exam (Psychiatric Residency In Training Examination), which measures acquisition of knowledge and skills well before residents sit for the formal specialty examinations of the American Board of Psychiatry and Neurology (which also are a measure of clinical/academic progress). Presentation of cases, performance in rounds, and scores on personal quizzes by teachers further quantify this dimension. From these data the heads of training programs then plan modifications of their training programs year by year.

As for research, documentation of change can include new projects started, proposals submitted, grants received, papers published, presentations given, and university academic advancement approved.

5. The concept of *no decline* is vital to combat slippage, which is ordinarily a natural phenomenon of organizational life. Except under unusual circumstances, if goals and aims are not reiterated and kept high by management, the second law of organizational thermodynamics prevails—that is, the goals gradually recede from mind, become dim, and may be forgotten. Among the mechanisms found useful to reenergize goal activities is *periodic feedback* of progress to all hands involved in goal formulation and implementation. Once goals are achieved, adequate recognition is given to all who helped.

Implementation of Change: Concepts and Techniques

"Where progressive institutional change is desired, a central variable often is the administrator's attitude towards *organizational creativity.*"[18] Considerable creative energy seems always to exist in the ranks of workers, ready to come forth if proper conditions are provided. Many workers are bursting with ideas for change; some possess potentialities of which they are hardly aware. Further, the release of this potential heightens morale, dedication, and loyalty to the system. Many examples exist of how a new leader can inspire a stagnant system to new heights of accomplishment simply by using the right key to unlock creative effort. How is this done?

Merely indicating to staff that creative effort is valued by administration, and that administration is aware that a great deal of latent creativity exists in the organization, does make a difference. It may have to be repeated many times, but soon personnel will test out administration's sincerity by offering ideas and suggestions. How the organization reacts to those ideas and suggestions also makes a difference. As with the good teacher who assumes that contributions to discussions offered by a student are inherently useful, so it is with contributions from institutional staff. Their suggestions, carefully considered and shaped and modified by additional inputs, are given practical trial wherever possible. The best reward to many workers is simply that care and attention has been given by higher-ups to their ideas, and that their thinking can make them a more important part of the facility. If such rewards can then be augmented by formal acknowledgment—financial recognition, or job advancement—so much the better.

To what extent, I ask, do administrators view release of the creative participation of workers as one of their primary responsibilities? For it is one of the surest roads to higher morale and favorable institutional change.

Pace of Change

How fast or slow should change be? Is it more advantageous to press forward hard, or to do it in leisurely manner? Much depends on the personality and style of the administrator.

The advantages of *moving swiftly* are manifold. It demonstrates that the organization is activistic; management does more than talk. Workers who have been used to much talk but little action are bounced out of their lethargy. A true atmosphere of action separates those who are forward-looking from those who are content with the status quo. Outsiders become interested in an institution in motion, where vital things may be happening. Applications for jobs increase.

But for many people, change is anxiety provoking, particularly if they cannot see exactly what their future roles may be. Absenteeism, substance abuse, psychosomatic illness, outspoken hostility, and thoughts of moving elsewhere may be forthcoming. Predictions of disaster and failure are common. Appeals to outside powers to stop disturbing new trends may be made. Grievances may be filed, and the unions may be asked to intervene.

These fears catapult the administrator into rounds of "administrative therapy" meetings with individuals and groups who feel hard hit. In these sessions, the administrator undertakes to allay anxieties and help people adapt to new realities. But anxiety cannot always be reduced to zero, and the ability of some to adapt to change is limited. Yet the process of change cannot be allowed to depend on the endless resistance of some recalcitrant individuals. There *is* a price to pay, for change (particularly rapid change) can hurt. Moreover, it may be true that some folks are happier in an organization that demands less of them.

On the other hand, *going slow* causes minimal disruption of staff and makes little demand on their adaptive powers. If, however, the pace is so slow as to amount to virtual stagnation, survival may be imperiled, and opportunities to do more for patients, families, and community may be lost.

One variation on the fast/slow theme, from my experience at Boston State Hospital, is worth mentioning.

Case Illustration

Unitization at a State Hospital

In the 1960s, a powerful innovation in the form of the restructuring of large hospitals was being advanced. It was called *unitization*.[19] In the typical large state hospital of that time, all admissions were received into one unit or building, which was relatively heavily staffed. After rapid diagnosis and treatment, the patients were discharged to transitional facilities, to the community, or transferred to the chronic wards. The ratio of the actual number of acute beds to chronic beds at that time was on the order of 200 to 2,000. In the chronic units, staffing was very thin, therapeutic activity with individual cases minimal, duration of hospitalization long, and discharges few.

Unitization—one of the great upheavals a hospital can experience—means radical departure from an essentially pyramidal hospital structure to subdivision of the hospital into (in this case) four highly autonomous units, each with its director and staff, *each receiving patients from a predemarcated population area, and each serving both acute and chronic patients from those areas.*

Without going into the details of the reorganization, suffice it to say that the pros and cons of unitization were discussed in many quarters, with great vigor and intensity, for many months, without a final conclusion or specific plan of action. Yet the administration, acting the role of "willing to be convinced," kept the discussion going, insisting that the issues be resolved on their merits, not by emotionalism, and that a move would be made only when a significantly large majority of those involved would back it up and see that it was accomplished.

The point is that unitization—a complex, all-embracing change—requires that most of the staff work out and accept significant changes in their roles. At times, frustration was at such a pitch it seemed it would be better to abandon the project altogether.

However, as a result of management keeping discussions alive, eventually most of the staff really wanted unitization—and some said that the administration, with its foot-dragging, was the chief obstacle to its realization. This was the turning point. Apparently, as discussion continued and emotionalism abated, the merits of the plan received more rational consideration. At the same time, the administrator felt he now had a sufficient mandate from his staff to proceed with implementation of the idea, with a good chance for ultimate success. Soon a detailed plan was drawn up, and the hospital organization was restructured in accord with the unitization concept.

Unitization in this case proved to be a boon in that it gave more individuals opportunities to assume responsibility and show what they could do. It diminished the sharp distinction between acute and chronic patients and the tendency to neglect the latter, and it linked each new unit to a catchment area. This, in turn, forced staff to view its mission in terms of serving a defined population, to mobilize community resources to meet those needs, to encourage use of volunteers and paraprofessionals, and to employ epidemiologic research to help chart its future course.

Here an important lesson seemed to be that where changes are overwhelming, reservations numerous, and outcome uncertain, long gestation is a necessity. That staff eventually prodded administration to do something illustrates that in this case the drive for change did not come only from top command but also from an increasingly strong base of involved employees. The "troops" had argued for so long that eventually they were fed up with debate and simply bursting with the need for action.

Other Observations Applying to System Change

Without challenges an organization tends to slow down, become entrenched, and ossify. The ensuing rigidities, in turn, make change even more difficult. It is desirable that leaders adopt the principle of *progressive expectations,* which means the introduction of challenges for change at strategic intervals that will perpetuate the mood for change and direct energies into fruitful channels. These ideas may come from any source. They come from within if channels are open, communication free, and new ideas and programs suggested by staff seen as a virtue. They may come from outside, particularly if visits to other leading institutions are encouraged. Often what one's own institution has accomplished is seen to have value elsewhere, and what seemed difficult or impossible to achieve at home is found elsewhere to be both feasible and practical.

(For example, when unitization was being considered in the above example, visits to Clarinda State Hospital in Iowa,[20] Fort Logan in Colorado,[21] and Kansas State Hospital[22] convinced the staff that the idea was not a mirage and that the final results could be very positive.)

Emphasis on progressive change, with its opening of communication channels, leads to a deemphasis on hierarchy and control and a definitive change in the culture of the organization, for entrenched power bases tend to thaw and the structural rigidities of the institution interfere less with its appropriate functions. As participation is more widespread, delegation of planning, decision making, and implementation becomes easier. Individuals who formerly saw their roles in very narrow terms find their minds opening up to larger hospital goals.

Bench Strength

In industry, a shortage of manpower can be readily made up by increases in entry salaries, stepped-up advertisement, or specialized inducements and emoluments. In many mental hospitals (especially those remote from universities or training centers) where salary structures are rigid and emoluments cannot be multiplied, the "bench" is thin or empty. This bench strength, in a manner of speaking, determines in part the administrator's strength, for if employees cannot be easily replaced they may respond by foot-dragging when change is expected. Thus, the name of the game is to cultivate retention internally of those who are indispensable, and to cultivate relationships outside with those who may replace, in timely fashion, the recalcitrant ones. Only thus can an administrator achieve full authority over his organization, and enjoy the flexibility and breadth of maneuverability necessary for positive cultural change.

Executive Mastery of the System: Seven Principles

Since the executive cannot master all that is going on in the system, the realistic challenge then is to try to gain mastery over the most important activities, functions, and information necessary to plan and crystallize policy and to delegate its implementation.

1. The first principle is that the executive cannot cloister himself in his office, surrounded by secretaries and assistants who, in the course of time, isolate him from his workers and the dynamic activities of his organization. In times past, a great deal was heard about span of control and the assumption that one could not deal effectively with more than six to eight subordinates. On the contrary, I submit that the executive has several arcs of contact emanating from his office—certainly an inner group that works with him intimately, and then other groups with less frequent contacts. But there is much ebb and flow in this configuration. Persons in the second or third outer arcs may move in and out of range, depending on their needs and the needs of the system. The executive office cannot be closed to new information, cannot depend entirely on the reports of an inner circle, and must be curious to see for itself what is going on—without embarrassment, one hastens to add, to the formal chain of command. Flexibility, not rigidity; freedom, not constraint; and firsthand observation, not just filtered reports.

Thus, periodic freedom from the palace guards must become an accepted modus operandi, and visits down the line should be expected. Administration by walking around is a good idea. At the same time, large mass meetings, small group meetings, and many one-to-one sessions should be used to keep in touch.

2. The second principle is that attention is given to those parts of the organization, or those functional units, that appear to have the greatest needs. This, obviously, must allow for shifting priorities that reflect the urgency of needs of different parts of the system. Thus, today it is ward coverage, tomorrow it is a new legislative mandate regarding rights of patients, and yesterday it was providing for the smooth entry into the work force of a new recruit. The number of glitches in system functioning cannot be perfectly predicted, so that "putting out fires" is a commonly expected experience in today's organizational life. An important caveat is that surface problems that appear to involve one area may reflect deeper tensions that involve the whole system. The administrator, therefore, must be wary of organizational scapegoating—that is, the displacement of distress upon problems that are not necessarily at the core of the difficulty.

3. A third principle is to shape the informational flow so as to give maximum information with the smallest number of "bytes." Personnel have a habit of loading down the chief with long reports or extensive reading matter. They should be encouraged to put nothing on his desk that does not have an executive summary. Précis writing up and down the line leads to more exact, more cogent, more parsimonious thinking. In addition, as is well-known, modern technology now permits a sophisticated grasp of information through the use of computerized management information systems (MIS) that can give almost instant pictures of personnel, patients, and budget.

4. A fourth principle is to make worker morale an important consider-

ation for all personnel. Good morale and happy workers mean fewer errors, less absenteeism, fewer grievances, less foot-dragging, and more creative solutions to knotty problems. It goes without saying that the morale of the leader himself is an important stimulus to the morale of the workers. "The institution," said Emerson, "is the lengthened shadow of the man."[23]

5. A fifth principle relates to the basic conception the administrator has with respect to the giving–receiving aspects of his role. Put in bottom-line terms, do the people work for him, or does he work for them? Both parties are presumably pursuing common institutional goals, but in relation to those goals, who gives and who receives? If the administrator needs praise, adoration, centrality in all things, indulgence, or lots of attention, he may not long be an asset. Instead, he should be thinking how he can help others with *their* self-esteem, their need for recognition and validation. No administrator should boast of the multitude under his supervision, but of the multitude he serves.

6. That accountability must match authority, and vice versa, is an old axiom. Accountability must also be accompanied by adequate resources to do the job. We do not necessarily expect that accountability, authority, and resources overlap perfectly, but to the extent that accountability may exceed authority and resources, stress is inevitable. Under such imbalance, the responsible executive not only views the situation as unfair, but also he becomes concerned about the threat of litigation should quality of care sag.

7. The last principle of mastery is based on the fact that the hospital, in addition to all its internal networks, has numerous relationships to outside agencies, and that two-way communication with all these agencies and facilities may influence the health and vitality of the organization and sometimes even its survival. In attempting to adapt to both inner and outer complexities, changing with time, the administrator is like the famous juggler who keeps many plates in the air twirling upon many sticks; the juggler runs from one to the other, seeing that they all remain aloft and twirling without a single one falling and breaking.

Summary and Comments

Inevitably, with time, institutions change. In today's climate of heavy competition, tight resources, and changing social demands, organizations are changing faster than ever—some phasing up or down significantly or even phasing out. Those that survive experience a considerable change in mission as well as in methods to achieve their goals.

Aims and goals are easier to define in industries where the profit motive rules the manufacture of a tangible product. In mental health facilities, the product is harder to define. Aims and goals, nevertheless, are the sine qua nons in evaluating the merits of an organization, and whether its disturbances are healthy or dysphoric (as discussed earlier in this chapter).

Targets of accomplishment should be delineated periodically (at least annually) and upgraded in relation to both short- and long-term timetables. Broad and general guidelines emanate from the top, within the framework of which flesh-and-bones details arise from a broad base of participation, every department's goals (and wishes) included. Budget figures, attached to specific objectives, too, are derived from top-down and bottom-up planning. Once goals are accepted and appear viable, the object is to prevent what has been called "goal slippage."

To prevent slippage, goals must be realistic and attainable, evoke the personal interest of workers, and be acceptable to a sufficient number of workers so as to make achievement possible. More importantly, means of measurement must be at hand. The concept of "no decline" should be inculcated into staff by periodic feedback of progress and interventions to maintain unslackened output.

Organizational creativity is a concept useful to management. It maintains that the work force almost always possesses potentialities not fully realized within the system, but which can be encouraged and released to good advantage by proper attention from administration.

How fast or slow should change be? Moving too swiftly has obvious advantages in that it increases output and fosters a climate of activism. In turn, this encourages creativity inside and draws attention of outsiders to a "system in motion," where vital things may be happening. However, anxiety and tensions may be provoked in those who cannot adapt.

Moving slowly, on the other hand, may encourage status quo stagnation and a loss of vital opportunities in a competitive market. The principle of "progressive expectations" has been discussed, in which change is introduced at strategic intervals, associated with progressive opening of channels of communication, new ideas from a broader base, and reduction of institutional rigidities.

Finally, this section ended with seven principles related to executive mastery of the system.

PRACTICAL INTERVENTIONS: ILLUSTRATIONS

What intervention strategies and tactics are available to administrators dealing with events that are troublesome? Actually, an abundance of mechanisms has been used, some of which are outlined here. They are limited primarily by the creative imagination of the administrator. A standard inventory of such interventions and systematic studies of their effectiveness in specific situations is much needed. Current validation of the effectiveness of various interventions is based primarily on the experience of seasoned administrators.

The following examples are selected with the optimistic view of what *can* be done in a variety of situations by the means at hand. They are not meant to convey the impression that the problems presented are necessarily isolated or disconnected from deeper issues in the system, or that they can be easily handled by a *mot juste* delivered by the administrator. In fact, every problem may be suspected of being a manifestation of deeper trends, and the solution of the one may lead to the discovery of, or even create, other problems. As the administrator gains increasing understanding of the interlocking nature of the system's parts and of the more remote consequences of his intervention, he begins to operate with greater wisdom and effectiveness. The two key system phenomena that face the administrator at all times are complexity and interdependence of functions.

The two most common interventions used in problem solving are the *face-to-face interview* and the *group meeting*.

Case Illustrations

Face-to-Face Interviews

ILLUSTRATION A: An administrator found it necessary to call on the carpet a physician who was reported to have been irritable, impatient, and impolite with visitors, referring physicians, and even superiors. Attempts to handle this at the level where it arose (always the preferred alternative) had failed.

The psychiatrist in question, head of a service unit, complained bitterly that orders had been given by a superior that he found difficult to carry out. Toward the end of a long discussion, the psychiatrist made clear several problems: He was suffering from migraine and gastric ulcer; he resented the cold, detached way he had been handled by his supervisor; and he was frightened that he would be downgraded and eventually fired from his job because he was not getting along. He admitted that his irritability was a long-standing problem based on early familial coping styles modeled on his parents, who were always fighting and bickering.

Reassurance that his job was not in immediate jeopardy, and a recommendation that he speak frankly to his superiors about his problems in interpersonal relationships, seemed acceptable. Also, it was suggested that immediate apologies were in order to those who had taken offense at his abruptness, irritability, and apparent lack of respect. A further recommendation that he consult a therapist for his problems was considered, but not followed up. (He was already in the care of an internist for migraine and ulcer.)

Happily, this one session of paternal-administrative "therapy" was sufficient to help this psychiatrist change his course. He continued his work and, freed of fear of reprisal for his poor behavior, often performed brilliantly.

ILLUSTRATION B: A staff doctor covering the emergency service at night ran into a very experienced but officious nurse who treated the doctor abominably and insisted that the latter's medication prescriptions were all wrong. The staff doctor refused to work nights any longer unless treated with more respect. Other night-time-covering doctors concurred that the nurse in question was a problem.

The service chief and the supervising nurse together agreed to meet with the offending nurse. A lively discussion ended with the offending nurse's sudden and sober appreciation of the realities of life (i.e., no doctor coverage equals no emergency service equals no need for nurses). Improvement followed.

In passing, it should be noted that the inability of the two parties to communicate with each other violated a cardinal principle of cooperation and collaboration—namely, that whatever the personal feelings involved, "thou must work harmoniously together for the good of the patient." Yet a simple problem of rudeness and lack of respect by a nurse for a doctor may hide deeper problems, such as a struggle for dominance and control between the nursing hierarchy and the medical chiefs of service. Indeed, in this case the larger quarrel was then a fact of organizational life, destined to be worked out eventually at a higher level.

Group Meetings

Scheduled group meetings of every description are ongoing throughout the institution, part of its normal "metabolism." Included are executive and professional councils, ward rounds, colloquia, grand rounds, cross-discipline meetings within the hospital, and meetings with outside agencies. However, there are also groups that are *not* regularly scheduled, but called together specifically to handle a difficult problem.

Persons invited to one of these informal groups are carefully selected. They represent different points of view related to a functional impasse.

Case Illustration

Treating the Patient Overload

A group consists of emergency room personnel, together with personnel from acute wards to which emergency patients are normally transferred. The issue: available ward beds were slowly disappearing, emergency ward was plugged up with patients overstaying their legal limit.

After much heated discussion, the following solutions were achieved: (a) greater respect and understanding by each party of the problems and trials faced by the other in the normal course of their work; (b) a recommendation, which was accepted, that discharges before noon of patients on the receiving acute wards (rather than late afternoon or evening) would help greatly to relieve the peak emergency room overload; (c) a recommendation, also accepted, to urge police to hold back cases they pick up until a very heavy emergency service overload could be whittled down; and (d) an agreement that the group would meet at intervals to monitor events and check up on the implementation of strategies suggested. (The problem, however, was a recurring one, and additional work on it was required at intervals.)

Job Changes

Inevitably, in any organization, square pegs are trying to accommodate themselves to round holes. Many personnel could do better if job functions or job environments were changed.

Case Illustrations

Fitting Talents to Job

ILLUSTRATION A: A very able and experienced doctor finds himself in a consultation/liaison job but eyes longingly a position as head of an acute ward. He likes the idea of developing his own ward team over a long time, rather than the hit-and-run character of the consultation/liaison role.

When such transfer is eventually arranged, his team-building talents manifest themselves superbly in a ward where team morale had sagged before.

ILLUSTRATION B: Emergency service personnel had been saddled for some time with the job of "gatekeepers" for a mobile PET (psychiatric emergency team) unit. Over time, the gatekeeping function expanded enormously until it invaded normal emergency room functioning. As a solution, emergency service personnel were encouraged to formulate a petition signed by all. This petition, enclosed with a letter from the administration to the central department, explained that the expanded gatekeeper function was not compatible with the ever-increasing emergency caseload.

The gatekeeper function was transferred by the central office to another hospital.

Constructive Evaluation of Job Performance

Periodic evaluations of personnel performance, if properly conducted, help personnel to see themselves as supervisors see them. The problem with these evaluations is that they tend to deteriorate into cover-ups, which give the whole evaluation program a bad name. Unless something truly damaging is mentioned about an employee's performance, the employee has no need to change his ways. The raters, however, are often so close to or dependent on those they rate as to surrender desirable objectivity. And since their ratings must be shared with the workers, there is that much more reason to suppress or minimize negative evaluations. Continuous input from the personnel office, therefore, is necessary to assist evaluators in exercising objective judgment and in working through their resistance to voicing critical comments. When these matters are taken care of, the exercise can then be an eye-opener for the worker and can place the supraordinate–subordinate relationship on a more realistic, honest basis. Vital to a good performance evaluation system is the necessity of providing help to a deficient worker in a way that will enhance his self-esteem, build trust and respect, and open up the possibility of improved performance and ultimate promotion.

Overload Reduction

In an era of austerity, management is often in the position of wanting or expecting personnel to maintain or even increase units of service while manpower is reduced. Reduction of units of service is tantamount to reduced revenue; therefore, on the theory that there may be fat in any system (or that creative people will find new ways of maintaining their work load), staff may be asked to do more with less.

However, sooner or later, both quality of care and work-load units will surely suffer if reductions in staff are repeated. The further consequences are absenteeism, resignation or early retirement, lowered standards of performance, compromise of professional integrity, difficulty in finding replacements, and a poor reputation of the institution in the community.

This is where the administrator shows his true mettle. Painstaking study of staff attitudes and morale will be necessary to determine how far staff will cooperate without organizing an overt or covert rebellion. Good judgment is also necessary to determine at what point quality of care must not be permitted to deteriorate further. Then the administrator needs the strength to take a proper stand against further cutbacks, and to develop ways to bring work loads and worker cooperation in line with quality standards.

Develop New Challenges

When things get dull and staff is restless, when truculence and foot-dragging begin to be manifest, it may be time for a new challenge. A few good "blue sky" sessions may uncover ideas that tap latent interests. In the course of time, an organization tends to plateau unless new and interesting tasks are taken on. A long plateau often precedes a further downturn in interest and creativity.

New challenges are as many as the imagination of workers and administrators can invent. Perhaps it would be well to add a new teaching affiliation to the department by developing a liaison with another professional school. How about a conference on forensic psychiatry, or on the effects of the homeless epidemic on treatment programs? A cross-discipline grand rounds to bring psychiatry closer to other medical specialties? A new outpatient service for geriatric patients?

As indicated above, when staff is in a restless, querulous mood, it is useful to bring them together to discuss what is on their minds and to make an accurate diagnosis of causes of institutional malaise. More than one session may be necessary. As malaise evaporates, creative ideas come forth. A unifying theme can bind the free energy and direct it profitably outward.

Sanctions

In the case of a negative, uncooperative, or disruptive employee who does not correct behavior even after a reasonable time, it may be necessary to depart from the positive approaches discussed above and, in some cases, apply sanctions. However regrettable, the administration must face the fact that sometimes an employee is too great a drag. Sanctions are of varying severity, selected to suit the problem presented. First, the employee is assigned to a supervisor or mentor who will *discuss* his problems with him, on the hopeful assumption that additional understanding will make him a happier person and a better worker.

The next level is that of *reprimand* or admonishment. In this situation the superior discusses the employee's problems in greater detail; if it is clear that his behavior has been out of line, a strong recommendation is made for immediate corrective action. A detailed statement about the reprimand or admonishment is introduced into the record, but there is no mention that the worker's future is insecure.

Although the organization is interested in its people and wishes to help them, it should be understood that the organization exists formally as a therapeutic institution for patients, not for staff. Staff persons whose neurotic or character problems go too deep must seek outside help. They cannot make a career out of subordinating the organization to their regressive needs.

A further step is *suspension,* with or without pay, for a period calculated to fit the magnitude of the infraction. This is to allow time for reflection upon alleged behavior that threatens job tenure.

Discharge or *firing* is the ultimate punishment. It is not pleasant to go through and should be rare. It requires careful thought and preparation; one should discuss procedures in detail with knowledgeable personnel consultants. It may also be wise in some cases to consult an attorney. Two questions that should be in the administrator's mind are:

1. What type of preparation is required to make sure the discharge or firing does not backfire?
2. What will be the effect on the total system?

A serious mistake is to underestimate the amount of documentation necessary to support termination of an employee, particularly if the case should come before higher authority or a labor relations board. Often there is little in the record that substantiates a decision to discharge. Labor relations boards have strong feelings about due process; as often as not, they rule in favor of the employee. A ruling against administration can result in a serious loss of face. If the employee has mobilized a great deal of support from friends and from labor, the effectiveness of an administrator in the case of a decision against him may be seriously compromised.

Employees in danger of losing their jobs will do many things to thwart management. They appeal to labor, consult lawyers, complain to the press and powerful political figures, make countercharges, and try to blow the whistle on administration by dredging up all sorts of accusations. Staff members look on this drama with interest and astonishment, wondering if their own security of employment is threatened if they take sides. The affair may be blown up disproportionately if an action against an employee becomes a rallying point for other, perhaps widespread discontents. In a civil-service environment, where employees have many protections, discharge should be attempted only under the gravest circumstances.

Having outlined the possible negative results of discharging an inadequate employee, I must now mention that sometimes the procedure can be smooth and without dire consequences. An employee may recognize his inadequacies and realize the job is not for him. He may abhor the idea of a fight against management. Sometimes documentation is so strong, as in some cases of alcoholism, mental disorder, and drug addiction, that the correctness of the executive's position is self-evident. Sometimes the employee possesses sufficient good feelings about the institution and his supervisors that he accepts the discharge without further recrimination.

Finally, before firing anyone, think of appointing a committee to evaluate the questionable employee and to advise on procedures. Such a committee cannot take over the responsibility of the officer charged with making the final decision, but it may bolster his judgment and point out ways of strengthening his case.

Case Illustrations of System Pathology and Treatment

In the course of working with psychiatric residents in six different training programs over 50 years, I have met with a number who have adopted a casual attitude toward their professional responsibilities. Medicine is a very demanding profession, requiring the strictest attention to patients' welfare, and some of the rules of responsibilities toward patients are not easy to follow, especially if one is tired and sleepy. Examples of typical infractions follow.

Case 1

How to Handle Negligent Residents

ILLUSTRATION A: A resident fails to show up in time to relieve his classmate of duties at the change of shift. This is not only a personal failing but has a bad system effect in that the resident who is deserted faces the frustrating necessity of staying on the job indefinitely or until relief can be arranged. Nurses, social workers, and attendants are disturbed, and patients may be left without medical supervision at a time when the ward may be in turmoil.

If no adequate excuse is advanced by the resident, on his second infraction a board hearing may be called to explore what can be done, or even to recommend dismissal.

ILLUSTRATION B: Residents are frequently delinquent in finishing up records on time. Sometimes, at the end of their training period, they go elsewhere, leaving records undone. Writing up records is a chore that few cherish; however, standard-setting bodies (patients' rights groups or JCAHO) take a dim view of sloppy or unfinished records. For some residents, this habit of postponement may be very stubborn, and possibly a remnant of adolescent rebellion.

Several courses of action may be effective:

1. Reprimand and/or admonition.
2. Deny vacations until records are up to snuff.
3. Send the delinquent resident to court on behalf of a patient who is under adjudication for continued involuntary detention. There the resident may learn what the public defender or the judge expects in the way of a written record on which they make a determination of critical patients' rights.
4. Deny promotion from one residency training year to the next.
5. In some jurisdictions, pay can be withheld—usually a most effective sanction.

Case 2

The Dangerously Low Census

In a university psychiatric hospital, during a period of general economic recession, the ward census had fallen well below the break-even point. Although this university hospital receives almost a third of its funds from the university to support clinical teaching and research, the remaining two-thirds must be made up by revenues from other sources—Medicare and Medicaid, private third-party payers, or direct personal reimbursement out of the client's pocket.

Needless to say, a too-low bed occupancy rate that continues for a protracted period depletes reserves and forces management to borrow, cut back services, close wards, or file for bankruptcy. With a continuing low census, training programs may lack a sufficient supply of patients of diverse pathology to satisfy training requirements.

What factors conspired to bring the vaunted university hospital to this predicament? Only a few years ago, the university hospital had enough discretionary clinical training support to admit almost anyone it pleased, regardless of ability to pay, Now, with escalation of costs, clinical training support is sufficient to pay for only one-third of the patients. Another factor was that during the course of the recession, other hospitals, particularly those in the private sector, had stepped up their public relations and advertising so as to command a larger market share, thus drawing patients away from the university. Still another factor was that university hospital management had become complacent. They had lost touch with market dynamics and had assumed that the university, with its great research reputation and its success with complicated tertiary care, would always have a crowd at its doors. For a long time, it must be added, referring physicians had not been privileged to treat patients they referred; thus, referring a private patient into the university psychiatric hospital in effect meant not only loss of a client but also loss of income. This long-standing policy was based on the assumption that outside physicians writing orders for patients in the wards would diminish the residents' autonomy in treating patients and, therefore, weaken the training experience.

It soon became apparent that nothing less than a major reorganization would save the hospital. After much discussion, the following measures were instituted:

1. A public relations firm was hired to awaken the community to the advantages of this hospital. Radio broadcasts, news releases, and thousands of

brochures were disseminated. Specific targets of development were the geriatric and adolescent services.

2. New outside signage programs were undertaken to attract the attention of auto and foot traffic, and to make it easier for referred patients to find their way into the hospital.

3. Parking facilities were improved.

4. A speakers' bureau was organized, and free courses (plus lunch) offered to both professional and lay groups on subjects of interest.

5. Referring physicians' goodwill was cultivated as never before, and ward-treating privileges for a selected group of community psychiatrists (who would also participate in teaching) was instituted.

6. Cutbacks in nursing staff to accord with fluctuations in bed occupancy became necessary. A hold was placed on annual salary increases, and all programs were mandated to produce a given savings in expenditures.

The above measures and others helped greatly to meet the challenge, and as a happy result, the hospital did not go under. Most important, however, was the realization that complacency concerning the hospital's ability to attract patients had to become a thing of the past. Hospital management from here on would have to run scared and struggle against others in the arena for its share of the health market.

Case 3

Emergency Room Treatment Staff Are under Stress

You cannot run a hospital without engineers, without food services, without supplies and equipment—and you also cannot run a hospital without doctors, nurses, social workers, and other frontline treatment personnel. Perhaps because they are highest paid and at the top of the professional heap, doctors in particular may be regarded by some employees as being "stuck up," pompous, or impressed with their own importance, but the whole frontline treatment team may seem overly convinced of their own value simply because they are directly concerned with the treatment of emergent patients.

Like all other personnel, the direct care team, too, needs attention and understanding from administrators. The stresses and strains in the operating room can be immense. In public hospitals today, work is often overwhelming. So many things have to go right to make the workday satisfying. Often, professionals struggle with themselves because the overload forces them to compromise their ideals of satisfactory service. The high sense of responsibility for every detail of the patient's treatment and the high vulnerability to criticism and litigation should anything go wrong are a constant source of distress to frontline caregivers.

ILLUSTRATION: The emergency service staff, apprehensive that some aggressive patients may attack them, has asked for panic buttons in all interview rooms. The panic button would activate a red light outside the door and also a light in the nurses' station. Help could then be quickly mobilized. A need for additional security officers was also expressed by the emergency service staff in a special petition to the chief of psychiatry, which he quickly conveyed to the hospital director. The accompanying note read: "I send you . . . a plea from the emergency staff in the department of psychiatry . . . asking for installation of panic buttons in all relevant rooms and areas. We point out that injuries to staff in the psychiatry department have been found to be four times greater than in other departments. . . . In the opinion of counsel, we are sitting ducks for legal action if any injury occurs either to our staff or patients. This is a very serious matter." The outcome was unexpected. Within a short time a plan (which had lain dormant for a year) for doubling the size of the emergency service department was activated, and panic buttons were installed as part of that renovation.

Summary and Comments

A systematic study and taxonomy of all organizational disturbances, interventions, and outcomes is a wonderful challenge for students of administration. Lacking such, in this section I have presented and illustrated a variety of intervention strategies available to the administrator today.

Face-to-face interviews (individual or group) with staff members in trouble are the most commonly employed technique to resolve stress and conflict. Job changes frequently alleviate problems of the square peg–round hole type. Reduction in overload is important in this era of curtailment of support manpower while trying to maintain quality and units of service. New challenges may counter institutional malaise and release staff creativity, provided that time and attention are given to identifying underlying causes of malaise and to mobilizing staff interest and morale.

Should corrective measures be necessary to handle difficult workers, available sanctions (in ascending severity) include discussion, reprimand or admonishment, suspension, and discharge or firing. The last sanction, firing, should be undertaken only under the severest necessity, and always with the advice of personnel experts and/or legal counsel.

REFERENCES

1. Bertalanffy LV: General systems theory. General Systems I:1–10, 1956. Reprinted from Main Currents in Modern Thought 71:75, 1955
2. Metcalf HC, Urwick L (eds): Dynamic Administration: The Collected Papers of Mary Parker Follett. New York, Harper & Bros., 1942
3. Kets de Vries MFR (ed): The Irrational Executive: Psychoanalytic Explorations in Management. New York, International Universities Press, 1984
4. Greenblatt M: The psychiatrist as social system clinician, in Greenblatt M, Levinson DJ, Williams RH (eds): The Patient and the Mental Hospital. Glencoe, Illinois, Free Press, 1957, pp 317–326
5. Virtanen R: Claude Bernard and His Place in the History of Ideas. Lincoln, Nebraska, University of Nebraska Press, 1960
6. Miller JG: Living Systems. New York, McGraw-Hill, 1978. See Chapter 10, The Organization, pp 595–745
7. Virtanen R: Claude Bernard and His Place in the History of Ideas. Lincoln, Nebraska, University of Nebraska Press, 1960.
8. Levinson H, with Molinare J, Spohn AG: Organizational Diagnosis. Cambridge, Harvard University Press, 1972

9. Kets de Vries MFR (ed): The Irrational Executive: Psychoanalytic Explorations in Management. New York, International Universities Press, 1984
10. Weber M (translated and edited by Henderson AM, Parsons T): The Theory of Social and Economic Organisation. New York, Free Press, 1947
11. Barnard CI: The Functions of the Executive. Cambridge, Harvard University Press, 1938
12. Miller EJ, Rice AK: Systems of Organization. The Control of Tasks and Sentient Boundaries. London, Tavistock, 1967
13. Sayre WS: Principles of administration—1. Hospitals 30:34–35, 92, 1956
14. Hodgson, RC, Levinson DJ, Zaleznik A: The Executive Role Constellation. Cambridge, Harvard University, Division of Research, Graduate School of Business Administration, 1965
15. Greenblatt M, Sharaf MR, Stone EM: Within the institution, Chapter 1 in Greenblatt M, Sharaf MR, Stone EM, Dynamics of Institutional Change. Pittsburgh, Pennsylvania, University of Pittsburgh Press, 1971, pp 3–22
16. Ollson DE: Management by Objective. Palo Alto, California, Pacific Books, 1968
17. Greenblatt M, York RH, Brown EL: From Custodial to Therapeutic Patient Care in Mental Hospitals. New York, Russell Sage Foundation, 1955, pp 155–156
18. Greenblatt M, Sharaf MR, Stone EM: Within the institution, Chapter 1 in Greenblatt M, Sharaf MR, Stone EM, Dynamics of Institutional Change. Pittsburgh, Pennsylvania, University of Pittsburgh Press, 1971, p 3
19. Greenblatt M, Sharaf MR, Stone EM: Decentralization through unitization, Chapter 4 in Greenblatt M, Sharaf MR, Stone EM, Dynamics of Institutional Change. Pittsburgh, Pennsylvania, University of Pittsburgh Press, 1971, pp 62–85
20. Garcia LB: The Clarinda plan: An ecological approach to hospital organization. Ment Hosp 11:30–31, 1960
21. Bonn E, Kraft A: The Fort Logan mental health center: Genesis and development. J Fort Logan Ment Health Center 1:17–27, 1963
22. Jackson GW, Smith FV: A proposal for mental hospital organization: The Kansas plan. Ment Hosp 12;5–8, 1967
23. Emerson RW: Self-reliance, in Emerson RW: Essays and English Traits. New York, PF Collier & Son, 1909

Entering and Leaving the System*

Before a mental health professional applies for a chief administrative position, he or she should ask: Do I really want the job? Am I ready for it? To answer these questions, one must know a great deal about the position; then one must assess and analyze one's motivation and capacities, including the ability to think in terms of a total system, to work in sometimes ambiguous situations, to relate to multiple persons and organizational functions, to tolerate criticism and frustration, and to sustain large outputs of energy over time. Most importantly, one must ask oneself: What are the organization's goals and expectations, and are they achievable within the framework of my God-given talents?

To answer the above, one must raise further questions: What is the pattern of governance of the organization, and how well can I fit into it? Who appoints the administrator, and to what extent is the appointee beholden to the appointing authority? To select an example from my personal experience, if one is appointed as commissioner by the governor of a state, the length of the administrator's stay in office is likely to be determined by the governor, who can remove his appointee at will. In addition, the administrator's term is likely to expire at the end of the governor's term in office. This makes the appointee the governor's subordinate, a part of the executive branch of government—in a word, a *political*-professional person. He is fair game for crit-

*This chapter is a considerable development of material contained in Chapter 15, Politics of Administration, by Milton Greenblatt, in *Psychiatric Administration*, edited by John A. Talbott and Seymour R. Kaplan. New York, Grune & Stratton, 1982.

icism and attacks from the opposite party (whatever his personal affiliation), and always fair game for the press and any public or private agency that cares to investigate him or his operation. Obviously, this is not a position for someone interested in job security. If one wants freedom from public scrutiny and public criticism, such a position should be avoided at all costs. On the other hand, if one is something of a gambler, not easily wounded, and able to enjoy the rough-and-tumble of the political arena, such a job may be appealing.

GOVERNANCE

The pattern of governance within the institution usually revolves around the relationship between the administrator and his board. Boards are of two polar types: advisory, and policy making. Generally, *advisory* boards do not appoint personnel; they meet less frequently and exert less power than policy boards. However, inasmuch as advisory board members usually represent diverse interests and a variety of constituencies, and often have powerful connections, they can exert a great deal of informal influence over organizational policy and personnel appointments. (I remember one state hospital board that included a close friend of the governor, a friend of the cardinal, a physician with strong ties to the state medical organization, several prominent businessmen, and representatives of powerful minority groups. They were very conscious of their informal strength, and they used it.)

Case Illustration

Confrontation between a Superintendent and a Board Member

In a large eastern state hospital, the board of directors consisted of seven members appointed by the governor. They, in turn, *appointed* the superintendent from a list of three eligible candidates submitted by the commissioner of mental health. They also had the authority to *initiate* removal of a superintendent (which became final, however, only when approved by the commissioner). Curiously, between those two points—one of approval and the other of dismissal—they were essentially an advisory board.

At one time in its history, a new member—a very intelligent, well-educated, and successful businesswoman and entrepreneur—began to dominate the board soon after her appointment. It was not long before she made it clear that she expected the board to take a more definitive role in policy. One of her first projects was to declare that the hospital, which had an abundance of geriatric cases, should concentrate entirely on geriatric research and thus make a great reputation for itself in that field. She rammed this concept through by majority vote of the board, and then announced to the superintendent that he was expected to implement the ideas as soon as possible.

The superintendent, however, who had considerable experience in research, felt that the idea was good, but for the immediate future impracticable. The few investigators engaged in research in the hospital were deeply immersed in problems of their own choosing that they had been pursuing for years. They were not about to abandon their direction to satisfy the whim of a new board member, and since no new funds were available to start a geriatric research program, it appeared that a change at this time was unfeasible. The superintendent explained his views in detail. He was startled by the peremptory tone of the new board member, and by the implications that the board was taking over policy and program direction that belonged to him.

At the next board meeting, a heated showdown occurred wherein the superintendent had to outline his view of his authority against the insistence of some board members that ultimate policy and direction were their prerogative. This meeting ended with the new board member leaving in a huff, declaring she would consult a lawyer and take the matter up with the commissioner of mental health, her friend.

This controversy, fortunately, cooled rapidly. The board member did not show up for six months. It was assumed that she had discussed the relative powers and prerogatives with lawyers and the commissioner and learned that she was in the wrong. As a matter of fact, the superintendent had a firm grasp of the extent and limits of his authority from research done prior to his appointment; also, he had previously checked with the commissioner, who had assured him that he would give no ground to the board member but instead would try to get her to accept the realities with good grace.

When the new board member returned, her attitude had changed considerably. She then became a most helpful, valuable, and affable partner in the total hospital enterprise.

A *policy board* may appoint personnel, including the administrator. It also may have the authority to terminate such appointments. It formulates policies that the administrator, functioning mainly as an executive secretary, carries out. The policy board has ultimate responsibility for the work and welfare of the institution. If it is to feel secure in its own responsibilities, it must have confidence at all times in the abilities and effectiveness of the chief administrative officer. Policy boards often work their will by appointing subcommittees to investigate and oversee various functions of the institution.

Case Illustration

Limiting the Power of State Hospital Boards

My experience as superintendent of a state hospital and then commissioner of the state mental health system convinced me that the powers of the state hospital boards should be changed. As noted in the previous example, by law they had the authority to appoint the superintendent from a list of three candidates submitted by the commissioner. Removal of a superintendent could only be initiated by vote of the hospital board. However, during his tenure the superintendent was directly responsible for his performance on a day-to-day basis to the commissioner of mental health, with the board essentially advisory. The boards generally were composed of laymen, were appointed by the governor, and met monthly; they were not in close contact with hospital activities, nor did they have the professional know-how to run a large mental institution.

At that time, finding good superintendents was not an easy job. Salaries were low, and although housing on hospital grounds was supplied at low cost, families were reluctant to rear their children on a mental hospital campus. Also, responsibilities of superintendents were becoming more burdensome, without a concomitant increase in budgetary support or other rewards. Private practice was far more lucrative and far less constrained by rules, regulations, and the adverse public image of a state mental institution. Although the boards, as a rule, contributed nil to the recruitment of hospital superintendents, they nevertheless made the final choice.

A second problem was that, since only the board could initiate removal of a superintendent, the commissioner was left with the intolerable situation that however inadequate a superintendent might be in the prosecution of his job, if he had ingratiated himself with his board, he would be impossible to remove. Thus, a commissioner could be left responsible for the actions of an inadequate employee without authority to correct the situation. It was obvious that in this case responsibility and authority had to be brought closer together.

A change in the law was, therefore, effected through the efforts of departmental legal staff and friendly legislators such that the commissioner, with advice and counsel, now became the deciding authority on both appointment and removal of superintendents. In the beginning, many board members resented the change—indeed, a good deal of discussion and argumentation went on for many months both before and after the new law went into effect. Eventually, to their everlasting credit, the majority saw the virtues in the change and accepted the new state of affairs with good grace.

Patterns of governance do vary. Thus, the aspiring administrator must learn the precise characteristics of authority and command in the institution he wishes to join. Knowing such, does he really want the job, can he live with it, or must he reject it?

Concerning the general functions of hospital boards in relation to the institutions they represent, the following may be helpful:

1. Boards may *legitimate* the work of the institution by contributing funds or matériel, offering volunteer services, interpreting the work of the institution to the community, and supporting the institution in times of attack.
2. Boards may carry out *auditing or investigatory functions* by reviewing programs, progress, budgets, appointments, promotions, and relationships inside and outside the institution, as well as complaints, grievances, and class or job actions.
3. Boards may exert a *directing or controlling function* by assisting in the formulation of policy, and by planning and supervising its implementation.

It is important to remember that whatever the agenda of the board at any particular time, the board presents a set of expectations to the administrator that if fulfilled assures him good standing, but if unfulfilled can lead to stress and strain. It also is well to remember that many boards, whether primarily advisory or policy setting, tend over time to shift emphasis from legitimation of the work of the hospital to auditing and control functions. Individual members of the board, as they become more secure and knowledgeable, want to understand more fully the reasons for administrative decisions and actions, expecting to become more involved in future decisions and actions. Wise administrators acknowledge that board members may possess valuable knowledge and experience in many aspects of administration and, therefore, will seek out these persons for advice and counsel.

The relationship between the director of the organization and his board is critical to the success of the enterprise. Functionally, the director may sit with the board, inform the board, and join in discussions (with or without voting). Other possibilities are that the director may function as moderator or chairperson of the board; or the board may have its own agenda, calling upon the director for information or clarification but without his involvement in deliberations and final decisions. Whatever the pattern, it is likely that the director's voice will have great influence in board proceedings. The director's experience in group dynamics can be of value in facilitating board activity, just as his knowledge of interpersonal dynamics can help him deal successfully with the different personalities on the board.

Clark's[1] summary of the dynamics of boards in action offers helpful suggestions for the director/administrator's role. Clark points to the need for active recruiting and orientation of new members, for only good members make good boards. Effective board training is more than just "a tour and a brochure." Personality differences of board members and problem behaviors may be anticipated; "such behaviors include the monopolist, the self-righteous moralist, the special-interest pleader, the hostile-aggressive member, the clown, and the silent-withdrawn nonparticipatory member." Effective group leadership means not only dealing skillfully with personal characteristics and conflicts, but also providing facilitation, clarification, support, and understanding where and when needed.

Group cohesiveness and loyalty can be cultivated even in the midst of conflict, for conflict is not necessarily negative. Indeed, avoidance of conflict may at times be more destructive than nonavoidance. Often, resolution of conflict results in greater respect and understanding between conflicting parties. A further note, readily confirmed from experience, is that a hardworking group feels more adequate than a group that sits around, argues about abstractions, and makes "wise" decisions. Here the administrator can evoke interest and involvement by identifying important in-hospital management issues that need thought and probing, and by asking for help in specific areas: budget, recruiting of staff, public relations, community development, donations of matériel, fund-raising, and elucidation of administrative problems that require creative analysis and special expertise. Formation of committees with well-defined missions, gathering of data, and reporting results in formal meetings provide grist for the mill. These strategies bring director and board together in mutual tasks and define the type of board members needed in the future.

CONSTITUENCIES

The constituencies to be served are special and unique to every organization. The commissioner of the department of mental health in a large industrial state, for example, at a minimum must seek and maintain the goodwill of the governor, the legislature, the attorney general, the state auditor, the citizens' lobby, the university and professional communities, labor organizations, and the mental health department itself—all in addition to the sick patients and their families. Beyond that, the commissioner must also be interested in the goodwill of federal agencies that administer programs such as Medicare and Medicaid, foundations, private contributors, the National Institute of Mental Health (NIMH), and JCAHO.

Every top administrator is surrounded by a circle of agencies with which he must interact. As from the center of a wheel, spokes emanate from the mental health administrative office to a variety of other offices or agencies. The two-way communication between any and all elements in this model constitutes the essence of administrative life (see Chapter 10).

MANAGEMENT SUCCESSION

Assuming all goes well and a new leader is appointed, he finds himself immediately involved in the many problems of management succession. Management succession may be defined as the assumption by one executive of a position held by another. It is one of the most familiar and significant events in an organization's history, yet the phenomenon has received relatively little systematic research attention. Its significance is succinctly stated by Redlich:[2] "Succession denotes the transmission of status, power, possession and its symbols from one person to another. It is a most important event in the social sphere, analogous in some ways to birth and death in the biological sphere."

In a recent meeting of top-level executives in the mental health field, all the executives in attendance had held two or more major posts during their careers. Many had experienced three or four major successions, and one had experienced no less than six major successions in a career that spanned four decades. Usually, a given succession creates a domino effect—that is, the successor, having vacated one office to fill another, leaves a vacancy that must be filled, and this in turn creates a series of openings down the line to be filled by a series of successors. Organizational disruption, therefore, may occur at many levels. In fact, if the successor has been chosen from another system, more than one organization may be involved. Only rarely is this process minimized or avoided (as in the unusual case where an executive builds an organization from scratch, recruiting all his staff into newly created, never-before-occupied posts).

It is important to recognize that although succession to high office in the political sphere, in our country, is by election, succession in medical institutions is usually by appointment. The chief executive officer of a mental health facility is usually not ushered into office by a democratic process. And once ensconced, his role may resemble that of a benign executive rather than that of an elected official. He is expected to make final decisions in hiring and firing as well as on policies and procedures. He has final say in the formulation and allocation of the budget. From that point on, the degree to which he democratizes the functions of the institution depends on *his* delegation of his own authority. It should be pointed out that many staff members are vague (or ambivalent) on this point, unable to accept fully the director's role as final authority. Some believe that institutional functions should be decided by democratic vote, or by elected committees. The director, therefore, must often work to raise the organization's acceptance of the fact that it is ultimately a managed system in which he is the leader, and not a pure democracy.

Hierarchically speaking, below the level of the director are the heads of various divisions or services of the organization, who often bridge the directorial regimes and provide stability and continuity to organizational life. Some have seen several directors come and go. They may be wise in the ways of organizational politics and masters of the strategies of survival; through the years, they may have accumulated considerable influence. In the long run the director must win over these lieutenants and build a cohesive and smooth-running team where cooperation, mutual respect and support triumph over competition, personal aggrandizement, and protection of parochial power. His big problem is in the early months of succession when, although still woefully ignorant of the intimate workings of the system and not always confident as to whom to trust, he must nevertheless make critical decisions and take responsibility for them.

STAGES OF MANAGEMENT SUCCESSION

Two polar reactions of employees caught in the upheaval of succession have been identified. One, based on DuMaurier's *Rebecca*,[3] is the "Rebecca myth." DuMaurier's novel concerns a widower whose new wife is made unhappy by the excessive adulation of his first wife, Rebecca. The Rebecca myth as applied to management succession[4,5] identifies an institutional ambience in which the employees mourn the passing of the old administrator and extol his virtues to the detriment of the new administrator. At the other extreme is the "messiah myth," in which the new administrator embodies the hopes of an organization that perhaps views the old administrator as having done a poor job. The new administrator, it is thought, will rescue the institution and every distressed employee from stresses and strains attributed to the former administrator's blunders. Between these extremes are many complex social system reactions to the phenomenon of succession.

Taking a longitudinal view, seven stages of succession have been suggested by Redlich:[6]

1. Anticipatory stage
2. Appointment
3. Inauguration
4. Honeymoon
5. Assertion of the new leader's personality, style, and programs
6. Working through of differences
7. Establishment of a new equilibrium

In the *anticipatory* stage, the Rebecca myth or the messiah myth may dominate, or a variety of expectations may prevail; overall, however, one notes considerable tension and free-floating institutional anxiety in the system, with much speculation as to who the successor will be and how that event will alter individuals' roles and happiness. Members of the organization share concerns and speculations as to what they might do if the new regime brings with it much personal discomfort. Some who have become attached to the goals and style of the predecessor and who feel the loss greatly may consider other jobs, but for the majority of employees a "wait and see" attitude prevails. At this time, however, rumor and fantasy are rife.

The identification and *appointment* of the successor gives relief to some and may increase the anxieties of others; however, it does introduce the factor of reality. Most employees look forward to meeting the new executive and accommodating themselves to a new style of leadership.

At the *inauguration* there is a show of solidarity and a spirit of optimism. Often the board or appointing authority makes an appearance in order to welcome the incumbent and to assure personnel that the succession will be smooth and their jobs secure. The appearance of the predecessor, who gives a warm welcome to his successor and calls upon his associates to help and support the new leader, helps greatly to legitimate the transfer of power.

A climate of optimism prevails through the *honeymoon* period—the early months of the successor's actual incumbency. It is a period of sizing up, testing, and learning that many of the disturbing anticipatory concerns were pure fantasy. Actually, the successor needs help and wants to make a good impression on everyone. There is a collective sigh of relief as employees realize that life can go on, and that their contribution is still valued.

Sooner or later the leader's *personality, style, and programs* require new adjustments by staff members. This may bring discomfort to some, evoke disagreements, or necessitate changes in roles and performance (which may be carried out reluctantly and with resistance). This is a period of locking horns, when institutional inertia begins to manifest itself, and when the incumbent's ability to tolerate resistance and deal with it in a patient, understanding way is put to the test. Before his goals and aspirations have been fully accepted, and before his relationships with key norm-setting individuals have matured, the new leader must *work through* many problems and resistances. (This dynamic process of resolution of institutional resistances can be compared with what goes on in individual psychotherapy where the client's defensive systems must be identified and then slowly unraveled.)

Eventually a *new equilibrium* is established; however, every organization must adapt to changing times, and all equilibria are, to some extent, unstable. Nevertheless, a sense of having passed through the acute stages of succession dawns, with the realization that new conditions are apt to continue for some time into the future.

RESEARCH ON EXECUTIVE SUCCESSION

Research on executive succession in the area of mental health is meager; consequently, we turn to business management for many insights. An interesting study by Kelly[7] (see the section below) on newly appointed CEOs appears to be relevant to management in general. It looks at management techniques and approaches from the point of view of the CEO trying to adapt to the challenges before him. It, therefore, complements what has been said above concerning the organization's reaction to a turnover.

How the New CEOs Perform

Although there are great variations in the way new CEOs perform, in general they move slowly in asserting their authority and establishing their imprint on the organization. They are first concerned with *establishing personal relations* with their new subordinates, stressing informality, and encouraging broad input. They avoid isolation; they want to know the people. Then comes an understanding of *organization structure*, both formal and informal, and knowledge of power relationships. (The new executive will intuit that many important informal aspects of the organization may not be revealed until later.) As a rule, attention to organizational structure precedes formulation of *strategies of change*.

Early in the succession period the CEO is thinking of forming a *management team*. It is important that the management team represent the best talent available. Thus, it may be necessary to look beyond the currently appointed administrative assistants and division heads to identify others who give evidence of great ability and originality. The team finally chosen may include new appointees as well as old leaders.

Should the new executive elect to seek advice and counsel from lower levels of the hierarchy, old leaders may resist use of their subordinates on a team where formerly the latter were excluded. If they now sit, advise, and plan on a more equal footing with their boss, this situation requires great sensitivity and understanding. Under conditions of deeply entrenched resistance, the new executive may choose to bide his time, waiting for the division head to accept the necessity for new talent and thinking—which, it may be argued, will not in any way weaken his position as operative head of his department. Or, the lower-level employees' managerial input may be sought on an ad hoc basis. Finally, time will be on the side of the new executive, for turnover of managerial employees is often accelerated when a new CEO takes over, and not infrequently the desired changes then occur in a more comfortable way.

As time goes on, the new CEO's influence begins to be felt more and more throughout the organization. Everywhere down the line, adjustments are made to the new person and his management style, often without formal instruction or direction. It is for him to decide the timing, breadth, and depth of changes; to try to calculate what will go over smoothly and what will be resisted; and to determine how to work things through without loss of morale, confidence, and loyalty. Changes that require new allocations of resources may be delayed by the necessity to wait for the next annual opportunity to reorganize the budget. This is very much the case in large organizations, particularly governmental organizations, where budgets are planned years ahead by authorities at higher levels.

Other Succession Studies

> The traditional perspective is that the course and impact of succession is a function of the individual leadership style or personality of the successor. A more recent perspective is to consider individual variables in combination with role and institutional variables.[8]

With these words, Kohler and Strauss introduce their critical review of the literature, as well as their own intensive interview study of executives. Their summary of succession studies indicates that succession is:

- More frequent in large versus small organizations[9]
- More difficult when the successor has been given a mandate for change[10]
- More difficult when the relationship between predecessor and successor is stormy[11]
- Better for an organization's subsequent performance if an outsider is the successor[12]
- More difficult when the characteristics of the successor do not match the needs of the institution in relating to a changing environment[13,14,15]

Kohler and Strauss also identify three classes of variables that affect succession:

- Relationship between predecessor and successor
- Key characteristics of the successor
- Organizational context factors

The duration and quality of each succession is related to whether the predecessor (a) died, (b) retired, (c) was forcibly removed, (d) resigned voluntarily, or (e) was promoted, transferred, or advanced. Whether or not the successor is different from the predecessor in age, sex, or race; whether he is hired with a specific mandate; whether he makes early changes in personnel and procedures; and whether the predecessor's tenure has been long or short—all of these may affect the period of transition in leadership. These factors have not as yet been studied systematically.

Long tenure of a predecessor permits interpersonal relations to deepen; ways of doing things therefore become entrenched, and the successor has a harder time effecting institutional change. A good relationship between predecessor and successor smooths the transition, whereas a poor relationship makes it difficult for staff members to transfer loyalties to the new leader.

The "hovering" phenomenon—wherein the predecessor hangs around familiar surroundings, engages the time and attention of former employees, or otherwise influences their performance—can be a disruptive force that delays the successor's ability to develop important staff relationships (see the section later in this chapter on "Reciprocal Tasks of the Entering and Exiting Executives").

When does the succession start and when does it end? Strauss and Kohler[16] report that, without exception, all of the 19 general hospital executives they interviewed identified a period of time (from 1 month to over 18) *before* they took office as part of the succession experience. This period, which averaged three months, included trips to the new hospital, relocating one's family, and negotiating final terms of employment. The average length of the total succession period was given as 11 months.

Feldman[17] surveyed members of five occupational groups in one 350-bed community hospital in relation to two possible end points: feeling accepted, and feeling competent. Achieving a feeling of acceptance required less time than developing a feeling of competence.

During the period of succession, what difficulties did the executives identify? According to Strauss and Kohler,[18] nearly two-thirds identified among the difficulties establishing one's own authority, stress between administrative and clinical divisions over turf and boundaries, and squabbles among service chiefs about priorities in the allocation of budgets and capital expenditures.

> Interestingly, the most frequent answer to our question about how these disagreements and difficulties were handled was that the executives said they *backed off and slowed down* [emphasis added] without giving up their point of view. In most instances they indicated they prevailed, and it was the rare executive who had done so by administrative fiat or by firing a subordinate.[19]

The technique of "backing off and slowing down" should be heavily underscored for several reasons. In the early phases of succession, before personal relationships have mellowed, insecurities and anxieties of either staff or the executive may intensify a need to defend one's position. If positions are held too rigidly, a battle may ensue, whereas slowing down may allow cooler reconsideration of the issues later. After all, what the parties usually want is that the issues be decided on their true merits. Backing off indicates that the executive, although higher in the hierarchy and possessing more authority, is not going to push anything through by force. He is opting for rationality and detachment. An analogy that comes to mind is when two motorists approach an intersection from different directions at approximately the same time. Who is entitled to proceed? The advice given by any state's department of motor vehicles is: Where the answer is in doubt, by all means yield—and never insist.

SUCCESSION PLANNING

We can learn something from the business world, where management succession is usually a major concern of two parties—the chief executive officer (CEO), and the chairman of the board. Not infrequently, the CEO is also chairman of the board. Studies[20] suggest that this consolidation may make administration more effective, eliminate disagreements, and present a unified corporate message to competitors and the public. (Succession to board chairmanship may also be a strategy employed to retain a successful CEO.)

Research[21] also suggests that top corporate management (i.e., CEO) turnover is a function primarily of three variables: return on invested assets, size of firm,[22] and retirement. But many other factors may operate, such as type of ownership, institutional environment, relationship with the board, capital-to-debt ratios, and salary and perquisite structure. Attractiveness of new job offers, and competitive uncertainty in the current marketplace, may motivate an executive to consider a change.

Systematic planning for succession is an increasing preoccupation of contemporary organizations and is obviously vital to their future welfare.[23,24,25,26] The benefits include continuity of management, identification of high-potential candidates, and satisfaction of employee advancement aspirations. Such planning requires a data base of information regarding desirable candidates, objective methods of evaluation, and a process of final selection by persons with both knowledge and good judgment. Three to five years of advanced planning may be required.

Case Illustration

Succession Planning in a Great Private Industry

Four years before the death of the head of a giant conglomerate in Orange County, California, plans for his succession had already been formalized. Assuming future waves of new managers, each 10 to 15 years younger than the previous wave, the planners aimed to identify and develop individuals who could occupy the 10 top positions in the organization in the foreseeable future. High-potential individuals were then given added responsibility in anticipation of roles they might eventually assume.

Since CEOs do not always succeed, and some 10% are actually fired[27]—half of these within the first three years—it is vital to choose the best available person, for the expense of succession may be costly in changing times, and attracting a new executive to follow one that has been fired may be difficult.

Family-held businesses are of particular interest, not only because over 90% of American companies are owned or controlled by families or have substantial family involvement[28] (and 8 out of 10 of them, it is estimated, court downfall if no plans for adequate management succession are made[29,30]), but also because succession in any organization may suffer from administrative inbreeding. A successful patriarch's finely balanced talents will inevitably suffer from the ravages of age or illness. Further, offspring do not necessarily have the talents of their forebears. A board is, therefore, in a favorable position to handle sibling rivalries and intergenerational conflicts.[31] It is obvious that in its final decision the board should be independent of the influence of the current CEO or other internal forces; however, a broad base of consultation should be invited so as to elicit input from those who have a stake in the future of the enterprise.

Often, a serious question that surfaces is whether the new executive should be an insider or an outsider.[32,33] Favoring the insider point of view is the assumption that the individual selected will have a greater knowledge of the organization and its resources, and thus will be able to use established social networks to help him do his job. The interim period during which the new executive has to gain mastery over the system, learn whom to trust, and make decisions often with inadequate knowledge is obviated. On the other hand, an outsider has a fresh perspective and may be able to take more decisive action, freed of entangling relationships and inherited personal bonds. When an enterprise is faltering, a new look is a necessity. A new executive may also revitalize the organization, adopt economies unencumbered by long-standing loyalties, increase stability, and in many cases, augment stockholders' confidence.[34] It is noteworthy that each year 10% to 15% of U.S. corporations choose a new CEO, and 80% to 85% choose them from outside.

Finally, however carefully the successor is chosen, it is generally recognized that at least 90% of his development occurs on the job. And whatever the problems the new manager may meet on the job (and they are sure to be numerous and complex), an unavoidable one has to do with the departing executive and whether the latter still retains a need for power and/or influence in the organizations he formerly headed[35] (see below).

CHOICE OF SUCCESSOR

An interesting sidelight on executive life comes from a paper by Gifford and Davidson in 1985.[36] Many executive officers in corporate ventures felt that their hospital's survival was threatened, or that they themselves were threatened, by the changing times, the high cost of care, increasing competition, and difficulties in keeping beds filled. To increase probabilities of survival, the CEOs stressed good staff relations and changes in board attitudes to favor more strategic planning. More efficient facilities, better access to capital, and more for-profit ventures were additional areas of concentration needed to beat the competition.

What role does the CEO play in choosing his successor? This question was asked in another study by Gifford and Davidson.[37] Here, corporate hospital executives were compared to noncorporate hospital executives. The interesting findings were that about one-third of corporate hospital CEOs had chosen their successors, compared to 18% of noncorporate hospital executives. Interestingly, nearly all CEOs planned to remain active after retirement. They projected either continued paying positions, new business ventures, or volunteering in some charitable work.

Should CEOs take responsibility in preparing members of their staff to fill their shoes? In this latter study, 71% of corporate CEOs were preparing someone to succeed them. Although the board or other appointing authority would finally decide, many executives felt that in the course of their tenure they should have attracted young talent of high quality and afforded them sufficient opportunities for growth so that at the very least these protégés could be seriously considered in the line of succession.

An interesting paper by Freund[38] reminds us that the CEO succession phenomenon can seriously threaten the tenure of the chief nursing officer (CNO). In a study of 250 university or affiliated hospitals, 12% of CNOs left within 12 months of a new CEO's appointment, and within a 10-year period, 40% of CNOs were asked to leave. Some CNOs were terminated for incompetence, many for political purposes. A new CEO wants a compatible CNO, and may find it easier to terminate someone with whom strong personal ties have not been forged. Freund concludes that CNO tenure and turnover are determined by "complex, multifactorial and interactive" factors. This is a reminder that meritorious service alone is not sufficient to guarantee continued tenure.

ON LEAVING THE ORGANIZATION

No matter how long or how well one serves an organization, sooner or later one must leave it. Just as a new executive may find it important to learn from and have the support of his predecessor, so an important factor for the departing executive is his relationship with his successor. One problem looms if and when the old executive has serious difficulty in separating himself physically or psychologically from the role he formerly occupied. This is the "hovering" phenomenon alluded to earlier in this chapter—he lingers or hovers, and in so doing may present problems for the incoming executive. The departing executive may try to influence former employees to remain loyal and responsive to him; on the other hand, he may help staff become responsive to the new executive and assist the latter in his transition into the new post. The narcissistic needs of the old executive at this critical juncture in his life may be hidden, unconscious, and/or denied. Both points in the executive's life—entry and departure—are stressful and demand maturity and self-understanding. It is important to recognize that deep emotional currents may be involved for which executives may at times need counseling.

Reciprocal Tasks of the Entering and Exiting Executives

Levinson and Klerman[39] published a thoughtful paper in 1967 on the tasks of ingoing and outgoing executives, as well as middle management. They view the administrator's role as that of a *clinician-executive* seeking to become a social system clinician. It is not clear in their paper how these two roles are related, or which is the predominant one in their view. (In Chapter 3, I emphasized the system clinician model as a primary perspective in relation to conceptualizing the core tasks and functions of an administrator.) Levinson and Klerman delineate succession role tasks as follows:

I. Role Tasks of the incoming clinician-executive
   A. Develop an integrated concept of the organization and its societal context.
   B. Become a social system clinician[40]
   C. Deal with problems of authority, power and influence
   D. Relate to professionals and personnel within the organization
   E. Relate to elements outside the organization
   F. Foster organizational growth
   G. Achieve new identity of clinician-executive
II. Tasks of the outgoing executive
   A. Organizational
      1. Prepare staff and community for the successor
      2. Orient successor to the organization
      3. Make self available for consultation
   B. Personal
      1. Separate
      2. Relocate
      3. Construct new identity
III. Tasks of middle management during an executive succession
   A. Realignment of interpersonal relationships
   B. Reassessment of aspirations
   C. Reevaluation of future
   D. Readjustment of work routines.

Personal Reflections on the Experiences of the Departing Executive

The experiences of the departing executive may be divided into three phases: (a) the preretirement lame-duck phase, (b) the ceremonial phase, and (c) the retirement phase.

The Lame-Duck Period

Picture the situations for executives about to leave their jobs. There are many patterns. After long and faithful service, one executive looks forward to retirement as a new opportunity to enjoy life. Perhaps he has prepared himself in terms of hobbies, friends, plans for travel, and closer relations with his family. He welcomes the years ahead.

Another executive is going to a new and challenging job—upward in the social, professional, and financial scale. He thinks of new worlds to conquer. If he is fortunate enough to leave with colors flying and the warm regards of colleagues, he is indeed a happy man.

Still another executive may have suffered burnout from the stresses of harsh competition or repeated criticism from superiors. Perhaps he has sought other employment a step ahead of anticipated dismissal. Ambivalent feelings about his departure may be reflected in relationships with his colleagues. Their formal congratulations may convey underlying, unspoken messages: "Wish you had done better," "Glad you landed something worthwhile," or even "The organization will miss you (but may feel a sense of relief)."

There are other situations in which the downside is even more acute, as when an executive leaves for a job of lesser status, responsibility, or pay—a clear demotion. Or when he is summarily fired. Or where the job was his main interest and raison d'être, and he looks forward after retirement to an empty future, devoid of the excitement and challenge that was his daily fare.

This period of social and psychological separation from an organization in which one has played a prominent part, when a successor has been nominated or a search has begun, is often described as a lame-duck period. When does it begin and how does it progress?

Students of organizational dynamics can sometimes predict when an important person is "on the skids." In state government, those privy to the governor's plan may know when an appointee of the governor—one who is dependent upon his goodwill—may be out of favor and, therefore, destined to be cashiered. Only the date of termination or the appropriate circumstances for making it known may be uncertain. I refer here particularly to those persons whose tenure of service is "at the pleasure" of the appointing authority. The situation applies to state or country directors of health, where politics enters heavily into security of employment.

At some point along the road, the administrator who enters the lame-duck period begins to sense a change in attitude and behavior of those about him. Although there may be no diminution in his formal authority, he notes that his staff is not as responsive to him as formerly. Colleagues whom he expects to show up at one of his important conferences are occupied elsewhere. Latent hostilities may surface in veiled remarks or changed interpersonal attitudes. Even the personnel who are most loyal to him realize they must begin to think in terms of their future security and alignments. The sensitive equilibrium of interrelationships and support systems is breaking up. Until a successor is appointed and each person's future is clarified, the natives are restless. Can the lame-duck executive understand these natural reactions of his associates to the disruption of vital bonds? At the same time, can he deal with his own reactions to separation and loss of status? For many, this can be a very hard time.

Although no statutory provisions usually exist to lessen the new executive's responsibilities during this trying period, his burdens may be appreciably decreased. Some factional tensions may be diminished by the changes in the system. Power struggles in which he has been involved may be suspended, and projects that formerly seemed urgent may be put on hold.

The Ceremonial Period

The ceremonial period of retirement is usually short and emotional. The ceremony, so to speak, is the punctuation mark that ends the work sentence. It is the symbolic *rite de passage* that conducts the retiring person into his next role. In its most familiar form, it ushers the individual from the world of workers to the world of retirees. It helps both the retired person and his colleagues and friends handle their separation feelings.

In a typical case, there is a round of parties involving the small office group, the larger community of employees, and the group of intimate family members and friends. Customarily, testimonials make light of stresses and strains suffered in the past, forgive old peccadilloes, dramatize significant historical events, and humor personal quirks and aberrations. A laudatory speech by the head of the organization or a good friend and a response from the "decumbent" close the ceremonies. The exercises help denial of deeper, less happy feelings, including the uneasiness of not knowing exactly what lies ahead.

The executive who retires from a post at age 55 to take on another one higher in the social/organizational scale sees things quite differently from the one who retires at age 70 with no job in sight. The former has years of fruitful activity ahead, new challenges, and the exhilaration of moving from one success to perhaps another. The latter may experience a special syndrome that is called "decompression."

The Retirement: Decompression

Decompression may be a phenomenon peculiar to the parting executive. It is thought to be different from the familiar clinical depression, although feelings of depression and loss are present. It is different from burnout, which is commonly construed to be an anhedonic state affecting workers who have lost zest for their jobs. It is different from culture shock, although there is a transition from one state of social equilibrium to another. In decompression, the pressure is suddenly off, the individual is thrust from a life of high tension, centrality in the arena of action, high status, and considerable power into a life of markedly reduced activity, involvement, responsibility, and status. Its symptoms include bewilderment, relief, a sense of being lost (as well as a sense of loss), and a vague feeling of being closer to the end.

Retirement is a major life adjustment, fraught with mythology and beliefs. Some think that retirement is a perilous period, threatening health if not life. Friends warn the retiree to keep busy, find new employment, volunteer for some occupation. Health professionals say that retirement breeds inactivity, loss of muscle substance and tone, decalcification of bone, lowered immunity, reduced resistance to infection, and a tendency toward depression and hypochondriasis. Others say that retirement is a time for self-indulgence, a time to reap the rewards of a life of toil. It is an opportunity to become reacquainted with spouse, family, and friends, and to practice "intelligent hedonism," leavened by wisdom and maturity.

In a study of decompression[41] I noted that for a majority of departing executives there is a combination of attraction and repulsion for the situation left behind. As noted earlier, some cope with the stress by hovering—that is, by returning to the old scene, engaging the attention of old comrades in arms, and trying to recapture the former life-style.

Another coping style is to break fully and cleanly, leaving the future business of the organization to the men and women who have inherited it. The organization may well profit from the infusion of new blood; it may even do better under the new executive than under the old.

Case Illustration

The Successor and Predecessor Work Something Out

In one such "hovering" situation, the man of experience kept returning to converse with the secretaries and to bring them gifts. He collared his former associates for long chats in the corridors. He sat in on strategic conferences, where loyal henchmen tended to orient themselves to him rather than to his successor, who was not yet fully ensconced in the seat of power.

This difficult situation began to be resolved when the successor summoned the courage to point out that his predecessor was still acting as chief executive, although his authority had ended upon his retirement. The reader can well imagine that this was a moment of high drama. But to his everlasting credit, the former executive quickly sensed what was afoot and phased down both his influence and involvement, making it possible for the successor to get closer to his associates, return to his agenda, and consolidate his leadership role.

The new executive's task was a complicated one: to make it clear that although he was responsible for final decisions, his status was to a large extent that of a learner, dependent on those about him for advice and counsel. He wanted to take up the issues with the former executive without hurting his feelings, and at the same time leave open the option of calling upon him for support, wisdom, and counsel when needed.

These all-too-human situations depend for their resolution on the maturity, goodwill, and understanding of the involved parties. They illustrate well the human side of enterprise, which has become of increasing concern to modern managers and executives.

Case Illustration

Seven Steps to Nonsuccess as a Leader

In one large university-affiliated acute general teaching hospital, after a careful search, a new medical director was appointed whose credentials and experience were impressive. Unfortunately, over the course of the next six months, the administration, faculty, and employees of the hospital had reason to be surprised and appalled at the behavior of the new executive. Indeed, it was astonishing how many rules of good executive deportment, in the sensitive setting of having succeeded an esteemed predecessor, he managed to violate. Here follows a summary of an extraordinary record of negative achievement that may serve as an excellent guideline of what *not* to do when taking over a new and important function.

I. Be interpersonally abrasive.
   A. Talk, don't listen.
   B. Order, don't request.
   C. Ignore social amenities.
   D. Insult subordinates by criticizing their professions.
II. Devalue the accomplishments of the system and its participants.
   A. Blame the previous administration.
   B. Insinuate that the system has been severely compromised, mismanaged, and nonproductive in areas that are important for success.
III. Disregard current organizational structure.
   A. Bypass managers and go directly to their subordinates for information and to make changes.
   B. Ignore the managers and their suggestions.
   C. Impose a new informal organization and communication system without dismantling the old, so the two work at cross-purposes and create confusion.
IV. Overvalue certain individuals in the organization.
   A. Announce publicly who you believe are the most talented, capable, and productive individuals in the organization ("The five best faculty in this school are . . . "). This serves to insult and demoralize the remaining ambitious and hardworking contributors.
V. Make decisions for new appointments based on political associations.
   A. Promote the chairman of the search committee to a newly created assistantship, but don't announce it officially.
   B. Compliment profusely and in public members of the organization who shared in recruitment. Pay particular attention to those individuals who share your religious background.
VI. Wield power at the very onset.
   A. In response to comments intended to be humorous or reflect the human element in systems, get angry and declare such comments off-limits ("Don't ever tell that to a medical director!").

       B. Fire two of the assistants to the previous director. Promote others based on hearsay. Apologize only after subordinates are in tears.

VII. Demoralize the members of the organization.

       A. Create ad hoc advisory groups made up of nonmanagerial personnel.

       B. Announce at a meeting of managers the unvalidated complaints of their subordinates, which were gathered informally (some through the grapevine).

       C. Announce program cuts based on inadequate information and accounting, then reverse your decision.

       D. Wonder aloud why there seems to be general unrest, confusion, and anxiety throughout the system, and use this to confirm your views about people in the system you don't like.

Comment

Most puzzling was the fact that based on information obtained by the search committee and on the recommendations of those who knew him, the new administrator's behavior was totally unexpected. It would take careful research to find a satisfactory answer to that riddle. Suffice it to point out, however, that in the process of recruitment it is always desirable to probe beneath the surface. A brief telephone call to the recommenders may not penetrate the surface, but a longer face-to-face interview may reveal critical confidential material. A review of how the individual behaves under stress may be revealing. Remember that a good second-in-command may be an utter flop as "head honcho." But prediction is always difficult; few can claim that of their last ten appointments, not one is a disappointment or a flop. If 8 out of 10 new appointees are satisfactory workers, and one or two turn out to be stellar performers, an administrator should congratulate himself for a superior batting average.

In this case, it seemed the leopard changed his spots. Some anxiety about making an immediate favorable impression, a misreading of the nature of the organization, or an inordinate drive to put his stamp early upon the system may have propelled him into numerous faux pas. What we can learn from this example is that patience is often a primary virtue that a successor can possess in making relationships in a new milieu, that the system must be dealt with in toto and not by overemphasis on one component, and that sensitive understanding of the values and practices of the new organization (in both its formal and informal aspects) is vital. Further, developing strong and trusting relationships with staff should usually come *before* major policy changes.

Despite the possibility of a later reversal to more acceptable behaviors, one wonders about the reversibility of the feelings and attitudes of subordinates and superiors. The ripple effect may have far-reaching implications in the community, where the reputation of a school or hospital can be affected for a period significantly longer than the duration of the institution's tolerance for abrasive leadership.

SUMMARY AND COMMENTS

Before accepting an administrative position, the candidate wants to know who appoints him, to whom he is responsible, and what the pattern of governance of the institution is. Usually he must relate to some board or council. Boards may be advisory or policy making; in either case, good relations with board members are vital to the success of the enterprise, but in the former case the administrator's formal powers are much greater than in the latter. Recruitment and orientation of new members of the board may devolve, at least partly, upon the administrator. Their business meetings usually include agenda items prepared by him; his comments, advice, counsel, and plans for the institution are, under the best of circumstances, discussed openly by all.

When the new leader is appointed, he finds himself thrust into the processes of management succession. There are seven stages of management succession, each with its unique problems: (a) the anticipatory stage; (b) appointment; (c) inauguration; (d) honeymoon; (e) assertion of the new leader's personality, style, and programs; (f) working through of differences; and (g) establishment of a new equilibrium.

Personnel's reactions to the new executive vary greatly. Some reactions are in relation to their past experiences and affective ties with the predecessor; his personality, administrative style, and past successes in achieving institutional objectives and good morale are very important. Under some circumstances, they may mourn his departure and feel apprehensive about the new director (the Rebecca myth). Under other circumstances, they may feel that the new director will solve all the problems and heal all the wounds inflicted by the parting director (the messiah myth). In all circumstances, the relationship between the new director and predecessor is of very great interest to the many people who depend upon the institution and its leaders.

The strategies of the new director in taking hold of the organization include establishing good personal relations with subordinates and encouraging broad informational input; understanding organizational structure; and forming a management team. The predecessor is faced with the decision as to what is his best role in helping the enterprise. Influencing the course of action through his former colleagues still active in policy development, and hovering over the processes of governance, are two (among several) trends that should yield to sober reflection and mature wisdom.

The administrator may or may not be involved in succession planning, depending on the type of institution he represents, its appointing authority, board functions, and the goals and expectations of the organization as a whole. Search committees face the question whether the new chief should be an "insider" or an "outsider." Also, they must consider whether to favor consistency of philosophy and direction, or to select a person who offers an opportunity to break with tradition.

Once the administrator's career within the institution comes to a close, the administrator prepares to leave the organization, in effect to become a predecessor to a new executive. This can be a hard task, a mixed blessing, or a joyous event. Much depends on whether the departure is due to normal retirement, illness, or firing; on possible acceptance of another job at a higher or lower level; and on whether or not his mission with respect to the institution has been accomplished.

In any event, three phases in the retirement process may be identified. First is a lame-duck period in which there is personal and institutional reorientation to his new status, and in which some institutional tensions are mitigated and some projects are put on hold. A second stage is a ceremonial one featuring activities directed to allay individual and institutional separation anxieties, and to reward the retiree for what he has done. The third stage is that of actual retirement and facing the future.

Decompression, a phenomenon from which many retiring executives suffer, characterizes the sudden change from a job of high status, challenge, excitement, centrality, and power to a situation that may be much lower in these traits. It was prominently displayed in a population of retired state commissioners of mental health.

Retirement is a major life adjustment fraught with mythology and beliefs. It may be seen as a perilous period, threatening life and health, or it may be seen as a time to reap the rewards of a life of toil, and to practice intelligent hedonism leavened by wisdom and maturity.

REFERENCES

1. Clark ML: The board of directors as a small dynamic group: A review. Admin and Policy in Mental Health 16:89–98, 1988
2. Redlich FC: Problems of Succession. Presented at American Psychiatric Association annual meeting, Toronto, Canada, 1977 (unpublished)
3. DuMaurier D: Rebecca. New York, Doubleday, 1938
4. Gouldner AV: Patterns of Industrial Bureaucracy. Glencoe, Illinois, Free Press, 1954
5. Kotin J, Sharaf MR: Management succession and administrative style. Psychiatry 30:237–248, 1967
6. Redlich FC: Problems of Succession. Presented at American Psychiatric Association annual meeting, Toronto, Canada, 1977 (unpublished)
7. Kelly JN: Management transitions for newly appointed CEOs. Sloan Management Review 22:37–45, Fall 1980
8. Kohler T, Strauss G: Executive succession: Literature review and research issues. Admin in Ment Health 11:11–22, 1983
9. Grusky O: Corporate size, bureaucratization, and managerial succession. Amer J Sociology 67:263–269, 1961
10. Pickhardt C: Problems posed by a changing organizational membership. Organizational Dynamics 3:64–80, 1981
11. Greenblatt M: Management succession: Some major parameters. Admin in Ment Health 2:3–10, 1983
12. Brady GF, Helmich DL: The hospital administrator and organizational change: Do we recruit from outside? Hosp & Health Services Admin 7:53–62, 1981
13. Pfeffer J, Salancik GR: Organizational context and the characteristics and tenure of hospital administrators. Academy of Management J 20:74–88, 1977
14. Osborn RN, Jauch LR, Martin TN, Glueck WF: The event of CEO succession, performance, and environmental conditions. Academy of Management J 24:183–191, 1981

15. Brown MC: Administrative succession and organizational performance: The succession effect. Administrative Science Q 27:1–16, 1982
16. Strauss GD, Kohler T: Executive succession in health care organizations. Admin in Ment Health 11:23–35, 1983
17. Feldman DC: The role of initiation activities in socialization. Human Relations 30:977–990, 1977
18. Strauss GD, Kohler T: Executive succession in health care organizations. Admin in Ment Health 11:23–35, 1983
19. Strauss GD, Kohler T: Executive succession in health care organizations. Admin in Ment Health 11:23–35, 1983
20. Harrison JR, Torres DL, Kukalis S: The changing of the guard: Turnover and structural change in the top-management positions. Administrative Science Q 33:211–232, 1988
21. Harrison JR, Torres DL, Kukalis S: The changing of the guard: Turnover and structural change in the top-management positions. Administrative Science Q 33:211–232, 1988
22. Grusky O: Corporate size, bureaucratization, and managerial succession. Amer J Sociology 67:261–269, 1961
23. Pattan JE: Succession planning, 2: Management selection. Personnel 63:24–34, 1986
24. Moore KW: Thoughts on management succession planning. National Underwriter (Life/Health) 90:17, 37, Nov. 8, 1986
25. [No byline]: Succession planning in closely held firms: Begin now–the company's future depends on it. Small Business Report 9:52–58, 1984
26. [No byline]: Making management succession more a science than an art. Intl Management (UK) (Europe Edition) 39:61, 64, 1984
27. Vancil RF: How companies pick new CEOs. Fortune 117:74–79, Jan 4, 1988
28. Hamilton PW: The special problems of family businesses. D&B Reports 34:18–21, 1986
29. Morris DM: Family businesses: High-risk candidates for financial distress. Small Business Report 14:43–45, 1989
30. Ferguson T: Relative prosperity. Canadian Business 58:50–61, 1985
31. Bernstein M: When the CEO dies. Black Enterprise 18:299–302, 1988
32. Chung KH, Rogers RC, Lubatkin M, Owers JE: Do insiders make better CEOs than outsiders? Academy of Management Executives 1:325–331, 1987
33. Geber B: Should you build top executives . . . or buy them? Training 26:25–32, 1989
34. Reinganum MR: The effect of executive succession on stockholder wealth. Administrative Science Q 30:46–60, 1985
35. Sonnenfeld J: Unfinished business: Managing his retirement is a CEO's most critical task. Business Month 133:61–66, 1989
36. Gifford RD, Davidson N: Gone tomorrow? CEOs speak out on institutional survival. Trustee 38:33–37, May 1985
37. Gifford RD, Davidson N: Executive succession: Who decides? Hospitals 59:66–69, 1985
38. Freund CM: CEO succession and its relationship to CNO tenure. J Nurs Admin 17:27–30, 1987
39. Levinson DJ, Klerman GL: The clinician-executive. Some problematic issues for the psychiatrist in mental health organizations. Psychiatry 30:3–15, 1967
40. Greenblatt M: The psychiatrist as social system clinician. In Greenblatt M, Levinson DJ, Williams RH (eds): The Patient and the Mental Hospital. Glencoe, Illinois, Free Press, 1957, pp 317–323
41. Greenblatt M, Gaver KD, Sherwood E: After commissioner, what? Amer J Psychiatry 142:752–754, 1985

Internal Dynamics: Stresses and Strains

In any human system, stresses can arise—among individuals, between the individual and the group, among groups, and between the organization and outside agencies and institutions. These stresses may be mild, moderate, or acute. They may lead to temporary dysfunctions in relation to the goals of the enterprise, or they may lead to major disruptions, even breakdowns. Administrators, in their natural role as social system clinicians, become sensitive to these stresses, striving to diminish them and to ameliorate their negative impact upon the functioning of the organization. The health and welfare of systems depends on early diagnosis, prompt and effective intervention, and efforts to prevent recurrences.

In this chapter, I study stresses between the chief of staff and the director, between administrative and clinical divisions, between doctors and nurses, and among various members of the interdisciplinary team. Major stresses may arise as a result of outside forces, system ineffectiveness or inefficiencies, fiscal troubles, personnel shortages, the personality quirks and aberrations of workers or leaders, and/or racial or ethnic strains.

STRESS BETWEEN ADMINISTRATIVE AND CLINICAL DIVISIONS

Ultimately, the therapeutic relationship between the patient and his treating clinicians must be regarded as the primary task and raison d'être of any hospital or institution serving clients. Ideally, all other functions of a hospital should be subordinated to the requirements of this unique relationship. Why then do doctors and allied professionals and workers in many facilities complain that they are being treated like hired hands, that they have lost prestige, dedication, status, or power? Why do many doctors today say they are no longer encouraging their children to go into the field of medicine?

Increasingly, the fact is that administrators—more than any other group today—determine hospital policy, including the pattern and form of direct services to patients. They have final say in planning, and they control budgets. Rules and regulations stem from their offices. Regularly, they make critical decisions relating to the allocation of personnel, supplies, and equipment, as well as about the management of the physical plant. They have final responsibility for meeting the standards for food, safety, fire protection, patient rights, quality assurance, and local (as well as state and federal) laws and regulations, and they have the critical responsibility to meet the requirements of JCAHO and other standard-setting agencies.

Over the years, there has been a dramatic shift in the balance of power between administrative and clinical divisions. As hospitals have grown in size and complexity, budgets have expanded, patient beds have multiplied, staffs have increased, and new disciplines, technologies, and departments have proliferated. The subtle and elaborate teamwork necessary to get supplies to wards, to dispose of wastes, to recruit and train nurses and other therapeutic personnel, to handle risks, to raise funds, to carry out proper public relations, and to develop successful marketing strategies has given administrators problems never before imagined. Any serious slippage in efficiency or morale, any threat to accreditation, any bungling of public relations can precipitate a crisis—then, people quickly label the institution a "bureaucratic nightmare." Patients may stop seeking admission; if this continues, the institution is in danger of collapse and closure.

As the institution becomes more complex, the qualities of top management become more and more critical to success of the enterprise. Today, a physician with an interest (even an instinct) for leadership has difficulty handling the task. He was never trained in administrative science and art while in medical school; indeed, most physicians do not have a taste for administrative details. Why should they move away from patients, teaching, and research to take a job where a great deal of new information must be quickly assimilated, and job strains can be immense? Financial rewards are usually less than private practice, and the risks of public opprobrium can be great. In addition, the joys of warm relations with patients and families will have to be surrendered.

My experience as Commissioner of Mental Health in Massachusetts (1967–1973), during the period of rapid deinstitutionalization, was that psychiatric administrators were gradually replaced by nonmedical administrators in several areas. When regional administrative centers were established, seven in number, it was not possible to fill all the new slots created (for mental health administrators, retardation administrators, and forensic experts) with psychiatrists. They simply were not available at the salaries offered. Further, the very idea that regional administration would take them further away from patients and students was totally unattractive. Those slots, therefore, were filled by a variety of other personnel—psychologists, rehabilitators, persons trained in special education, and social workers with good administrative track records.

In some of the state mental hospitals, after the psychiatric superintendents retired, it was difficult also to replace them with physicians who showed promise as administrators. I was forced to seek the best I could find in other fields. In the schools for the retarded, I resorted to recruiting from the growing numbers of "mental healthers"—some of whom were very able and enthusiastic, and more than eager to accept a hospital leadership position (which for them actually offered more, rather than less, challenge and compensation than they had previously enjoyed).

This was in the late 1960s, when it was felt in many circles that to put nonpsychiatrists in power positions over mental health facilities was a dangerous precedent. Arguments over the relative merits of psychiatric versus nonpsychiatric leadership of treatment organizations pointed to the latter's lack of appreciation of medical professional values, and of the subtleties of the doctor–patient relationship, as a serious handicap. Also, it was argued that a nonmedical administrator would have a hard time exercising leadership over the large number of professional health workers who came from diverse fields. It was feared that purely economic considerations, plus overemphasis on information and accounting systems, would submerge the idealism and dedication of medically trained professionals.

These arguments waned during the 1970s and 1980s, due to the increasing number of management challenges critical to survival. Control and power over therapeutic institutions then largely shifted to professional administrators. Of the challenges facing administration from which physicians, for example, may recoil, I need only mention the fiscal strains from diminished third-party payments; the subsequent restrictions on freedom and flexibility of treatment programs; and the intensification of competition among various health providers. Today many beds are empty on wards of university, VA, and private hospitals—and many hospitals and facilities have gone under in the struggle.

To epitomize the changes that have occurred in the Department of Veterans Affairs, an example is in order.

Case Illustration

Shift in Balance of Power between Medical Chief of Staff and Nonmedical Director

In one VA hospital in the year 1973, the chief of staff (a surgeon) sat with the lay director and his staff and told them what was to be done. To a large extent, he established priorities of clinical and administrative activities, and gave general directions on the assumption that the primary function of the administrative apparatus of the hospital was to support the clinical operation. Twelve years later, with a new director (and a much larger administrative staff)—and a new chief of staff having replaced the old—the new chief was told by the director what to do in affairs that included quality assurance, preparation for JCAHO, reduction in expenditures for patient care, and techniques for increasing revenue (including changes in admission policy and review of diagnostic procedures so as to favor the most financially rewarding diagnostic groups). How the tide had turned!

The arrangement, quite familiar in the VA system, of a nonmedical director who is finally responsible for all actions and a medical chief of staff who is presumably the final expert in all matters related to the care and treatment of patients, can be fertile ground for stress and strain. In many overt and covert ways, the director may vitiate the program of the chief of staff—in the allocation of support among different programs, the balance of emphasis on research and teaching versus service, the support of intramural versus extramural programs, and a host of other decisions. Indeed, the director, by making himself unavailable, by failing to discuss major policies with the chief of staff, or by listening to other voices, can render the chief of staff impotent. I have seen instances where the director, threatened by an aggressive chief of staff, makes sure that the latter's recommendations are watered down or referred to unresponsive committees. Although the final powers of decision are essentially in the director's hands, continuous efforts to maintain goodwill and much time spent in communication are necessary if the organization is to benefit from a true partnership of talents at the top.

Whatever the contribution of the director to stress and strain, unilateral decisions on professional matters by the chief of staff, and/or failure to orient the director adequately on medical issues on which the director must give final consent, also can make the working relation a failure. One may be assured that the staff is highly sensitive to disagreements at the top, particularly personality clashes, struggles for power, and fights over turf. Some staff members will exaggerate in their minds the seriousness of the differences and the amount of bad feeling; and some, consciously or unconsciously, will contribute their own negative behaviors to the general tension.

How, indeed, can a director undermine the status and authority of the chief of staff? The following illustrations are drawn from real life:

- Rather than deal directly with the new chief of staff, a director who is dubious of the former's programs and style complains to his administrative assistant that the chief had made an announcement that should have been made by the director's office.
- In discussion with the chief of psychology, the director lets it be known that a program dear to the heart of the chief of staff will not go through.

The chief of staff knows of this conversation only on report from the psychologist.

- The director takes up policy problems mainly with the professional executive committee as a whole, thus minimizing the chief of staff's role as primary consultant on all professional matters.

On the other hand, how can the chief of staff contribute to deterioration of a working relationship?

- The chief of staff fails to clear program initiatives with the director through timely discussions in depth.
- The chief of staff consults with outside authority, such as dean's committee chairman or central office executives, without previous discussion with the director.

The question naturally arises as to whether these kinds of difficulties would be minimized if the director were a physician rather than a layman. Personality clashes and differences in style still could be manifest, but problems relating to the director's status among a group of strong-minded medical professionals might be mitigated. For decades it has been argued whether the conversion of a highly trained physician to a full-time administrator is a suitable use of talent. Can a retreaded physician be as good an administrator as a professionally trained executive in the health field? Considering the enormous amount of detail involved in modern administration (budget, personnel, physical plant, standards and accreditation, disaster planning, etc.), can the retreaded physician maintain his interest in administration, knowing that each year takes him further away from his collegial base? Perhaps the ultimate consideration is whether it is possible to run a huge organization, such as the VA system of 172 hospitals or a large state system (with a dozen or more hospitals and many ambulatory programs), without totally dedicated, trained professional (nonmedical) administrators at every level.

With every shift of power, there is, according to Galbraith,[1] an opposite assertion of power. In one case, the clinical staffs of the hospitals, exploring the possibilities of collective action to restore the power of the medical clinicians, formed a group to seek a greater hand in decisions affecting their welfare. This turned out to be a very potent move, for administration cannot afford to ignore a group of senior physicians who speak with one voice. Such meetings can bring favorable results over the course of time, although some sessions may be stormy. The deeper appreciation of the problems of both sides can result in greater respect and enhanced efficiency in caring for patients.

In the VA system, as indicated above, stress between a nonmedical professional manager and a medical chief of staff is not unfamiliar. In the state system of Massachusetts, I encountered instances where, for lack of available physicians, I appointed psychologists or social workers to top institutional directorships, but where top *clinical* positions were still occupied by physicians. In fact, the nonmedical directors were very appreciative of the expertise of the medical chiefs and gave them great sway. Under these conditions, for harmony to prevail, it is important that the medical chief *not* harbor strong ambitions to be the director; and, contrariwise, that the nonmedical director try to appreciate the limits of his medical knowledge.

In a university system with a very large department of psychiatry, I encountered a pattern of governance that was new to me but apparently not unknown in other university settings. Here the psychiatric hospital and clinics were in the hands of one psychiatrist, and the research and educational programs were in the hands of another. The overall institute directorship, with its relationships to neurology, the affiliating hospitals, space allocations, and academic appointments and promotions, was also governed by the latter physician, although the former (the hospital and clinics director) functioned as associate director of the institute. The institute director reported to the dean; the hospital and clinics director to the chancellor. The two budgets were essentially separated, although in some functions salaries were made up by contributions from both sources.

A very complicated arrangement, yes. Here we have the topmost functions headed by two psychiatrists—so, one would hope, no troubles should arise from the possession of different formal training backgrounds and different academic degrees. Unfortunately here, too, stresses arose as a result of different personal styles and differing views as to where the institute as a whole should be going. Needless to say, tensions between the two top figures were transmitted down the personnel line, causing the development of two antagonistic encampments and the choosing of sides by personnel. The lesson is that, whatever the arrangement, the seeds of discontent may be sown unless there is goodwill, flexibility, and friendly compatibility between the power figures.

Here one might ask about the wisdom and logic of separating hospitals and clinics from research and education. Are they not indissolubly united in any good department of psychiatry? How can training and education go on without excellent patient care? Research, education, and clinical care must be smoothly integrated in any teaching hospital, to be sure, but when the institute reaches a certain point of size and complexity, then perhaps it is not possible for a single individual to give proper attention to all its parts, for in many a university setting, administrators too are expected to produce creative research and scholarship.

With essentially independent budgets and domains of influence, can such a partnership work? The answer seems to be yes and no: yes when the two get along like good brothers, and no when personalities and ideologies clash. More and more the administrator of today, challenged to deal with changing complexity, different personalities, and conflicting pressures, needs to compromise, compromise, compromise.

Case Illustration

Stress between Clinicians and Administrators, or How Long Does It Take to Hang a Picture?

In this general hospital, the chief of psychiatry has a running battle with administration. He is not alone in this, but is probably more strident and persistent than other service chiefs.

When the chief of psychiatry asks for information, his claim is that his request is often ignored, or the response is delayed, or information given is often unreliable. For some time he has been urging the desirability of making the psychiatric wards more cheerful and homelike by adding pictures and plants and by repainting using a variety of colors. *A year and a half has gone by* without results, although 50 telephone calls have been made and many meetings held with personnel assigned to interior decorating, who kept saying something would soon be done. However, the real message was, "This is not important; other priorities in other departments are much more pressing." Then it became, "We have a plan for the whole hospital, but psychiatry's plan is on hold because of a lack of material to finish pictures already in stock. When such material arrives, your needs will receive first priority."

But the chief of psychiatry is not satisfied. First, the typical delay of months in responding is nettling; second, he feels his patients' needs should not be subordinated to an overall hospital policy that does not recognize the special sensibilities of mental patients to their physical environment. He quotes studies that show that patients' irritable behavior is modulated by a soft environment. A reduction in patient irritability means a reduction of assaults on nursing staff, the number of which has been much greater than in nonpsychiatric wards of the hospital.

He also points out that the offices of administrators are lined with pictures. Finally, he resents the aloof attitude of decision makers, the lack of any desire to search for new solutions. Any reasonable view, in his judgment, would conclude that there was little justification for an 18-month delay in hanging a picture.

This seemingly minor controversy is symptomatic of a chronic stress that exists between administrators and clinical service chiefs in many hospitals. It is familiar in VA hospitals, where directors, usually nonphysicians, are brought up through the VA system as professional administrators. They make final budgetary decisions that impact upon quality of care and professional standards. Their salaries are often less than those of physicians, although their position in the hierarchy is higher. Clinical specialists sometimes view them as sitting far back from the firing line where the patient load is sometimes overwhelming, where lives are at stake, and where great responsibilities are faced every day. There is resentment that over the years, as administrative problems of running an institution become more complex and detailed, physicians have lost ground to lay administrators; the balance of power has shifted radically toward the nonmedical side. Administrators are preoccupied with balancing the budget and overcoming the most recent cut in funds. Hanging pictures on the wards of mental patients is far from their thoughts. It is easy to assume rather that mental patients are usually "out of it," insensitive to their surroundings—and anyway, their stay in the hospital is generally short, an average of only 12 to 14 days.

What is to be done? Holding grudges is no answer. Erecting barriers, where the chief of psychiatry holds that administrators are impossibly rigid, and the administrators think the chief of psychiatry has no understanding of the hospital as a whole, is also no answer. Sooner or later, the parties must confront each other. The chief of psychiatry's case can be made infinitely stronger if he can persuade other chiefs of service to join him in the confrontation. In effect, the service chiefs have to come out with gut feelings ("You treat us like dirt"), citing instance and example. When confronted with such revelations of collective resentment, administrators are aghast and defensive. Emotional tides are let loose. Most important is to let the process continue until satisfactory rapprochement occurs; for if, as is sometimes the case, both sides become entrenched, nothing less than a blasting operation will change their ways.

Sometimes it is true that the persons involved cannot be moved from their bases. Frustration continues or may deepen. What then? The problem may move to a higher level; on rare occasions, they spill over into the courts. Often, as the emotional intensity dissipates, business continues but on a restrained note. The wages of nonhealed relationships are often paid in chronic morale problems, loss of staff, and difficulty in recruiting good replacements. It is tragically poor administration to allow such conditions to continue, but who should take the initiative for conciliation? Conciliation takes time, lots of time, particularly if bad feelings have been allowed to accumulate. For such impasses, administration must have skill in the art of diplomacy, for success in managing group relations has two bases: (a) self-understanding and self-control, and (b) experience in the dynamics of group relations.

> This impasse, in which service chiefs repeatedly urged administration to do something, and administration resisted by constant foot-dragging, was finally (partially) resolved in this instance by the service chief himself. Taking the bull by the horns, he advanced funds to staff members eager to proceed with ward beautification and willing to hang pictures by any means that would not damage walls. Should administration complain that the psychiatric service had proceeded without permission, or had defaced government property, the service chief made it clear he would take the blame and make restitution, if necessary. Thus, after almost three years, pictures began to appear on the walls, delighting both staff and patients. Unexpectedly, management then reimbursed the chief for advancing money and encouraged further efforts along the lines of ward beautification.

Probably a factor favoring the final resolution was a site visit to a new private psychiatric hospital, part of a successful chain, that had put much effort into interior decorating. Pictures, plants, flowers, and distinctive color schemes for many of the rooms charmed the visitors, one of whom was the administration liaison to the department of psychiatry. His report, I believe, helped turn administrators' attitudes in the more favorable direction.

Commentary: The Ward Environment

The ward environment is not something that can be left to chance; continuing work on it is necessary to keep it from stagnating. Both patients and staff behave better in an environment that speaks to them of order and beauty. Martin Orne's [2] felicitous phrase, "the demand characteristics of the environment," was never more apt than in its application to hospital patients. The decoration of one's home is a particularly interesting and satisfying indulgence of a family. On the ward, joint endeavors to improve the physical environment bring staff and patients together. At Massachusetts Mental Health Center, in the 1940s and 1950s, ward beautification became an interest of all parties. When patients and staff jointly collaborated in painting wall murals, they were never happier. Then, experts in interior design and art students visited frequently, offering aid and expert consultation.

Attention to the physical environment alone, it should be noted, is not enough. The *social* environment, related to and interwoven with the physical environment, is even more meaningful. Together they define the life of the "citizens of the ward"—staff and patients. The real question is: How can the time spent on the wards be of maximal benefit to these individuals?

Note on the Social Environment

In the 1940s and 1950s, stimulated in large measure by the Russell Sage Foundation (one of whose missions was the application of social science insights and methodologies to medical care), a number of studies of ward environment were initiated.[3] Maxwell Jones[4,5] at that time had popularized his particular approach to the development of the ward as a *therapeutic community*. In Boston, Levinson and his students developed the Custodial Mental Illness scale[6,7] (modeled on earlier work on the authoritarian personality[8]), which measured an individual's or institution's place on a so-called custodial–therapeutic dimension. Those at the custodial end were less inclined to changes in a therapeutic direction, and less interested in forming closer ties with patients. They saw the patients as different from themselves, and were more comfortable at a distance. Those who, according to the scale, were more therapeutically oriented could be relied upon to favor moves toward a therapeutic community. Proponents of patient government[9,10,11,12] greatly influenced the social therapeutic process at that time by stressing the patients' potential for participating in a democratic process, leading to a more normal, therapeutic ward life.

What useful concepts and practices emerged from this period?

1. A warm supporting physical/social environment can counter the "de-socialization" associated with the patient's withdrawal, disorganization, anxieties, and depressive tendencies.
2. Organization of ward life toward optimal healthy involvement requires active and continued support not only of ward leaders, *but also of medical and administrative authority.*
3. Continued support and in-service training are necessary to help ward staff adopt roles, concepts, and practices more consistent with a therapeutic community.
4. Instrumentalities to accomplish these ends include daily community group meetings with all "ward citizens" (à la Maxwell Jones), group and individual counseling, psychodrama, patient government, occupational therapy carried out on the ward rather than in remote occupational therapy departments, recreational activities mirroring what goes on in the community, and educational activities for all patients (not only younger clients).
5. Strongly recommended is the establishment, through discussion involving all ward citizens, of a *progressive set of expectations* (see "Institutional Change" in Chapter 3) as to how ward life can be improved. Such expectations must be flexible and appropriately tailored to fit the level of interest and ability of ward citizens at any given time. Thus, at one stage the ward community can promote beautification, at another psychodrama, at another patient government, and at another expression of artistic interests.
6. Particular emphasis should be directed to patients' assumption of responsibility for progressively higher levels of behavior and for sharing in group decisions.

Why an emphasis on social rehabilitation? In recent years, effective pharmacotherapy has shortened hospitalization time and shifted the emphasis to biological treatment. However, it is social competence that primarily determines the patient's ability to get along in the community. To counteract the "social breakdown syndrome," which Ernest Gruenberg[13] has described so perceptively, every opportunity for resocialization should be exploited during and after hospitalization. In a series of careful studies, Goldstein[14,15] has shown that the family milieu exerts an outstanding influence on the schizophrenic patient's ability to adapt, notwithstanding adequate treatment with neuroleptic medication.

Most pertinent are studies by Whitehead et al.,[16] Fairbanks et al.,[17] and McGuire et al.[18] of two wards at the VA Medical Center in the San Fernando Valley of Los Angeles. One ward was thoroughly changed in its physical appearance after soliciting recommendations from patients and staff, which were translated into a plan developed by a group of architectural students, then approved and financed by the VA central office. Patients and staff found the "new" ward a more pleasant place in which to live and work. A control ward, housing the same type of patients, was untouched. Before-and-after studies of ward behavior of the mentally ill patients revealed that in the renovated ward, aggressive outbursts were reduced, and the patients were more relaxed and tractable.

Case Illustration

Ban on "Therapeutic Outings"

The cases quoted above are proper examples of internal dynamics insofar as they arise and play out their course essentially within the boundaries of the organization. Herewith is a case illustrating a major stress that arose between clinical and administrative divisions and included as a major player an outside organization—the Professional Risk Management Group, an organization in contract with the hospital to provide consultation on risk management and lawsuit containment. Professional Risk Management (PRM) clearly states that it does not set hospital policy; in this instance, however, hospital administration took an opinion of PRM as if it were an order from some legally constituted and qualified higher authority, without consultation in depth with the department of psychiatry. Most distressing to the clinical division was the fact that in some ways it was being controlled in its treatment of patients by an outside group that was not clinically credentialed, hardly understood the impact of its rules on the system, and knew almost nothing about the patients who were affected.

It all started with a memo to the chief of psychiatry, signed by the hospital administrator and medical director, regarding off-site outings:

> In response to our inquiry regarding the hospital's liability during a psychiatric patient's leave or outing, Professional Risk Management responded that measures should be taken to reduce the County's exposure to lawsuits. It is their opinion that in-house activities provide the best control/supervision environment that greatly reduces the County's legal exposure to the usual allegations of failure to meet the community's standard of care or lack of supervision, and/or failure to warn individuals of potential risks.
>
> Therefore, to legally protect this facility we are adopting Professional Risk Management's recommendation and therefore must request from the Mental Health Department a revised policy and procedure on outings by our psychiatric inpatients (adolescents and adults) which permits only on-campus activities."

To discuss the memo, a large meeting was called including clinicians versed in adult and adolescent psychiatry, forensic specialists, mental health department administrators, and hospital administrators. Members of PRM were invited but failed to attend; however, they received a summary of the proceedings which made the following points:

1. The hospital had experienced *no* untoward incidents related to the use of therapeutic outings. Outing privileges were earned by patients based on a four-point scale combining reliability, responsibility, and safety; only individuals with the highest possible score were selected for the privilege. The

vast majority of selected patients were on voluntary status; a few were on temporary conservatorship. Staff supervision, consistent with staff–patient ratios elsewhere, was required on all outings.

Evidently, both PRM and hospital management were reacting to the conviction that mental patients were generally more dangerous than other people; they did not fully understand that the selection process was based on a very detailed knowledge of the patients' behavior, characteristics, and potentialities. It is a truism that the risk in treating patients can never be reduced to zero. Every intervention from medication to major surgery is a balance between benefits and risks. The danger of a bad happening during outings was certainly one of the smallest in the whole kingdom of medical risks, while the benefits could be very great.

2. Information collected from 10 local institutions revealed that all were prescribing therapeutic outings for their patients.* Selection was based on the patients' having already won a high level of privilege. A wide variety of community experiences was included (sports, movies, beaches, parks, picnics, shows, museums, hikes, etc.). Most of the patients were on voluntary status, and 7 of the 10 wards from which they were taken were locked-type wards.

3. Similarly, information from many hospitals *outside* Los Angeles revealed that all were using therapeutic outings enthusiastically and with success. Outings were deemed necessary to facilitate discharge planning, aftercare arrangements, home visits, and court visits, and to prevent rehospitalization. They provided valuable experience, too, for those suffering from "social breakdown syndrome" or anxieties that made them homebound.

4. Obvious to all experts was the fact that benefits greatly overweighed risks, and that treatment under the least restrictive arrangements was a legal imperative that cast a shadow on any ban on outings—especially for voluntary patients. Further, the ban was resisted by staff as an intrusion on their right to treat patients according to their best judgment. They bitterly resented legalistic interference from outside.

Happily, after considerable argument, administration reconsidered the ban and eventually rescinded the order. The lessons to be learned are that (a) boundaries between clinical and administrative divisions can be easily overstepped unless vigorously protected, and (b) every aspect of the life of the mental patient must be regarded as important. Administrative decisions based on generalized stereotyping of all mentally ill patients as dangerous and unpredictable discriminate most unfairly against those who have never belonged in this class.

STRESS BETWEEN DOCTOR AND NURSE

Traditionally, the doctor and the nurse work very closely together. The doctor works up the patient, writes his orders, and expects the nursing department to follow through with speed and exactitude. The nurse is dependent on the doctor's orders, but in all other functions is either independent or

---

*I am indebted to Susan Hussey, R.N., for this information.

works collaboratively with the doctor. The doctor comes and he goes, but the nursing service stays with the patient through the 24-hour day. The nurse depends on the doctor for his knowledge and leadership. Sometimes it is the other way around: A strong head nurse provides the ward leadership that is lacking when there is no full-time administrative psychiatrist, or one who is really "not in touch" with the milieu. The nurse also expects from the doctor a high degree of maturity, immediate response in times of crisis, and respect for the nurse as a loyal and dedicated colleague. The popular doctor admits he does not know it all, and asks for help with difficult cases; the know-it-alls are seen for the insecure individuals they are. The popular doctor is the one who "knows his stuff," is generous in his appreciation of the nurses' work, and is lighthearted or "fun to be with." The doctor who is aloof, rigid, controlling, or narcissistic is quickly diagnosed for these characteristics. Accommodation to these traits can become an important source of stress between the two professions.

Another source of stress arises from the fact that the nurses have several loyalties—a primary loyalty to the patient; loyalty to the doctor as head of the ward and giver of the plan related to the care and treatment of the patient; loyalty to the nursing hierarchy, which hires, fires, and sets standards of nursing practice (and takes care of all administrative details related to supplies, equipment, schedules of work, vacations, complaints and grievances, and administrative contacts with top hospitalwide management); and, finally, loyalty to the profession of nursing.

In numbers, the nursing department is by far the largest clinical division of the hospital, and much of its clout depends on this fact alone. In the current severe nursing shortage, the influence of the nursing service is significantly enhanced. Nurses may have the final say about whether a ward can stay open or must be closed, whether day and night coverage will be sufficient to satisfy JCAHO requirements, whether there are enough nurses available to handle the admission of a second or third violent patient, and when it is necessary to hire nurses off the registry because of a shortage of regularly employed nurses (despite the fact that registry nurses may be a heavier drain upon the treasury). Finally, the nursing hierarchy reports directly to the chief of staff or medical director, so at any time a nursing problem or complaint can be taken up directly with the top medical office—at the same organizational level to which the doctors of all services report.

Thus, a ward nurse, dissatisfied with her relations with her ward doctor, can make an end run with the greatest of ease simply by reporting her concerns up through her own hierarchy. It should also be stated that nurses are instructed not to follow slavishly all orders given by the doctor, but to state their opinions and feelings, particularly when they believe that the doctor is out of line (e.g., prescribing too large doses, coming to work intoxicated or possibly on drugs, being crude or impolite with patients or anyone else). They are, in a sense, therefore, also the watchdogs and conscience of the organization, with special emphasis on the behavior of physicians in the nurse–doctor relationship. In fact, the American Nurses Association code of ethics[19] states that the nurse acts to safeguard the client and the public when health care and safety are affected by incompetent, unethical, or illegal practices of *any* person.

A special case of potential strain in the nurse–doctor relationship applies to the training program for psychiatrists and, to an extent, to undergraduate physicians in their clinical clerkships. Young psychiatrists in training often come onto the ward looking for an opportunity to take on large responsibility for patients and ward leadership, only to find out that the nurse in charge knows far more about the patient and his treatment than does the resident in his first and sometimes even second and third years. While the resident psychiatrist is involved in a sharp upward growth-learning curve, the nurse maintains her strength in ward management and governance. The role of the resident as *student* learning from the experienced nurse becomes the appropriate one at this time and forevermore, for far beyond residency, the wise doctor will be asking nurses for their observations about patients and for their suggestions as to the best management of them.

Is the relationship between doctor and nurse a hierarchical one—the doctor superior to the nurse, a relationship of dominance and submission? Or is it a relationship of mutual interdependence between experts, each vital to the treatment of the patient? The same question, of course, might apply to the relationship between the doctor and any other member of the professional team. If the doctor is the leader, in what way can he lead so that the several expertises can be best blended together, and hierarchy and dominance do not get in the way?

With respect to the doctor–nurse relationship, there has been a radical change in recent decades.[20] Thirty years ago it was clearly hierarchical. Open disagreements were avoided at all costs. Nursing schools were tightly run, disciplined institutions; almost 90% of nursing students trained in hospital-run nursing schools where they were taught their place—clear subservience to doctors.

However, in the ensuing years, the public's view of physicians has changed. They are no longer deemed omnipotent. At the same time, nursing school enrollment has dropped, and a great nursing shortage has developed. The image of the nurse is now more that of a specially trained practitioner with independent duties and responsibilities. Consistent with the general civil rights movement, nurses want more autonomy and equal partnership in the health team. They are moving away from bedside nursing to specialty, teaching, and administrative positions.

Case Illustration

Stress between Doctor and Nurse and Its Resolution

Bill, the chief psychiatrist of an inpatient ward of acute patients, and Laura, the chief nurse, are having trouble. Bill is a highly regarded, highly experienced senior psychiatrist, whose great interest is teaching medical students. They come to his ward, four or five at a time, for six weeks' clinical rotation in their third or fourth years. Laura is a dedicated nurse, deeply involved with her patients' welfare, highly responsible, and profoundly imbued with the humanitarian ideals of the nursing profession. Each, as a person, is excellent in his or her own right, and each has great respect for the other. Why, then, are they having trouble?

Bill and Laura are summoned to the chief psychiatrist's office to talk things over. Laura says she doesn't believe that Bill sees all his patients, apparently leaving their diagnosis, care, and treatment to the medical students. Whatever supervision the students get is not visible, because their consultations take place together behind closed doors in an empty ward (for the reason that space is not available elsewhere). Further, students write orders that Laura believes sometimes are *not* countersigned by Bill. One such order was for a large dose of barbiturates for an alcoholic patient; Laura thinks the dose was excessive. She has already complained to her nursing supervisor about all of the above. Although she truly respects Bill for his intelligence, experience, and gentlemanly qualities, she is very unhappy about the way the ward is running.

Bill says that with rare exceptions he sees all the patients. Surely, that should be left to his judgment. His examinations of the patients may be taking place early in the morning when Laura is not on duty. Further, the dose of barbiturates prescribed for the alcoholic patient was fully discussed with the medical student. The nurse's question about dosage should have been brought to his attention first; his knowledge and experience with alcoholic patients is as great as anyone's in the hospital. Furthermore, the patient did just fine on the dose prescribed.

Bill describes his philosophy and approach to the training of medical students in their clinical clerkships. Briefly, he lets them assume a great deal of responsibility for patients, but gives them a great deal of close supervision. He teaches them the art of computer-assisted record keeping, according to a very effective system he has already devised. Indeed, with his own funds he has bought several small computers, which the students use during their clerkship with him. It teaches them to compress all essential information into carefully thought-out forms, leaving out nothing that is clinically relevant. Besides mastering a system of computer-assisted record keeping, at the end of their clerkship they have an original little library of all their own cases, useful as a personal reference at any future time or for preparation for the boards.

Commentary

This case is one of a legion of cases that has to do with the different personalities and needs of vitally important people in a system who, unfortunately, become estranged and alienated from each other in ways that sooner or later affect the welfare of patients. The prognosis for this kind of institutional pathology depends on many factors: the general maturity of the individuals involved; their ability to identify with institutional goals, as opposed to their personal needs; the depth of their anger with each other; the intensity and rigidity of projections of blame upon the other person; and, inevitably, their trust and respect for the senior officer who calls them into his office for face-to-face discussion.

Other matters that come into play have to do with perceptions of the principals' roles in the organization. If a nurse believes a doctor is neglecting patients, should she first talk it over in depth with the doctor or complain upward within the nursing organization? How does the doctor feel about having his authority brought to question by his head nurse? Is the doctor's role as ward leader—responsible for morale and support for all ward personnel—perceived as the primary one, or is teaching medical students, a role that he cherishes, given too high a priority? How can these two roles be blended?

Overall job satisfaction and job need are also to be considered, for when interpersonal difficulties go deep enough, personnel inevitably begin to think about quitting and seeking jobs with fewer headaches (and perhaps more pay).

Another factor to be considered is the pressure to obey rules and regulations—a point of great importance to administrators trying to meet legal, departmental, and accreditation standards—versus the pressure on individuals to utilize their peculiar styles in the performance of their work. In this case, it was necessary to impress on Bill that hospital rules required that each and every patient be seen personally by the physician in charge, and that his personal signature be affixed to all orders written by students, with as little delay as possible.

In this case, there was the advantage that both parties were mature individuals, respectful of the talents and needs of the other, and were not responding to any wells of anger stemming from deep and unresolved neurotic conflicts. In addition, they were both capable of self-criticism—the quality that is often a strong harbinger of success in resolving interpersonal disputes. Bill quickly caught on to the idea that he was desperately needed by the head nurse, and he immediately became much more visible, making sure that his contacts with *all* patients were duly recorded. Whereas before, the process of teaching was run almost as an independent enterprise, now he began to cultivate relationships between students and the head nurse and other members of the treatment team.

Concerning intervention techniques in episodes of this kind, the most effective instrumentality administrators possess is the face-to-face meeting between aggrieved parties. The intervention of the service chief is indicated only when it is clear that other measures have failed. Meeting with each one independently is not as powerful as bringing the distressed parties together. It is then that the real material comes out—the anger and the disappointment, the differential perception of roles, the constant irritation with one's job—and then, later, the respect and need for one another.

How long should these sessions last? Not everything can be accomplished in one session; several sessions may be required. But my experience is that time spent in these face-to-face meetings usually pays off abundantly in mutual understanding and regard, and in the formation of good working relationships. During the course of discussions, Bill's particular strategy for teaching medical students came in for considerable praise. Finally, since the chief of service seemed willing to spend as much time as needed to resolve the conflict, both parties felt that he understood their feelings and cared about their morale.

INTERPROFESSIONAL RIVALRY

In psychiatry we speak often of the therapeutic "team," and we believe that good teamwork is what offers the patient his greatest opportunities to overcome his illness. What is meant by the team? How does it work, and what are the problems that occur among the team professionals of differing training, and differing personalities, who yet must cooperate intimately for the good of the patient?

The therapeutic team in its earliest representation consisted of the doctor, acknowledged as the undisputed head of clinical operations, and the nurse, who functioned essentially as the doctor's handmaiden.[21] Later, social workers joined the team.[22] At first, social workers concentrated their efforts in the community, working with the family and community agencies to return the patient to his or her fullest functioning in society; but with the passage of time, they shifted their base of operations to a great extent to the institution— working with the family, to be sure, but also working closely and on an individual basis with the patient.

Psychologists then joined the team, first as testers of mental functioning using increasingly sophisticated instruments to diagnose brain damage and to delineate personality characteristics and aberrations. In more recent years, particularly after World War II and with the growth of the Department of Veterans Affairs, psychologists also moved closer to psychotherapy with the patient, in individual and small group relationships.

These two professions, social work and psychology, then began to challenge the physician's exclusive claim to the vaunted "specialty" of psychotherapy. In their schools and in their professional organizations, psychologists gave more and more prominence to *clinical* psychology as a subspecialty. It now is true that both psychiatric social work and clinical psychology are recognized by state licensing authorities for the purpose of psychotherapeutic practice, with the privilege of collecting fees directly from the patient or his insurers. The threat to the physician/psychiatrist's exclusive dominance in this area of psychotherapy has thusly been concluded by a resounding victory for these two professions—yet the psychiatrist continues to function in most hospitals as the so-called leader of the treatment team.

At this point a note on medical supremacy and resistance to change may be in order. Several decades ago, it was considered an effrontery for a nonpsychiatrist to attempt to practice psychotherapy in the Boston area. I remember a meeting of one of the learned societies when the issue of private practice of nonpsychiatrists came up. A friend of mine, a Ph.D. graduate of Harvard's Department of Social Relations, was most eager to hear the verdict.

He had undergone years of analysis, was very friendly with many psycho-therapists, and was in fact working in a mental hospital setting (where, in relation to his Ph.D. thesis, he had made substantial research contributions to an understanding of the sociodynamics of a mental hospital and of the influence of ethno-cultural factors on the etiology and treatment of mental illness). He had also done courageous work in almost single-handedly upgrading the therapeutic climate in a state hospital ward of geriatric patients who had for the most part been sadly neglected. In addition, he had considerable experience doing psychotherapy on hospital cases under psychiatric supervision.

The verdict of the learned psychiatrists was negative. Distinguished senior colleagues with national and international reputations pointed to the risks: The patient must be treated only by the best trained professionals; psychologists and social workers could not fully appreciate the relationship of psychiatric manifestations to medical and neurological disease; misdiagnosis would become common; brain tumors and other serious somatic complications would be overlooked. Somatic therapies should not ever be prescribed by nonmedical people. The fear was that a rush of quacks and charlatans into a field that required the utmost sensitivity and judgment would be encouraged.

Several decades later, we find clinical psychologists, family therapists, social workers, and pastoral counselors doing mental therapy on a large scale. Not only doing it, but claiming legitimacy through state licensure and by offering courses of instruction and training in psychotherapy that they themselves control. (Incidentally, my friend eventually established a private practice despite the disapproval of leading psychiatrists, although for years he felt he was a pariah, charged small fees, and took great pains that any somatic complaints of his patients were quickly referred to medical authorities.)

Clinical psychologists in particular have thrusted toward autonomy; they fought for independent reimbursement by third-party payers as soon as the era of insurance coverage began. They have asked for hospital admission privileges for their patients, and this has indeed been granted in some places. They have demanded freedom in the care and treatment of their hospitalized clients, using physicians and psychiatrists whenever consultation seemed to them indicated. They have asked for an increasing role in hospital governance, and for a place on the board of the Joint Commission on Accreditation of Healthcare Organizations. All this has taken place *pari passu* with increased utilization of psychologists and allied professionals as primary therapists for mental patients even in conservative hospitals, provided they were supervised by members of the medical/psychiatric hierarchy.

It must also be noted that when group and family therapy became established modalities, especially after World War II, psychologists and allied professionals quickly took to these fields and gained experience and expertise ahead of many psychiatrists. Probably not needing mention is the fact that in areas of research in mental health and behavioral science, which mushroomed vigorously after the 1940s, psychologists took strong hold because of their special training and know-how in experimental design and methodology. As of now, clinical psychologists as a group present a formidable political force on behalf of their interests, lobbying effectively at the state and national levels.

Organized psychiatry has resisted this intrusion at every level, despite the fact that it also claims that the need for mental health care and treatment is admittedly far greater than the present crop of psychiatrists can possibly supply. A strong postwar push, it should be noted, to train family practitioners in principles of mental health care and treatment was fostered by the federal government. And some state and federal mental hospitals, bereft of psychiatrists, have depended upon clinical psychologists and other nonmedical professionals to man their operations.

This background is necessary in order to understand the nature and depth of the rivalry between clinical psychologists and psychiatrists that is being acted out in various ways in many of our hospitals. In VA hospitals, psychologists established training programs, introduced group therapy, and carried out many functions when psychiatrists were not available. After World War II, psychologists, social workers, and rehabilitation workers were given considerable status as a way of attracting personnel. The VA has also tried to keep the several allied professional departments strong by giving them representation in the central office.

When the rehabilitation specialists arose in the 1940s and 1950s, their work as therapists and as vocational placement officers had to be wrested largely from the domain of social workers. Some social workers in those days who had gained particular expertise in this area and viewed it as "proper" social work were particularly hard hit by the loss. However, it was not long before rehabilitation therapists gained a firm foothold. Ambitious graduate schools soon evolved specialized training tracks for this group and began to confer specialty degrees.

Pastoral counselors also came forward in the postwar period (again associated with training programs in pastoral counseling offered by schools of theology), with new identified jobs assigned for pastoral counselors to work in institutions for the mentally ill. Inasmuch as the clergy from time immemorial have served as spiritual guides and helpers to troubled members of the flock and their families, it was therefore only natural that they were included in the growing therapeutic team.

More recently, as a result of a large increase in the rights of the mentally ill and a concomitant increase in legislation protecting these rights, a new class of *nurse-counselor* has arisen. These new professionals have the task of representing patients and staff in probable-cause hearings before court officers, who then determine whether patients should be retained in the institution involuntarily for further treatment or released. Where hearing officers and counselors (the latter functioning as representatives of staff) disagree, the issue may then be argued before the court. The patient, if aggrieved, may also have his day in court. Acute facilities that catered to severely ill patients, most of whom are held involuntarily beyond the initial 72-hour period of preliminary assessment, had become so overloaded by probable-cause hearings and court adjudications that it was deemed more efficient to create a new professional category than to require busy physicians to make themselves available at the call of the judicial system.

One possible basis for stress between the professions lies in the struggle for "patient turf," or, more delicately, in the establishment of *boundaries* between the professions in their efforts to help the patient. The patient is divided up: Neuropsychiatric overall assessment and team supervision is in the hands of the psychiatrist; psychological and neuropsychological testing, plus often individual and group therapy, are in the hands of psychologists; day-to-day ward supervision and ward organization are in the hands of the nurse; family relations and family therapy are in the hands of the social worker; work activities are in the hands of the rehabilitation specialist; legal relations are in the hands of the nurse counselor; and spiritual guidance is in the hands of the pastoral counselor. However, all hands are in actuality engaged in what has been called the *therapeutic use of the self*, and in addition they share the single common craft of trying to make the patient well.

In these latter respects, any one of the professionals might be superior to the others. For however much training a person has had, his actual therapeutic effectiveness may override all technical training considerations. Empathy, the capacity to identify with the deepest needs of the patients, warmth and affection, instinctive understanding of dynamics, and the ability to manage transferences often appear to express endowed aspects of the individual rather than learned characteristics. Thus, a primary task of the psychiatrist-leader is to recognize and utilize the particular talents of individual team members (especially in the assignment of the patient's primary therapist) without necessarily bowing to formal training or academic credentials.

When the interdisciplinary team operates, the level of participation of the disciplines is determined by three factors: (a) who is recognized as the leader of the team, (b) who is recognized as the primary therapist for the patient, and (c) how much participation of the various professionals in vital decisions affecting the patient is encouraged by the acknowledged team leader.

Usually, the psychiatrist is the leader of the team. However, often another team member becomes the primary therapist for a given patient and is afforded wide latitude in making decisions. This responsibility may fall to a nurse, a social worker, a psychologist, a rehabilitation worker, or a counselor. Still another member of the team may have an affinity for working with *groups* of patients, or a member of the team may feel especially equipped for a ward management role. However, to be the primary therapist, most important to the patient's welfare, is often the highest aspiration of a team member.

A common source of strife is over the supervision of therapeutic personnel, since this may be carried out by more than one person. An example of struggle over the "soul" of a psychologist is given; from the system's point of view, this is stress resulting from "double subordination."

Case Illustration

Battle between Psychology and Psychiatry

In a VA hospital, an ambitious psychiatrist in charge of a ward is anxious to improve the care of patients by more frequent meetings with therapeutic staff. He also wants it clearly understood that in times of heavy admissions, or when agitated, aggressive, violent or suicidal patients cause a crisis, all personnel should be ready to assist under his general direction. He would like all absences from the ward by any professionals, therefore, to be cleared with him.

"No," says the chief of psychology, who runs his own active program of in-service training and who utilizes his psychologists as trainers of young residents in psychology. The psychologists belong to him, he says. In the past, he has controlled their time by a master schedule that includes their supervision by senior psychologists and their obligations to teach and do research. He is concerned that psychiatry may invade his authority, particularly in recruitment, standard setting, assignment, and performance evaluations.

In some ways, recent history supported the chief psychologist's argument, for the psychiatry service for years had been relatively weak and ineffective. Psychiatric residents had been few and second-class. Psychologists, not psychiatrists, were mainly used as consultants to medicine and surgery. In effect, the psychiatry service had no organized consultation-liaison program at all. Space utilization was mainly at the recommendation of the chief of psychology. In a word, the status of psychiatry in this hospital was at that time well below that of psychology.

This became a cause célèbre. The ward chief almost came to blows with the chief of psychology. The latter called the VA central office chief of psychology for support. Each party independently pressed his case with the hospital chief of staff and with the director. The new chief of psychiatry, it should be noted, was, in a sense, partly responsible for the controversy because he had encouraged the ward psychiatrist to assert himself in the hope of gaining "appropriate" status for the department of psychiatry.

After a long series of stressful meetings, the details of which may be omitted in this discussion, the following guidelines were established:

1. Since the care and treatment of the patient was of central importance, the ward psychiatrist would be the arbiter of all decisions related to the patient's treatment and clinical welfare.
2. Insofar as possible, the schedule for use of the psychologist and that of the psychology service would be modified so that important exercises of the department of psychology would be respected.
3. The chief of psychology would have sway over hiring, evaluation, in-service training, academic functions, standards, and performance. He also would be responsible for administration related to vacation, sick leave, overtime, promotion, and so forth.
4. Any absence from duty of any professional from the ward would be cleared in advance with the ward psychiatrist.
5. As a matter of courtesy, new psychology recruits to a ward would be interviewed by the psychiatric chief of that ward, and new recruits in

psychiatry would be seen by the chief of psychology. Evaluations and recommendations would then be submitted to the appropriate service chief for final appointment.

6. The same general pattern would prevail in social work, nursing, rehabilitation, and so on.

The reader should note a distinctive feature of Veterans Affairs hospitals vis-à-vis hospitals in other jurisdictions. In the VA hospital, the so-called ancillary professions (psychology, social work, etc.) are not as such answerable to the chief of psychiatry, but rather to the chief of staff. In many state and county hospitals, as a rule, ancillary professionals (with the exception of nurses) are answerable to the chief of psychiatry. In the latter instance, turf disputes of the type mentioned above are, understandably, more easily settled.

Aside from the problem of multiple subordination of team members, there are numerous other ways characteristic of the mental hospital scene today in which smooth team operations can be disrupted. Consider the following, taken from real life:

1. The medical director changes a medication dosage or schedule without discussing it with the treating physician or the assigned professional team members.
2. The psychiatrist writes notes to the treating professional without face-to-face discussion, indicating exactly what should be done with the patient—an example of micromanagement, which is usually destructive of enthusiasm and creativity.
3. The treatment team resents the leadership style of the psychiatrist, assembles a dossier of his "errors," and sends it directly to the administrator.
4. One member of the team adopts the attitude that his insights are the correct ones, and that he gets better results with patients than all the others.
5. Residents who become primary therapists with a patient go on to other assignments without recognizing the dangers of abandoning the patient and without making a sensitive effort to realign the patient with another therapist.
6. A team member engages in "wildcat" therapy—that is, takes on patients or even families for treatment without clearance with the team leader.
7. The therapist's report of his therapy with patients is vague, lacks dynamic insights, shows repeated avoidance of conflict areas, is overly directive, and reflects anxiety caused by some of the patient's revelations. His awareness of transference/countertransference identification is superficial. Obviously, the person is not ready to engage in a long-term psychotherapeutic relationship.

There are numerous ways in which aspects of the function of a treatment team can go wrong. On the other hand, when things go right—when the members possess sufficient maturity, flexibility and willingness to learn— membership on the therapeutic team can be one of the great satisfactions of life in a psychiatric hospital.

RECRUITMENT OF MENTAL HEALTH PROFESSIONALS

In recruiting professionals to new vacancies, the aim is to try to get ever better-quality personnel. Recruitment is a technology all its own. To a large extent, administrators recruit administrators, surgeons recruit surgeons, nurses recruit nurses, and so on. One is thus in competition with homologous disciplines in other settings, and the competition may be fierce. Nowhere is this more true than in the competition for scarce nurses.

Various techniques of recruiting include word of mouth and advertising through journals and newsletters that are read by the professional group. Repeated advertisements are more effective than a single display. The cost of advertising is not negligible. Advertisements should be short and pithy, with proper use of white space. A common fallacy is to use too many words. Buzzwords are important—words like "high morale," "teamwork," "advancement," "good for children," "safe," "affordable housing," and "educational advantages." Salary is important, but the chance for a good life is also salient for many who are trying to get away from smog, pollution, congestion on the highways, long commutes, violence, gangs, and so forth. That an area is rated highly by environmentalists as "one of the better places to live" means a lot. In the future, out-migration from our great cities, whose glamour has sputtered because of overcrowding, crime, and drugs, is expected to increase.

Other recruiting devices include payment for travel for the candidate and his spouse or significant other. The candidate should be interviewed by several people and invited to join in selected group activities. In recruiting psychiatric residents, a common technique is to have the candidate talk privately with residents already in the program. When morale is high, this can be powerfully positive, but beware the angry, bitter resident whose dissatisfactions have not been adequately dealt with during the year.

A hospital child development center for use of children of employees can be a huge advantage. This center must be conducted in a professional manner, enhancing the growth and happiness of the youngsters. Employed parents should be welcome to visit their children during the day. Such a program can also be utilized to provide opportunities for students and trainees to learn about child development; this gives it an academic aura pleasing to parents. Availability of medical consultation in the event of sudden injury or illness is a must.

Many places provide educational leave and a stipend for travel at least once a year to enable the employee to keep pace with the advance of his profession. In-house seminars, colloquia, and personal supervision are further emoluments. In the long run, nothing takes the place of a happy environment where the individual is respected and appreciated; this becomes obvious to the candidate who keeps his eyes and ears open.

I have seen many a promising recruitment wrecked by a single detail. One very good person was lost because vacation time during the first year was inadequate; being with his family was very important to him. Another wanted research possibilities and formal "protected" research time, such as is promised in the VA and in universities. A scholarly type turned down a job because library facilities were meager. Another thought expectations were too high, and that he would be uncomfortable. He had a very clear view of his limitations. One man was sensitive to smog. Another found commuting time on the highway too long; he was fed up with traffic. One candidate may like the mountains, another the sea.

The Great Nursing Shortage

The nursing shortage is a phenomenon that has been brewing for a long time, but although discontents have been voiced repeatedly, the critical phase came upon us abruptly and with stunning severity.*[24] Hospitals had been using nurses at an extraordinarily high rate. The opening of new chains of psychiatric hospitals caused a drain on nurses almost everywhere. The Northeast was particularly hard hit, and acute inner-city public hospitals were soon in desperate trouble. New jobs for nurses were created in managed care and in administration. The insurance industry siphoned off a large number.

Many factors conspired to make nursing less attractive. The work was difficult, the responsibilities great and unrelenting and paperwork increasingly burdensome. Salaries fell to levels below that of other comparably trained occupational groups. As austerity reared its ugly head, nurses were asked to carry out duties formerly assigned to lower-level positions (i.e., the duties of practical nurses, aides, and escort personnel). Shorter lengths of stay and more rapid turnover of acute patients led in many cases to burnout. Work environment and advancement opportunities were neglected. Some states gave nurses opportunities to become independent practitioners, licensed to collect insurance payments for their services.

In addition to the above negative features were a drop in enrollment in master's programs in psychiatric mental health nursing, a decline in National

---

*In this section on the nursing shortage we utilize material presented in the panel[23] organized by John A. Talbott, M.D., Editor of *Hospital and Community Psychiatry,* with Linda Aiken, R.N., Ph.D.; Ann Marie Teresa Brooks, D.N.Sc., M.B.A.; Ellen Doerner, R.N.C., B.S.N.; and Eleanor M. White, Ph.D., R.N., at the 40th Institute on Hospital and Community Psychiatry, New Orleans, 1988.

Institute of Mental Health funding for graduate training, and a change in undergraduate curricula such that everyone received education in psychosocial aspects of illness, but specific exposure to psychiatric nursing was minimized. For example, the California examination for nursing licensure now does not include special emphasis on psychiatric nursing.

Thus, nursing lost much of its glamour, and alternative professions often seemed more desirable to prospective nurses. A few more years of schooling and they could become lawyers, or doctors, or Ph.D. psychologists; or they could go into business, running nursing homes or child development programs to relieve working mothers. Many decided that marriage and family were more desirable choices, with the knowledge that whenever the family exchequer was low, they could be readily employed as registry nurses—with incomes exceeding regularly employed nurses, and relative freedom to come and go as they wished.

The administrator's problem is how to deal with such a crisis that not only threatens maintenance of work load and therefore revenue, but restricts expansion of services. To be sure, some nurses want to remain at the bedside and will stay if a ward secretary is provided, or if an aide also works under their direct supervision. Such an aide could support the nurse in much the same way as a physician's assistant supports the physician in charge of the ward. Opportunities for professional development, special educational programs, and career-ladder advancement must be explored. Many are eager to learn more about psychopharmacology, psychodynamics and psychotherapy, and community psychiatry, and nurses are pleased if they can take courses jointly with psychiatric residents. Seminars and colloquia should be open to them both as attendees and as presenters. One will find that nurses' understanding of patients they work with is both intuitive and dynamic, and their presentations often as skilled as the best of the psychiatric residents in training.

Nurses appreciate being involved in governance of their unit and in the selection of their unit chief. They need a feeling of greater autonomy and some control. Above all, they need a feeling that the physician head of the unit and the administrators above him accept them as full partners and value their judgment and opinions. They need an opportunity to rededicate themselves to caring for the sick in the manner that excited their compassion and idealism when they decided on nursing as a career in the first place.

The administrator must explore not only opportunities for advancement but also ways in which non-nursing functions, piled on nurses by unexpected exigencies, may be taken over by others. Some shifts are so overloaded with details of record keeping and administration that one more pair of willing hands becomes the instant cure for aggravation and burnout. Students, either paid or as volunteers, prove to be very helpful in this regard. Those majoring in the humanities—psychology, sociology, or anthropology—find the ward an exciting place. Those majoring in organizational psychology, management, or the like will find the ward a system worthy of study. Night coverage may be a lot easier for an apprehensive female nurse who has a strapping young male student assisting her, particularly if she has to control aggressive, impulsive patients who evoke continuing concerns about safety—hers and that of her patients. We tend to underestimate the hazards nurses and other ward workers face, as well as the long-term effects of such tensions on their ability and willingness to stay on the job.

Upward mobility is very important, not only for relief of the tensions described above, but also to provide the rewards for good work that every conscientious worker desires. Promotion upward to higher clinical administrative or educational responsibilities is one avenue. An interesting option, mentioned earlier, is promotion to the new position of nurse-counselor.

Finally, because salaries have been low and conditions of work have deteriorated progressively, nurses have been forced into collective action. The ultimate weapon is, of course, the strike, usually organized and implemented under the direction of the nurses' union. Where nurses have had the courage to strike, they have usually caught the attention of legislators and the public and have won improvements in salary and working conditions.

The strike is a disaster that weighs heavily upon the administrator, for it challenges his ability to keep services running and tries his conscience. Whereas his sympathies may be with the strikers, his prime responsibility is to maintain services for sick patients. The striking nurses are similarly conflicted. Those nurses who remain on the ward because they are unwilling to leave sick patients become embittered against those on the picket line who have "deserted" the sick.

Important to the administrator is the realization that collective action by organized units within the hospital is a thing of the present; more such events may be expected in the future, as mental hospitals continue to feel the pinch of competition and shortages of vital personnel.

EMOTIONAL PROBLEMS OF WORKERS

Human organizations are the creations of individuals who band together to accomplish work that cannot be achieved effectively alone. In modern society, mechanisms for the satisfaction of the individual worker's needs become important, for since the days of Roethlisberger and McGregor, we have learned that the happiness of individual workers has a causal relationship to overall productivity. To what extent can modern psychiatry and behavioral science help us understand the individual in his organizational context?

A normal individual's potentiality for happiness is enhanced if he is in a milieu that gratifies his needs for safety, belonging, and self-actualization. Unfortunately, many workers are not easy to satisfy, because they bring considerable neurotic baggage to the workplace. A small number have had longstanding emotional disturbances that have impaired their efficiency and effectiveness. As an example, suppose that the secretary of a department head in a government hospital has a deeply held paranoid view that there is "rampant evil" at all levels of the institution. Although her relations with other workers are poor, she manages to stay on, protected from the "evil" system by her ability to work within the written rules. Other workers give her a wide berth, resent her low productivity, and blame management for not finding a way to fire her. In private industry, such a person would be quickly dismissed, but in government circles they have tenure and are difficult to dislodge.

On the other hand, a larger number of people may suffer from neurotic tensions in their outside lives, but have moderate to good success in the work situation. Often they are emotionally deprived persons, depressed, anxious, and sometimes caught in difficult psychosocial tangles. Divorce, lack of family support, children in trouble with the law, and financial distress are familiar. For these people, the opportunity to come to work on a regular basis, to share their troubles with others, to belong to a stable group, and to produce something they are proud of is a blessing. For them, work is therapy. Their transference to the group, or to the organization, may be the sustaining element in their lives.

Many individuals find the hierarchical system of the organization, and the opportunity to rise above others, much to their liking. It fits their need for power and dominance, and their desires—often largely unconscious—to subjugate or control others. Job success may actually deepen such pathological drives and delay a truly realistic perspective of themselves and their effect on the organization.[25]

Quirks and Aberrations of Executives

The supervisory and executive branches of an organization are not immune to personality aberrations. Kernberg[26] approaches this topic along clinical lines. The *schizoid* head of a department conveys the impression that no one is in charge. There may be considerable ambiguity in the delegation of authority, which puts a strain on those staff members who need definitive structure for the performance of their duties.

The *obsessive* leader favors orderliness, precision, clarity, and control, with clear lines of authority and precise job descriptions. Carried too far, an obsessive character may lead to perfectionism and overcontrol of subordinates to the point of sadistic destructiveness. In the *paranoid* leader, the need to control becomes paramount. He projects his hostility onto coworkers and subordinates or manifests his paranoid position by grandiose trends that foist unreasonable expectations for productivity upon the group.

The *narcissistic* leader overevaluates himself, is overdependent upon external admiration, and must be the center of all events. Carried to its worst expression, this leader expects submissiveness from his staff, yet at the same time hungers for love and affection and gives favors to those who admire him the most. He keeps decision making ultimately in his own hands. Underlying this personality constellation is insecurity, shallowness, and an inability to place organizational objectives above narcissistic needs.

The *sexist* leader assumes that women are subordinate to men, that the sexes are endowed with sharply differentiated natural abilities, or that roles and functions are best assigned on a gender basis—thus, doctors should predominantly be men, and nurses should be women. Male nurses are out of place; therefore, there must be something wrong with them. Women doctors are not fit for certain "macho" specialties such as orthopedics, surgery, or urology. Because of changes accompanying the menstrual cycle, such leaders suggest, many women are subject to mood swings that affect their stability and judgment. One physician, when confronted by a sharp difference of opinion from one of his nurses, said that she was probably "at that time of the month," and that maybe he should consult her boyfriend.

Another manifestation of sexism is the assumption that women basically like to be treated as sex objects, and that the way to a good relationship is to compliment them often for their appeal to the male libido. This bias, especially if held by major administrators, may pervade the organization, leading to unfair appointments and promotions and an institutionalized feeling that women are second-class citizens, with attendant morale problems and grievances.

Harry Levinson[27] brings to the study of management an acute psychoanalytic sense of how personality traits, slightly exaggerated, may interfere with a manager's effectiveness. He deals with anxiety and guilt as follows: *Ego anxiety* refers to the threat of overwhelming loss from outside (such as loss of job) or fear of physical disaster. *Id anxiety* refers to threat of being overwhelmed by one's own aggressive or sexual impulses. *Superego anxiety* refers to the fear of not living up to expectations from without (the introjected ego ideals), with subsequent loss of self-esteem. How the superego forms within the mental apparatus determines to a considerable extent how the individual relates to authority, as well as the pattern of expectations the individual imparts to subordinates.

Guilt can be an extraordinarily important factor in management if the leader unconsciously or consciously projects it onto situations requiring sensitive executive judgments.[28,29] Where guilt intrudes into relations with individuals, it is difficult to make decisions most appropriate to the larger group. Many situations may evoke guilt—for example, where there is a misdirected concern about an employee with long service, the manager may not be able to tell that employee about the latter's deteriorating performance. An aging, loyal, lonely spinster secretary, in effect married to her job, who becomes increasingly irritable and discourteous to other employees may cry when her shortcomings are pointed out, making further confrontations impossible due to the manager's guilt. A younger executive advanced to position of authority over older men may feel guilty over vanquishing older competitors, and may be unable to discuss with them their mutual feelings about this issue, or even to ask their advice before making final decisions. A new leader may be unconsciously afraid to be stronger than the man he has replaced; he may turn to a committee in an effort to allay guilt and thus avoid issuing direct orders to his predecessor.

Aggression and anger become problematic when an executive feels undue pressure from subordinates to pursue a line of action he is reluctant to take. He may cave in to their demands and suffer the price of chronic resentment, or become unduly authoritarian and demanding of his own way without adequate "working through" to achieve their acceptance or to arrive at a compromise. Such a situation can lead to impulsive firing, with a subsequent chain of undesirable consequences.

The success or failure of an executive depends on a balance of forces within his nature such that no one trait is so exaggerated or rigidified as to make it difficult to relate to the great variety of personalities within the organization. In addition, he must adapt to changing goals and crises within the organization and to a variety of pressures from outside. That is why it is sometimes difficult to predict, even after the most careful assessment, who will do well in an executive job. And that is why it is difficult to generalize about the qualities needed for executive success, even for those who have demonstrated success in other environments.

Characteristics of Successful Executives*

Given the fact that leadership involves a complexity of talents that must be held within a subtle balance such as to keep the organization and the individuals optimally in tune with each other, do successful leaders have something in common? Yes, says William Henry,[30] based on a study of over 100 business executives in various types of business houses. First, successful executives show high drive and achievement desire; they must always accomplish something in order to be happy. They all have strong mobility drives, a need to move continually upward and to accumulate the rewards of their accomplishments. They view authority as a helpful force, not as a destructive or prohibiting force. They have a high degree of ability to organize unstructured situations and to see the implications of their plans. Decisiveness is a further trait, an ability to come to a conclusion after weighing alternatives.

Successful executives, says Henry, have a firm and well-defined sense of self-identity. Activity and aggression are usefully channeled into struggles for status and prestige. These executives are also strongly oriented to immediate realities. They look to superiors with a feeling of personal attachment, as symbols of their achievement desires; they look on subordinates in a detached and impersonal way, although they are generally sympathetic with many of

---

*See Chapter 52, Administrative Psychiatry, by Milton Greenblatt, in *Comprehensive Textbook of Psychiatry/IV*, edited by Harold I. Kaplan and Benjamin J. Sadock. Baltimore, Williams & Wilkins, 1985, pp 2007–2015; esp. p 2014 Success and Failure in the Role as Administrator.

them. Ties to family of origin are attenuated to the point that they function as "their own man." Ties to the mother are more completely broken than to the father, who is regarded as a helpful but not restraining figure.

The successful executive, in summary, represents values highly regarded by middle-class American society: they are achievement oriented, activistic, self-directed, and independent, and they look for rewards of status, prestige, and property.

Much effort has gone into the task of defining and predicting the successful executive. Common experience tells us that they come in many shapes and sizes, that there are many effective styles of management and many personality types behind these effective styles. However, one problem that has been less studied has to do with the identification and measurement of success in managing systems. Successful management during a period of buildup may be different than during a period of retrenchment. Success in one area of endeavor may be incompatible with success in another. Sometimes budgetary or social/political factors make progress in any direction extremely difficult. And sometimes, particularly in times of severe retrenchment, simply taking a stand on principles of extraordinary importance is more laudable than continuation in office and compromise of professional integrity.

DISCRIMINATION IN THE MENTAL HOSPITAL

With the progressive cutbacks in funds suffered by so many institutions in recent years, even county hospitals try to keep their programs going by favoring those with third-party coverage. This is discrimination on the basis of economics and social status. Discrimination on the basis of color was practiced in Alabama until 1971; before 1971, blacks and whites were unintegrated, each race having its own building. Commissioner Stonewall Stickney managed to integrate the patients during the transition from one governor to another. However, simply by having black and white patients closer together in the same building does not end discrimination; in fact, in some ways it may make it sharper.

Subtle forms of discrimination may be practiced by staff, for some patients are more attractive than others, and some invite rejection and neglect as a result of "bad" behavior. The preferred patient may receive attention and kindness that is denied to the nonpreferred patient. What follows is an example of racism in a mental hospital in the Midwest.

Case Illustration

Racism in a Public Mental Hospital

Dr. S, a female Pakistani, works as a ward psychiatrist in a state mental hospital. Because of her brown skin, she seems to avoid being caught up in the racial biases she observes. She also claims to be objective insofar as her upbringing was essentially devoid of color bias. Dr. S says that racial prejudice on the ward is manifested particularly by the aides, whose education is essentially high school level. Professional staff members—nurses, social workers, psychologists, physicians—may react to the prejudices, but by and large do not activate it themselves.

She notes that whenever black staff members have to deal with white patients, or vice versa, people support their own race and question the motives of the other. This is manifested particularly when a patient of one race has to be secluded on an emergency basis. Blacks appear to resent orders from white more than vice versa. Even lighthearted comments on race differences by whites can be taken seriously by blacks. On the other hand, whites are sensitive to, and resentful of, loud or boisterous behaviors of blacks.

Dr. S describes an instance in which she withheld the ground privileges of a black psychotic woman who was hostile and delusional. The blacks questioned her judgment: Why shouldn't this patient have ground privileges? They interpreted her decision as a manifestation of discrimination against blacks.

Another story is that of a black patient who, on weekend pass, shot and killed two white men in a bar, one of whom worked in the hospital's forensic unit. When the black patient was returned to the hospital, the black aides refused to check him for drugs and weapons, saying they would take his word that he had no contraband on his person. Later, marijuana and other drugs were found in his locker. The white staff expressed great concern that this patient might well have the means and motivation to shoot white workers.

In those wards where the treatment team is all white, racial problems are most severe. When, for example, a white physician enters the nurses' station, the white nurse will frequently stand up and give her seat to the physician. Blacks will not.

Commentary

Prejudice and discrimination have not been studied enough on mental hospital wards, although it is well-known that favoritism toward patients is often demonstrated by staff members. This came out strongly in studies of an all-white ward by Morimoto and others[31] in 1954. If, for example, a patient and staff person shared the same interests and skills, they were likely to get along better than if their interests and skills were different. Further, it appeared that those patients who got the most attention were likely to do better than those that were neglected. In a study of spontaneous groupings among patients on an acute ward, it was found that clique formation among patients could be very strong.[32] In this study, it seemed that the sociodynamics of the ward responded closely to the behavior of a young, attractive sociopathic lady, named Ruth. Patients who were not accepted into Ruth's clique could become very isolated. Overall ward interaction rates fluctuated positively with the interaction rates of the clique, but negatively with the interaction rates of the isolates. When the leading clique member (Ruth) was transferred to another ward, in this case a ward for "better" patients, the other clique members would soon be found on the new ward. In a ward with both black and white patients, Kellam and Chassan[33] found that interaction rates of black and white patients often moved in opposite directions.

Obviously, powerful social dynamics lurk beneath the surface and may be expressed in exaggerated form in a racially mixed ward. If we understood them more fully, we might be able to make more intelligent assignments of patients to rooms where two, three, or four persons must live together. Pierce[34] has called attention to what he calls "microaggressions." These are seemingly small slights and rejections that are not necessarily visible on the surface, but are nevertheless hurtful to those who are sensitive to them. Many well-educated and well-meaning professionals may practice these microaggressions, often quite unconsciously. It takes insight and penetration to uncover them. Stanton and Schwartz[35] in 1954 opened our eyes to the effects of so-called pathological triangles—namely, the deterioration in behavior of patients when two staff persons responsible for their treatment are at odds with each other. Their hostilities may be largely beneath the surface, yet when they are identified, exposed, and worked through, tensions disappear and the patients improve.

The famous social anthropologist Esther Lucile Brown,[36] referring to her observations on the acute wards of state hospitals, sensed an enormous area for social exploration and potential therapeutic interventions in the social biases that patients bring from the outside. Much more research is obviously needed before these social factors can be sensitively employed clinically for the patients' benefit.

ABSENTEEISM

In these days of austerity, every means of controlling costs and increasing productivity must be explored. Absenteeism has long been a problem in all organizations. In health facilities, absenteeism cuts into units of service, forces added work responsibilities upon the colleagues of the absentee, impairs morale, and—to complete the vicious circle—leads to more absenteeism. A steady rise in absenteeism has been reported, despite rigorous efforts to control it.

"The cost of employee absenteeism nationwide has been estimated at $40 billion per year."[37] Today, many hospital beds in the United States are empty, and many hospitals have been forced to close. Particularly in hospitals with marginal financial viability, where there is a great need to provide high quality care and treatment for every patient, absentee staff members are sorely missed.

Employees who call in sick may be suffering from an illness that truly prevents them from working. An employee who contracts acute coryza, even without severe systemic manifestations, and is concerned about exposing others and perhaps causing a small epidemic in the workplace may, therefore, remain at home. Some employees, however, although minimally indisposed or not sick at all, may want to take a day off, charging it to "illness" rather than vacation or other leave time. Such "illness" days are not uncommon on either Fridays or Mondays. In such a case, a suspicion that the employee may be expanding his weekend holidays does come to mind. When such suspicions arise, it is reasonable to ask for confirmation by an outside physician. However, this may not always help: In one instance in our experience, the employee claimed absence due to "migraine" and/or "gastritis"—both diagnoses that depend very much on subjective reports.

Employees may call in sick just before the start of their shift. This is particularly unsettling during a staff shortage, when ward coverage may fall below standards. An emphasis on morale, professionalism, and loyalty to the service and one's colleagues may counteract this nefarious practice.

In an effort to determine the best way to reduce absenteeism, Markowich[38] sampled 1,200 human resource executives to determine which of seven absentee-control programs they were using and to rate these programs' effectiveness in reducing absenteeism. Programs were categorized as to whether they offered rewards for good attendance (personal recognition or bonus), disciplinary control (disciplinary action, year-end review), or a mixed consequence system such as a *paid leave bank*. A paid leave bank combines days off for sickness, vacation, personal time, and legal holidays in a single benefit (with a buy-back option), but the amount of sick time included in the paid leave bank is less than what is traditionally granted. This program aims to eliminate incentives to be sick, and makes the employee responsible for his own leave program. In effect, employees who abuse time for illegitimate illness are forced to dip into either vacation time or personal time allowed for real illness. In this study, the paid leave program offered the most promise of reducing absenteeism and increasing productivity.

SUMMARY AND COMMENTS

Stresses and strains may occur at any level of the organization and among any individuals or groups. It is the task of the administrator, as social system clinician, to anticipate and diagnose these stresses and strains at the earliest moment, and thus to practice prevention and early intervention and to forestall recurrences.

Because of the dramatic shift that has occurred in the balance of power between administrative and clinical divisions, considerable stress occurs at this juncture. Physicians have been edged out of top executive jobs in favor of specially trained nonphysician administrators. Stress between the nonmedical professional manager and the medical chief of staff does occur, and chiefs of service often resent the role or style of nonmedical managers, particularly in decisions involving the allocation of scarce goods and services. Administrators can keep rancor and bitterness at a minimum by frequent meetings with clinical chiefs, inviting participation in difficult decisions before disagreements move to higher authority. Several case illustrations in this chapter emphasized the severity of the discord that can ensue.

Stress between doctors and nurses—two highly interdependent professional groups—arises when boundaries are not clear, when personalities clash, when doctors overemphasize hierarchical differences, when nurses are not respected, and when nurses report treatment orders or practices of doctors that they consider out of line. It should be noted that nurse–doctor relationships have undergone radical changes in recent decades—from the subservience of nurses to doctors to a more equal status relationship where each is regarded as an indispensable specialist in his or her own area.

Interprofessional rivalries may arise when the multidisciplinary team approach is the common mode in treatment of patients. Here the problem centers around the relationship of the team leader, usually the doctor, with another discipline representative on the team who may be the primary therapist for the given patient.

The recruitment of mental health professionals, particularly those in short supply (such as nurses), is a significant source of distress. As the supply of nurses dwindles, it happens that their authority increases—they often determine which wards may stay open and which closed, or they assert their clout through collective actions (sometimes strikes), demanding higher wages, better work conditions, and so forth. Here the administrator must explore causes of disgruntlement, and reasons behind grievances; he must consider work loads, cases of burnout, and opportunities for educational and professional development.

Further internal stresses and strains arise from the emotional problems of workers, as well as the quirks and aberrations of executives. Each worker brings a baggage of needs and wishes to the workplace, often gaining satisfaction from his work but sometimes foisting poorly resolved neurotic character deviations upon the environment. Temperaments of executives that cause distress in the organization have been analyzed under the headings of schizoid, obsessive, narcissistic, and sexist attitudes; mechanisms for handling anxiety, guilt, aggression, and anger have also been studied. This has given further insight into the characteristics of successful versus unsuccessful executives.

Discrimination in the hospital exists in a variety of forms. Some patients are preferred by staff workers, some are not. Differential empathic reactions may play a role in who gets well. Racist biases show up in the ward, sometimes in exaggerated forms, altering delivery of treatment to patients and even affecting safety and security.

Finally, absenteeism is a stress phenomenon in all organizations. Much of it is related to morale and job satisfaction. Absenteeism can be very costly, as it cuts into units of service, revenue, and profit margins. The administrator is at great pains to discover the factors affecting absenteeism and ways to mitigate its negative effects.

REFERENCES

1. Galbraith JK: The Anatomy of Power. Boston, Houghton Mifflin, 1983
2. Orne MT: On the social psychology of the psychological experiment: With particular reference to demand characteristics and their implications. Amer Psychologist 17:776–783, 1962
3. Greenblatt M, York RH, Brown EL: From Custodial to Therapeutic Patient Care in Mental Hospitals: Explorations in Social Treatment. New York, Russell Sage Foundation 1955. See Chapter 5, Resocialization, pp 106–131; also Chapter 6, Patient Government, pp 132–146; also Chapter 7, Development of Therapeutic Potential of Personnel, pp 147–199; and Chapter 21, Social Treatment: Emerging Guideposts to Social Treatment, pp 416–423
4. Jones M: The Therapeutic Community. New York, Basic Books, 1953
5. Jones M: Beyond the Therapeutic Community: Social Learning and Social Psychiatry. New Haven, Yale University Press, 1968
6. Gilbert DC, Levinson DJ: "Custodialism" and "humanism" in mental hospital structure and in staff ideology, in Greenblatt M, Levinson DJ, Williams RH (eds): The Patient and the Mental Hospital: Contributions of Research in the Science of Social Behavior. Glencoe, Illinois, Free Press, 1957, pp 20–35
7. Gilbert DC: Ideologies Concerning Mental Illness: A Sociopsychological Study of Mental Hospital Personnel. Unpublished doctoral dissertation, Radcliffe College, 1954
8. Adorno TW, Frenkel-Brunswik E, Levinson DJ, et al: The Authoritarian Personality. New York, Harper, 1950
9. Bockoven JS: Moral Treatment in Community Mental Health. New York, Springer, 1972, p 127 et seq
10. Roberts L: Group meetings in a therapeutic community, in Denber HCB (ed): Research Conference on Therapeutic Community. Springfield, Illinois, Charles C Thomas, 1960, pp 129–146
11. Hyde RW, Solomon HC: Patient government: A new form of group therapy. Digest of Neurol & Psychiatry 18:207–218, 1950
12. Manasse GO: Patient government: History, structure and ethics. Amer J Social Psychiatry 1:9–16, 1981
13. Gruenberg EM: The social breakdown syndrome and its prevention, in Caplan G (ed): American Handbook of Psychiatry, Vol. 2. New York, Basic Books, 1974, p 697
14. Goldstein MJ: Psychosocial treatment of schizophrenia, in Schultz SC, Tamminga CA (eds): Schizophrenia: Scientific Progress. New York, Oxford University Press, 1989, pp 318–324
15. Miklowitz DJ, Goldstein MJ, Nuechterlein HK, Snyder KS, Mintz J: Family factors and the course of bipolar affective disorder. Archives of General Psychiatry 45:225–231, 1988
16. Whitehead CC, Polsky RH, Crookshank C, et al: Objective and subjective evaluation of psychiatric ward design. Amer J Psychiatry 141:639–644, 1984
17. Fairbanks LA, McGuire MT, Cole SR, et al: The ethological study of four psychiatric wards: Patient, staff and system behaviors. J Psychiatr Res 13:193–209, 1977
18. McGuire MT, Fairbanks LA, Cole SR, et al: The ethological study of four psychiatric wards: Behavior changes associated with new staff and new patients. J Psychiatr Res 13:211–244, 1977
19. American Nurses Association: Code for Nurses with Interpretive Statements. ANA Publication Code G-56 25M9/76. Kansas City, Missouri, American Nurses Association, 1976
20. Stein LI, Watts DT, Howell T: Sounding board—the doctor–nurse game revisited. NE J Med 322:546–549, 1990
21. Stein LI, Watts DT, Howell T: Sounding board—the doctor–nurse game revisited. NE J Med 322:546–549, 1990, p 547
22. Cannon IM: On the Social Frontier of Medicine: Pioneering in Medical Social Service. Cambridge, Harvard University Press, 1952
23. [No byline]: The nursing shortage and psychiatry. Hosp & Community Psychiatry 40:393–396, 1989
24. [No byline]: JCAHO study: NY hospitals with deficiencies exceed the national average. AHA News, 25:3, Issue No. 21, May 22, 1989
25. Lobier D: Irrational behavior in bureaucracy, in Kets de Vries MFR (ed): The Irrational Executive: Psychoanalytic Explorations in Management. New York, International Universities Press, 1984

26. Kernberg O: Regression in organizational leadership, in Kets de Vries MFR (ed): The Irrational Executive: Psychoanalytic Explorations in Management. New York, International Universities Press, 1984
27. Levinson H, Weinbaum L: The impact of organizational leadership, in Kets de Vries MFR (ed): The Irrational Executive: Psychoanalytic Explorations in Management. New York, International Universities Press, 1984
28. Levinson H: Management by guilt, in Kets de Vries MFR (ed): The Irrational Executive: Psychoanalytic Explorations in Management. New York, International Universities Press, 1984, pp 132–152
29. Levinson H: Anger, guilt, and executive action. Think 10–14, March-April 1964
30. Henry WE: The business executive: The psychodynamics of a social role, in Kets de Vries MFR (ed): The Irrational Executive: Psychoanalytic Explorations in Management. New York, International Universities Press, 1984
31. Morimoto FR, Baker TS, Greenblatt M: Similarity of socializing interests as a factor in selection and rejection of psychiatric patients. J Nerv & Ment Dis 120:56–61, 1954
32. Kegeles SS, Hyde RW, Greenblatt M: Sociometric network on an acute psychiatric ward. Group Psychotherapy V:91–110, 1952
33. Kellam SG, Chassan JB: Social context and symptom fluctuation. Psychiatry 25:370–381, 1962
34. Pierce CM: Personal communication
35. Stanton AH, Schwartz MS: The Mental Hospital. New York, Basic Books, 1954
36. Brown EL: Personal communication
37. Markowich MM: How to reduce absenteeism: A comparative analysis. Hosp & Health Services Admin 34:213–227, Summer 1989, p 214
38. Markowich MM: How to reduce absenteeism: A comparative analysis. Hosp & Health Services Admin 34:213–227, Summer 1989

6

Human Resource Management

HUMAN RESOURCE MANAGEMENT*

Wolf[1] has stated it succinctly: Human resource management is more than hiring, firing, record keeping, and picnics. It "designs and implements support systems and structures to maximize the productivity of the employee in a positive work environment." It involves recruitment, selection, orientation, and assignment of the employee, and placement in a fair system with consistent policies and procedures. Opportunities to obtain work-related consultation when needed, and recourse to mediation and grievance systems, should be available. Administration should also be committed to the health and welfare of employees, their protection against risks and hazards, and the further development of their knowledge and skills.

The employee's compensation should be based on fair classification, and repeated evaluation of performance on the job. He should have opportunities to consult with superiors to correct shortcomings or deficiencies, and thus to open up possible future promotional opportunities. Compensation—whether direct, deferred, or bonus type—should consider provisions for salary savings, health protection, and retirement. Management concerns itself also with planning for the proper coordination of jobs and functions in any given unit. The changing business environment calls for feedback loops from marketing surveys to workshop activities. This implies periodic surveys of workers' productivity, continuous team building, in-service training, restructuring of goals, and efforts to sustain and improve morale.

*For much of the section on Human Resource Management, I am indebted to expert knowledge generously shared by Charles J. Canales, Personnel Officer for Los Angeles County–Olive View Medical Center.

With the growth of civil service legislation designed to assure workers security of employment, nondiscrimination, grievance rights, and the right to organize and strike, management–employee relations has become an art as well as a science. For this large responsibility, the concept of human resource management is very apt. Possibly the most important element in human resource management, if we take seriously Theory Z and the Japanese model (see Chapter 2) as well as reports of the most successful American businesses, is the nature and meaning of employee participation in the affairs of the organization.

Employment Interview

The laws are quite clear in this area and should be thoroughly understood. In California, the law strictly prohibits discrimination in hiring, promotions, and working conditions based on race, religious creed, color, national origin, ancestry, physical handicap, medical condition, marital status, sex, or age.[2,3] A biased interview can lead to a complaint of discrimination. Questions regarding birth date or dates of attendance or completion of high school, which might establish a candidate as over age 40, are not permissible. Lawful aliens who are legally eligible to work may not be discriminated against on the basis of citizenship. Questions regarding the applicant's current or past assets, liabilities, or credit rating;[4] organizations to which the applicant belongs; marital status, pregnancy, or child care status all may be considered potentially discriminatory.[5] Even inquiries about arrest records[6,7] or convictions,[8,9] unless they are clearly factors that disqualify an individual for the particular job, may be considered irrelevant.

The courts have identified the concept of "business necessity,"[10,11,12,13] which can be used as justification for discrimination only if the safe and efficient operation of the business is imperiled and no alternative policies with less discriminatory impact can be formulated.

Administration must make reasonable accommodations for its employees in two major areas. The first is religion: The law allows no bias or discrimination on the basis of religious preference. However, one can discuss religion in the workplace provided it does not interfere with work or use space otherwise employed for business purposes. The second is that of physical or mental impairment limiting life activities in orthopedic, speech, or visual areas. Palsy, learning disabilities, AIDS or AIDS-related complex (ARC), tuberculosis, and alcohol recovery likewise may not be cited per se as reasons for not hiring someone. In both of these areas, however, demonstration by the employer of undue hardship may sometimes prevail against the requirement of reasonable accommodation.

Sexual Harassment

Unlawful sexual harassment may take many forms: verbal, visual, or physical; threats and demands; or retaliation for having reported harassment.

The victim may file a grievance or complaint with the Civil Service Commission, or the complainant may receive consultation from the Office of Affirmative Action Compliance (OAAC). The person claiming sexual harassment should tell the harasser that his behavior is unwelcome, keep a log, and write a letter to the harasser with a copy to the supervisor, in addition to informing the supervisor of the problem.[14]

In preventing sexual harassment, management—particularly middle management—should pay attention to the way individuals interact, and should be aware of the impact of what they say or do on other persons' attitudes, performance, and self-esteem. Do not assume that employees probably enjoy sexually oriented jokes or comments, or being touched or stared at; or that they will necessarily tell you when they are offended. Above all, managers must be models of the type of behavior expected of employees. Finally, do not retaliate against anyone who files a complaint of sexual harassment.

Sexual harassment takes two forms: quid pro quo (i.e., sexual favors expected, or demanded, in return for employment or promotion),[15] and hostile environment (i.e., leering, touching, showing offensive pictures, or using offensive language).[16] Sexual harassment may be experienced when the victim is confronted by unsolicited or unwelcome advances. Even if the victim has participated to an extent in the sexual contact, but compliance was not freely given, that action may still be judged harassment.[17]

If potentially offensive behavior is observed, the suspected person should be counseled immediately as to the possible inappropriateness of his behavior, and all offending material should be removed immediately. The incident should then be discussed calmly and objectively with the complainant and referred to the appropriate personnel officer for careful investigation and recommendations for proper disciplinary action. Confidentiality should be maintained throughout.[18]

Discrimination

The federal courts have identified two basic forms of discrimination—namely, disparate treatment and disparate impact.[19] *Disparate treatment* is situational discrimination against a person because of race, sex, religion, or the like. *Disparate impact* involves a seemingly natural employment practice that, in actuality, has a discriminatory impact upon a protected group. In the disparate treatment case, the moving party must first prove a prima facie case of discrimination, then the burden shifts to the employer to articulate some work-related reason for his action; then the burden shifts back to the employee to show that the articulated reason is not the real reason for the action. In the disparate impact case, the moving party must first show that the employer's practice creates a disproportionate action pattern *against a group* of employees or applicants. The figures submitted to bolster the case of disparate impact on groups must have statistical significance. Then the responding party must show a job-related reason for the practice; finally, the moving party must prove that some alternative practice could achieve the same objective without discriminatory impact.

When a suit is filed, the plaintiff usually claims membership in a protected group—often a minority group, although women recently have been added to the list. Recently also, the courts have required not just allegations but measurable documentation of discrimination. It is also important to realize that percentages of minority individuals in any agency, corporation, or hospital need not be the same as percentages in the outside population; the percentages should be related to *what is available in the job market*. For example, if there are only 4 Hispanic psychiatrists out of 100 in the community, then 4% or more Hispanic psychiatrists employed in the agency would presumably be sufficient to counter a charge of disparate impact, regardless of the fact that the percentage of Hispanics in the general population may be much higher.[20]

Human Resource Utilization

After recruiting, selecting, orienting, and placing the individual employee into an appropriate work setting, the many work units in the institution must be coordinated and adapted to the changing demands of the environment. It would be well if the resources of a mental hospital could be adapted to the *needs* of a population; but unfortunately, in recent years that which the hospital is able to offer seems increasingly to deviate from what the population truly needs. Mental hospitals today are holding patients for fewer days, treating more acute illnesses, and using pharmacotherapy more and psychotherapy less. More patients seem to be committed and fewer are voluntary. More suffer from substance abuse; and more patients, especially adolescents, are self-destructive. And as budgets are cut, there are fewer opportunities for long-term follow-up.

The needs of patients were better met when more were admitted voluntarily and treated by carefully selected modalities—including psychotherapy, group therapy, family therapy, social, occupational and educational rehabilitation—in addition to pharmacotherapy. They were afforded day care and night care; assiduous follow-up helped them sustain psychological gains and avoid rehospitalization, achieve a home in the community, and placement in a job.

The needs of populations were also better met when, in some advanced programs, the prevalence and incidence of defined populations were determined by epidemiologic studies, and efforts made to meet needs through hospital outreach, mobilization of paraprofessionals and volunteers in the community, and judicious use of community facilities such as day care, halfway houses, apartment cooperatives, and sheltered workshops.

Under present conditions, however, reality dictates that the human resources of the hospital be organized to meet the daily pressing patterns of *demand*. This requires flexible control of human resources as follows:

1. *Numbers of staff persons in the different units may be changed* upward or downward, and the mix of the various disciplines in the unit modified to fit demands. Several examples come to mind: (a) The emergency room, increasingly overloaded, calls for more doctors and nurses. (b) The CAO (chief administrative officer) imposes a reduction in beds in the hospital, together with a freeze on hiring and a ban on filling vacancies, with exceptions only under extraordinary circumstances. Some employees may be placed on part-time status or let go.

Another example: (c) A new method of obtaining financial credit for service units in an overburdened emergency room makes it possible to hire additional medical caseworkers. Or group therapy in the outpatient unit virtually displaces individual therapy because of the need to reach more patients without an increase in staff.

2. *The tasks of the units may be redesigned.* For example, an acute adult service with 21-day average stay may be whittled down to a 12- to 14-day average simply because insurance is inadequate to cover long-stay patients. A chronically overloaded emergency room may petition referring police officers (whose referrals normally receive first attention) to hold patients back whenever all emergency beds are occupied and a backlog of critically ill patients has developed.

3. *New units may be phased in and old ones phased out.* For example, an adolescent unit may be created to answer desperate community demands that had finally resulted in a specific legislative initiative. A consultation/liaison unit may be created after expert testimony indicates that if it is well run, it may pay for itself; at the same time, the consultation/liaison unit enriches the training program. On the other hand, a day-care program may be phased out altogether when a new cycle of cost containment is set in motion. Or the inauguration of a new obstetrical unit may reveal a whole new clientele of mothers who need specialized psychological help both before and after childbirth.

4. Human resources management for the total complement of workers in a given organization involves *relating fiscal realities to changing community demands*. It includes efforts to avoid labor problems that play upon adversarial relations, entail lengthy and expensive negotiations, and lead to job actions or strikes. Human resource management must also pay attention to new legislation dealing with privacy, discrimination, the handicapped, and sexual harassment.

Administrators should note that legislation in 1985 (the U.S. Consolidated Omnibus Budget Reconsideration Act, or COBRA)[21] mandated that employers offer continuance of medical, dental, vision, and prescription coverage to employees who terminate or who work reduced hours (only employers with less than 20 employees are exempt from COBRA). Legislation in 1986 (the Immigration Reform Act)[22] mandated that the employer verify citizenship of all employees, hiring only authorized aliens (except domestic workers in private homes). Finally, businesses that receive federal funds must have a policy that all workplaces are free from illegal use, possession, or distribution of controlled substances by officers or employees.[23]

EXTERNAL FACTORS: THE PLATEAU PHENOMENON

Two basic functions in human resource management are recruitment and retention of employees. Managers are always searching for people to replace those who quit or retire. They hope that the new recruits will be at least as good as the persons replaced—if possible, better. Otherwise, the organization will obviously suffer a deterioration in the quality of its manpower, and often a concomitant increase in clinical and/or administrative problems—for good employees tend to solve problems, and poor employees tend to create them.

In order to upgrade human resources, it helps if the market for good employees is favorable. It was shown in Chapter 5 ("The Great Nursing Shortage") how a nationwide shortage of nurses crippled the operations of many hospitals.

Administrators are eager to correct any factors that make recruitment and retention difficult. Within the limits of reality, they try to adjust wages and make jobs more attractive. This is easier in private organizations than in large public systems where a wage raise for one category of personnel may require millions of dollars and quickly set off a round of budget-straining demands from other echelons. Administrators can improve conditions of work and cultivate better working relations between different occupational levels. They can offer special inducements such as educational leave, seminars, retreats, and greater involvement in decisions affecting employees' work lives. Without a pool of talent, however, the administrator is heavily handicapped.

Still other negative factors affecting recruitment and retention are quite beyond administrators' control. For example, growing urban congestion, traffic jams, crime, gangs, violence, and drug dealing make the cities undesirable places in which to work and bring up children. Sensitive people may not tolerate the summer smog. In many communities, public schools are below par, and private schools financially out of reach. Inclement weather may drive workers from one place to another.

These factors add to the restlessness that afflicts labor in our country—whereas in Japan, by contrast, workers are often tied to a particular industry for life. The tradition of movement, and the search for promotion, is very strong here. In America, an individual works and studies, acquires a particular set of skills, and then seeks to sell those skills to the highest bidder. In Japan, manager–worker relationships are more paternalistic, workers are more loyal to their companies, labor is not so strong, and personnel turnover rates are therefore not nearly as high as in the United States (see "William G. Ouchi: Theory Z" in Chapter 2).

In the past, promotions in industry were more common than they are today. In a penetrating paper, Bardwick[24] calls attention to a phenomenon she has identified as *plateauing*—the decrease, especially in the last few decades, in the number of opportunities to move upward in an organization. From 1950 to 1975, it is noted, when corporations increased by 56%, the nation experienced the most phenomenal period of economic expansion in its history. At that time, finding trained people to fill slots, particularly in middle management, was very difficult. However, when the expansion slowed and the demand for educated, qualified people correspondingly declined, many employees reached a plateau in their careers. Upward mobility became difficult or impossible, and many became frustrated, disappointed, and bored. For those whose commitment to work and organizational advancement had been very great, the later years of their careers were particularly hard. This general trend, says Bardwick, was greatly aggravated by the recession of 1982, which increased world competition and forced many organizations to trim the ranks of their employees, particularly in middle management.

In mental health, developments have been parallel. The heyday of building and staffing community mental health centers at government expense is over. The bonanza of profits from privatization of mental health services has turned into increasingly intense competition and narrower profit margins. For some time, a general climate of sharply reduced federal and state expenditures for mental health has prevailed. Today, austerity is the national mood. The following brief example is typical of the frustrations of one faithful psychiatrist.

Case Illustration

Unrewarded, He Leaves

Dr. O has reached middle age without advancement in a government hospital. Twice he was passed over for the position of clinical director, although he had served at a lower position satisfactorily for 15 years. Regarded as a fine clinician and teacher, he unfortunately was not selected for executive responsibility. Further, in this particular institution, the number of leadership jobs had recently been cut down. Disappointed, Dr. O decided to go into private practice, where he found opportunities for income enhancement, and yet was retained on faculty because of his rare teaching abilities. The plateau phenomenon in this case contributed largely to his career change.

MIDDLE MANAGEMENT*

Between top-level administration and the clinicians who work directly with patients are the middle managers. Middle managers increase in numbers and importance as organizations grow larger and more complex. Although

*Information for this section is drawn in part from John F. Talbot, Middle Managers in Mental Health: A Study of Management Tasks.[25]

this group is the vital intermediary in any organization between planning and policy (on the one hand) and the final "marketable product" (on the other), the boundaries of middle management are often ambiguous. Differential perception of the tasks of middle management can lead to misunderstandings, stress, and inefficiency.

One can look at middle management as embracing three levels of functioning. *Upper* middle managers include those close to top managers, who are consulted in many policy and planning questions and whose realm of supervision embraces several departments or divisions. *Lower* middle managers include those personnel close to the level of direct care and who, in fact, may now and again be drawn into direct care, as during shortages of primary caregivers. *Middle* middle managers are those who supervise units of direct caregivers.

An example: In one hospital, the psychology group is so small that the chief of psychology spends much of his time working with patients. However, he also arranges schedules, recruits staff, supervises their work, handles personnel problems, and attends departmentwide planning meetings. In the same hospital, the social work service is much larger; here the chief does no line work at all, but supervises all his social workers, attends to administrative details, and serves on planning committees.

The director of clinical operations, a psychiatrist, makes regular rounds on all inpatient, outpatient, and emergency services, outlines work schedules for all psychiatrists, adjudicates interstaff problems, consults on all problem patients, and arranges for adequate night coverage on all wards. He also confers daily with the overall head of the department and helps him with goal formulation, as well as with planning and implementation of those goals.

In this view, the chief psychologist is a part-time lower middle manager, but also a frontline service worker; the chief social worker is middle middle management; and the director of clinical operations is upper middle management as well as chief consultant to upper management.

Where do middle managers come from? Mainly from direct clinical care ranks, although some, to be sure, come through transfer from middle management elsewhere. Ewalt[26] calls attention to the shift in concepts and values of those who traverse this pathway. Since this can be a difficult road, the individual may need help in transition to his new role.

Since middle managers are dependent for their success on acceptance and support from top management as well as from staff clinicians, differing expectations of performance from these groups may create problems. Middle managers actually must interact with several constituencies: supervisors, subordinates, peers, and outside groups. Because of the rapidly changing environment and sharper competition, and the strategic position of middle management in the organization, the tasks of middle management are changing. Marketing, program development and evaluation, quality assurance, utilization review, and public relations are receiving greater emphasis.

Feldman[27] expatiates on the psychological problems of middle management arising from the fact that professionalism per se breeds ideology that in some respects is counter to good management, to wit: (a) a great need for autonomy, and thus an antagonism to rules, regulations, and demands for conformity; (b) an inflated self-image and sense of entitlement arising from long years of study and sacrifice together with the ego gratification from patients who see them as wonderful and all-powerful; and (c) divided organizational loyalties, with strong ties to professional values and standards often at variance with organizational values and standards. Middle managers find that their desire to be in good rapport with the clinical staffs from whose ranks they have just emerged may conflict with their new mandate to supervise and evaluate their colleagues' work. This in turn conflicts with the need to be liked, and evokes feelings of personal loss of intimate relationships they had enjoyed with clinical colleagues. Rather new and different is the necessity to rely on other people rather than oneself to carry out necessary tasks. And previously alien values like efficiency, budgets, costs, rules, orders, and performance are now demanding of interest and cathexis.

In Talbot's[28] study, middle managers were found to have received significantly less training than upper managers. The principal tasks for which middle managers felt the most need for training were hiring, training of subordinates, running meetings, monitoring daily work flow, and organizing record-keeping systems. Formal management training or a degree in management made them feel more competent, particularly if it emphasized marketing, use of computers, and budgeting.

How should middle management personnel be trained? It is suggested that training should be performed in-house as far as possible, be tailored to meet the unique characteristics of the group, and include both didactic exercises and case studies. It should deal with the personal problems related to role shifts, the formation of new loyalties, and the handling of conflicts resulting from the new posture toward former colleagues. Feldman also suggests that training should include a period in the hospital as a pseudopatient. This would tend to immunize the manager from the numbing effects of distance from the client's world, yet foster identification with the larger, impersonal system.

END RUNS AND REVERSE END RUNS*

At this point, let us shift our thinking to several recurring phenomena that may have negative effects on human systems. Space permits highlighting only a few—namely, end runs, closed and broken dyads, multiple subordination, and hidden beliefs and practices. End runs are considered first and in some detail because of their high prevalence in many systems, their ubiquitous threat, and their potentially damaging effects.

An individual who attempts to influence higher authority without going

*This section, with few changes, taken from my paper, " 'End Runs' and 'Reverse End Runs': A Note on Organizational Dynamics," *American Journal of Social Psychiatry, 6,* 114–119, 1986. Reprinted with permission.[29]

through the chain of command is said to be performing an "end run." (The analogy is probably borrowed from football, where end runs accomplished around the defensive line may yield highly prized yardage.) In organizations where work and responsibilities are divided, and a defined chain of command exists, the end run is often regarded as undesirable and disruptive. *Although it is one of the most frequent and recurring events in any management system, its manifestations have not been fully described.*

The background in which the end run occurs is all-important. In military systems, hierarchy is clearly defined, and communications are written or verbal commands. Communications downward are often far more important than communications upward. A "tight organization" prevails (to use Kotin and Sharaf's phrase).[30,31] The decision makers do not regularly share their thinking with the person in the front line; they justify themselves primarily to their superiors. Power is concentrated at the top; the structure is autocratic and pyramidal. In such a system, an end run is frowned upon, may be bitterly resented, and may even lead to punitive measures.

In contrast, consider a typical academic or university system. Chains of command exist, but the ambience is loose, informal—more open and less punitive. Communications upward are encouraged. In a university almost everyone, instructors included, is in some sense a student. An open mind and a climate conducive to free thinking, argument, persuasion, and even dissent are encouraged. Since ideas, concepts, and creative activity may arise at any level, intellectual doors are open. And since hierarchy, authority, and control are underemphasized in the academic atmosphere of informality, an end run is not so often viewed as disruptive. It is accepted as part of an open communication system that is basic to the free exchange of ideas.

The significance of the end run, therefore, depends to a large extent on the nature of the organization. What is regarded as pathological in one system may be regarded as benign in another. In terms of organizational perception and reaction, only end runs experienced as disruptive to the goals of the organization or the accepted way of doing things may be classified as pathological.

What are the major parameters involved in an end run, and how do end runs turn out to be pathological for a given system? There are many facets worth considering.

1. First, the concepts and/or motivations of the "runner" are important. He may be ignorant or uninformed as to how the system works, or have little respect for his superior(s). He may seek personal (sometimes departmental or even organizational) gains through attempts to alter and/or manipulate the system. He may possess—or fancy he possesses—a special relationship with a person at an upper level that justifies his actions, or he may believe that the superior officer he runs to will welcome his communication. He may be unaware of the effect of his end run on the organization, or he may be counting on a reaction within the organization that will enhance his plans.

A common reason for the end run is personal aggrandizement. American society puts a great premium on bettering oneself. From childhood, upward mobility is stressed; and a hierarchical system provides a ladder to climb. Big business tries to swallow up its competition. Aggressive, imaginative executives able to outwit competitors, enlarge markets, and make profits are in demand.

The runner who wants to climb the ladder quickly is hyperalert to opportunities to gain favor with high-level decision makers. Especially if endowed with energy, ambition, and talent, he may see himself as a very valuable person with more to offer the company than other workers at his level, and maybe more than his immediate boss. Perhaps his tactics have already succeeded in getting him a promotion. A common belief is that if one masters the game, one's star can rise meteorically. In Budd Schulberg's novel *What Makes Sammy Run?*,[32] Sammy, the quintessential end runner, was a for a long time successful at this game.

However, we must not overlook the possibility that the end run, even if regarded as disruptive, may have mitigating or even healthy components. At least from the standpoint of the runner, it may seem necessary and justified. Sometimes the immediate superior is too controlling, too bureaucratic, lacking in flexibility, or lacking in appreciation of the runner's abilities, needs, and drives. The superior may be experienced as oppressive, as standing in the way of the subordinate's healthy growth and advancement. Or the system itself may be experienced as sticky, unyielding, and insensitive to special talents. Under these conditions, the individual becomes restless, impatient of restraints and delays. His choices appear to be either to mark time and show that he is a person of great value or to open up communication to the higher command by means of an end run. (He can also, of course, resign from the company, seeking recognition and reward elsewhere.)

2. The bypassed officer's reaction to the end run will depend largely on the importance he attaches to line authority and to keeping information within proper channels. He may see the end run as a relatively benign act of a person inexperienced in institutional procedures, or he may see it as an attack upon his competence, judgment, and efficiency. He will be anxious to hear his superior's views on the matter. If, however, he only hears about it from the runner himself, or from other workers in the system, his fantasies may run riot. The possibilities of demoralization then are great.

If the bypassed executive has a close, secure, and trusting relationship with *his* superior officer, the end run bothers him little or not at all. His superior officer will soon convey to him its contents, and quickly it will be decided what is to be done about it. How different if that relationship is distant or strained, or if his superior officer is new to the system and has not yet decided whom to trust. How different also if the bypassed person, too, is new to the system and does not know how much confidence his boss has in him.

If the bypassed officer has a strong sense that organizational functioning should follow structural lines, he will resent the end run. If this view is consonant with that of his boss, he is safe; but if his views on the sanctity of channels are discordant with those of his boss, the end runner might achieve more compatibility with higher authority than is desirable from the officer's standpoint. It is not inconceivable that the superior may be tolerant of end runs and, under certain conditions, may even welcome them.

Most people in responsible positions have pride in the way they are doing their jobs, and satisfaction in the orderly control of their sphere of responsibility. The end run can disturb peace and harmony. The distressed (i.e., bypassed) executive says to himself, "Perhaps I am remiss in not keeping my subordinates happy; perhaps he is troubling my busy superior with trivial business when I should be keeping him in line; perhaps he is undermining my superior's confidence in me and my work."

The bypassed executive is the man in the middle—for the moment impotent, angry with the runner and uneasy about his own standing with his chief. If all is done behind his back, he may be deeply grieved when he hears about it. If it is done openly—that is, the subordinate says he is going to go over the executive's head with some potentially hurtful news—he can at least prepare a rebuttal, or check the potential damage by a swift outflanking maneuver to his superior.

This situation can cause much pain and suffering, for nothing is more disturbing than the feeling that there is an enemy at large. Even a little malevolence loose in a peaceful organization can contaminate the atmosphere, destroy peace of mind, and impair efficiency.

3. The superior officer, the target of the end run, is in many respects the controlling element in this drama. Unlike the bypassed person, his role is not threatened. Calmly, he can examine the issues; it is an opportunity for the exercise of his wisdom.

Much depends on his feelings about his employees, his confidence in his assistants, and his attitude about system structure and function. If he is the "open door" type, encouraging any employee to come to him, he may view the end run as an opportunity to learn about his staff and to help them with their problems. There are many advantages to an open-door policy. It makes the staff feel that the boss is available, interested, and willing to listen. It reduces the feeling of oppressive structure and hierarchy. Some individuals, knowing the door is open and that help is at hand, may show more initiative in solving problems by themselves. Or, considerate of the boss's time, some may be more selective of the problems they bring to him for advice and counsel. Others test out the policy of the open door to see if it is an actuality, and upon finding that the boss is indeed willing to discuss even those matters they feared were trivial, they are reassured and comforted by the opportunity to communicate. They retire to their desks with morale heightened. The wise superior, knowing that the problem presented to him is often an opening wedge to deeper matters, realizes that an employee down the line has much to teach him about morale, work, and productivity, and that a little time spent forming a good personal relationship can pay heavy dividends in the long run.

But many people with high-level authority and responsibility are very busy; they handle their business through secretarial gatekeepers and tend to protect themselves by the "closed door." They need privacy, or they feel that communications shared with anyone in their office demand great discretion—that if any part of their business is overheard, the information may be misused.

The officer with the open-door policy may welcome a visit from the worker. The officer who favors a closed-door policy is often the one who instructs his secretary to direct lower-level "operatives" back to their supervisors, who in turn will make whatever report is necessary. In this case, the end run is nipped in the bud essentially before it happens, whereas in the former case, the executive himself contributes to the end run: He has accepted the problem into his own hands.

It is not difficult to visualize conditions in which the end run is viewed as at least the partial solution to the problems of an administrator entering a new system.

> When a new administrator of a large organization takes over, he is usually given a structure with inherited department heads and their subordinates, some of whom may not favor either his plans or his methods of achieving change. He must decide how much to recognize their authority in all matters pertaining to subordinates or how much to permit direct communication between lower-level staff and his office. It is a double-edged sword. On the one hand, if he allows all communication to be screened first through the department head, it may be difficult to know what is going on below that executive's level. On the other hand, if he permits subordinates to communicate directly with him, the effect on the department may be devastating. This is especially true when a top lieutenant has had the full confidence and trust of previous administrators.[33]

A new administrator, who may come from outside and not from the ranks of the institution he now heads, who feels a need to learn as quickly as possible what is going on at lower levels, or who has reason to suspect that all is not well (or even that there is a cover-up) may not only allow but encourage access to the front office. Communication between himself and other levels may be viewed as a means of quick transmission of information with a minimum of red tape. This active opening of doors—which may, in fact, take the form of initiating direct contact with underlings, bypassing some executives—constitutes a "reverse end run."

Recently, violation of hierarchical barriers has been given a certain legitimacy, especially as a result of the distrust of political leaders since the Watergate scandal. In 1978, the federal government passed a law protecting so-called whistle-blowers.[34] The law recognizes that in a complex social system, power becomes concentrated at the top; hence, it is a right of good citizens to watchdog the powerful ones entrusted with huge resources and with final decision making. Thus, a top administrator, responding to the public's interest in morality and efficiency, may resort more often to the reverse end run. He gambles that any ill effects from bypassing some of his executives will be more than offset by reducing the threat of whistle-blowing and subsequent investigations resulting therefrom.

Apart from the effect of end runs or reverse end runs on the morale of a bypassed person, two special problems may be identified. Employees, always fascinated by the ebb and flow of power, may surmise that the department head in question has suffered a fall in his superior's esteem, that his authority has been weakened, and so they may treat him with less respect. Indeed, if end runs have been tolerated or welcomed by his superior, this *does* diminish his authority, and he may find it more difficult to do his job. Word spreads fast that he may be on the skids, and that one shouldn't hitch one's wagon to a falling star. In such an event, unless the superior officer takes quick and effective action to restore morale, not only will he have a spreading problem on his hands, but also the morale problems of that department will ultimately affect organizational goals.

A final problem may be even more distressing. If the department head feels both vulnerable and betrayed, he may fight back by undermining his superior. He may feel he has been undermined by end runs that his superior has tolerated without sufficient consultation with him. As a result, he may fail to report upward, withhold vital information, or embarrass his superior by distorting messages. Or he may fail to fulfill his decision-making responsibilities, passing it on to higher levels, as if to say, "If they don't trust me, let them do the job themselves."

Variations

An imaginative runner may use other tactics than those described above, often with unhappy consequences.

1. He may commit the sin of outright mendacity. In this variation, he may obtain the approval of his superior to go to higher authority with some problem, but once there he may deliver a diabolical message—namely, he denigrates the supervisor he has bypassed, perhaps even distorting facts and inventing stories. Once unmasked, this employee should have a short life in the organization.

2. The runner may recruit another person to his cause. That person may be someone really high up (for example, a member of the board of directors) who may, indeed, be able to exert considerable influence on administration. The bypassed supervisor may then be powerless to assert himself—unless in a showdown, he, too, has powerful friends in high places. The top administrator may now find it difficult to act in accord with his best judgment, or to protect a blameless department head.

3. The runner may have influence outside the organization—possibly a politician or bureaucrat who, in part, determines the destiny of the institution. In governmental institutions, a mayor, a governor, or the chairman of the legislative ways and means committee can exert decisive pressure. Consider, for example, what can happen if the superintendent of a hospital in a

given state is related to the governor by marriage and chooses to undermine his commissioner of mental health (who, as luck would have it, is not appointed by that governor). This can lead to a collision course with dire consequences for the tenure of the commissioner, the management of the system, and the recruitment of new talent to the enterprise.

Dynamics

Why are some people given to making end runs and others not? Is the motivation to make end runs based on unconscious or conscious mechanisms? In the case of end runners, three conflict areas may be considered: (a) unresolved narcissistic drives, (b) problems with authority, and (c) problems related to sibling rivalry.

The child's original *narcissism*, with its demands for instant gratification, omnipotence, and a need to be central, is gradually attenuated by reality and by the teachings of his parents. He learns to respect others, to share, to cooperate, and to check aggressivity. But basic narcissism may be too strong, the curbing of impulses may be too weak, and restraint may require too much effort. The mother who instills in her child that he is superior, will dominate others, and must overcome all opposition may be preparing the child for end runs in his later years.

The *conflict with authority* has many roots. One is the inability to accept harsh repression of instinctive drives. The parent who brutally crushes narcissistic needs may evoke so much anger in the youngster that he constantly battles authority in order to rectify earlier humiliations and defeats. Another is ambivalent identification with authority as a consequence of inadequate love or conditional approval from parents. A third dynamic arises from the fact that our social and political systems are viewed by millions as uncaring, oppressive, and unfair; this is particularly true for the poor, the underserved, and the chronically emotionally deprived.

Sibling rivalry activates narcissistic wounds when an individual is forced to share his treasured, but inadequate, affectional supplies with another. A newcomer into the family takes one's parents away, and never again does one have the security of their undivided attention and affection. If the competitor is viewed as more handsome, intelligent, or lovable, the sibling who is relegated to second fiddle abhors this position the rest of his life. The urge to overcome the narcissistic wound, if necessary by stepping on the bodies of rivals, may become irresistible and thus an end runner is born.

Still another dynamic may operate. If authority figures—parents or other important adults—were constantly at odds with one another, quarreling, and forcing the child to choose among them, or if they used the child in a game of vengeance, the child may develop the countertactic of playing one against the other for his own purposes—still another breeding ground for the development of a future system manipulator.

Thus, some of the energy leading to repetitive and destructive end running may arise from deeper dynamic conflicts that are not readily available to consciousness without special assistance.

Treatment

Many end runs that are benign or based on ignorance may be automatically corrected by the workings of the system. The end runner soon learns that what he has done is "not done around here," and he quickly suppresses that behavior. When end runs are repetitive and do create significant disturbances in the system, what is to be done then? The following guidelines are suggested:

I. The two upper-level managers meet as soon as possible and make sure that they agree on the facts in the case, as some runners are especially talented in dividing "parental figures" through confused messages.

II. The managers evaluate carefully whether or not this person is worth cultivating as a continuing member of the organization.

III. The immediate supervisor (the bypassed officer) then meets in closed session with the runner and counsels him to the effect that:

A. The end run has been found unacceptable and should be abandoned as soon as possible.

B. The top officer (the target of the end run) has been consulted and is in total agreement.

C. The end-run type of behavior is hurtful to the employee's chances of growth in the company.

D. If the immediate superior (the interviewer) is seen as indifferent to the needs of the runner—inaccessible or hostile—it would be good to discuss this in detail in order to increase mutual respect and understanding and harmony in working together.

E. The runner is wanted in the company and has a good future, if these kinds of disruptive behavior can be moderated.

F. The meeting will be kept confidential.

Note that the superior (bypassed) officer, although inviting a frank discussion of the incident(s) and perhaps suggesting that the employee seek counsel, does not play therapist even if equipped to do so by training and expertise. That is left to another counselor, provided that the runner elects to ask for help.

CLOSED DYADS AND BROKEN DYADS

Two recurring phenomena with negative impact on a system are closed dyads and broken dyads. Classically, a *closed* dyad occurs when two members of staff, by conscious or unconscious agreement, limit their important communications to each other, neglecting the community in which they work. They may slip into this situation gradually, seeking mutual support and reinforcement for attitudes that they regard as alien to the general culture or that, if generally known, might be detrimental to their standing in the organization. For example, suppose two workers share a strong feeling of dislike for their superior. They keep this secret but seek in every way, openly or by innuendo, to slow down his program, embarrass him personally, and hasten his departure. This is a form of sabotage found in every organization. If it involves persons with important responsibilities for the functioning of the system, it can cripple the effectiveness of management and lead to its downfall. If it spreads to more and more people, it may signal a palace revolt. It may do more harm when covert than if it came to open expression. The following is another example of this phenomenon.

Case Illustration

Husband and Wife Team Is above It All

Two psychologists (who happen to be husband and wife) adopt a superior and critical attitude toward almost everything that is going on. Reports to the ward doctor on their group therapy with patients are an exercise in withholding, as if to say, "Who is he to question us?" They are disdainful of physician efforts to get started in research. Nothing seems to meet their rigid criteria for methodology and statistical refinement. (Indeed, their training in design, methodology, and statistical analysis *is* superior to that of the psychiatrist.) They are particularly hard on psychiatric residents struggling to learn the art of applying appropriate research methods to clinical problems of everyday life. These two "superintellectuals" could be extremely helpful if they could simply stop their cozy tête-à-têtes and open up to their coworkers.

A variation on the theme occurs when a ward staff member forms a closed dyad with a patient. Together they form a twosome against the world.

Case Illustration

A Private Affair

An alliance formed between a young nurse and a handsome depressed lad with psychopathic tendencies. They seduced each other into a closed dyad with strong romantic overtones. Individual and group therapy attempted by ward personnel with the patient was filtered and reinterpreted by the nurse. She even winked when alcohol was smuggled in by his cronies. It was some time before ward management caught on to the spirit of the thing. The nurse was called on the carpet and exposed for highly unethical behavior. The patient, seeing the game was up, began to cooperate more willingly in therapy and soon left the hospital much improved. It is unknown what happened to this dyad after the patient's discharge; however, the nurse stayed on, considerably humbled.

The example above brings out that romantic attachments between employees and patients can and do exist and may influence treatment outcome. Decades before the birth of the liberal, egalitarian philosophy of ward life, nurses and attendants were often forbidden to form close alliances, let alone romantic attachments. At one time, a nurse reported as dating a recently discharged patient could have been dismissed summarily.

It is perhaps relevant to note in this context that in Maxwell Jones's therapeutic community, only group therapy was practiced. One-to-one therapeutic dyads were dismissed as too costly; also, it was felt that it might be better if "confidential information" were shared with the whole ward. His model was utilized in many hospitals after World War II, and played a prominent role in the deemphasis of authoritarianism, hierarchy, and control that typified that era.

Case Illustration

A Secret Conspiracy

Another dyad consisted of the secretary of the service chief of Hospital A, and the director of psychiatric training of the combined program involving both Hospital A and Hospital B. The secretary and the training director are friends. He tells her a great deal about Hospital B's attitude and plans for the integrated program, some of which could be of importance to her boss (but is kept secret from him). When the existence of the secretive aspect of this dyad becomes known to Hospital A, the secretary is left with the choice of (a) going underground or resigning, or (b) telling the training director and her boss that all "secret" communications to her related to the joint program would in the future be conveyed to her chief because it was her professional obligation as his employee.

The *broken* dyad is essentially the converse of the closed dyad. In the broken dyad, communication between two individuals in a system who are estranged from each other is sharply diminished or broken off altogether. Not infrequently, this involves individuals who are important to two different programs of an institution; for example, a service chief thinks the assistant administrator is a "horse's ass" and will have nothing to do with him. Open factional strife under such circumstances cannot be far from the surface.

Case Illustration

"We Are Not on Speaking Terms"

An executive secretary of the chief of staff, when asked to deliver a letter to the secretary of the chief of psychiatry, remarked, "I am sorry, could you get someone else to do it? We are not on speaking terms." This extraordinary statement suddenly gave the chief of staff a glimpse into possible hidden system pathology, which he undertook to correct immediately. He imagined what might happen in a time of crisis—as in an earthquake, fire, or bombing—if information flow depended on adolescent grudges between important staff members.

These examples of system pathology, as the reader will note, are reciprocally related. When a dyad is closed, communication outward is reduced. When a dyad is broken, communication between involved parties may be minimal, hostile, or suppressed. In either case, the desirable open and easy exchange of information that leads to good morale and effective functioning is seriously impaired.

MULTIPLE SUBORDINATION

Difficulties may ensue as a result of multiple subordinations; in this, an individual who is beholden to more than one department head takes advantage of his position by playing one manager against the other. Whatever work he owes one department but would like to avoid, he neglects on the basis that the other department demands his time. If his obligations are to two bosses, each at different levels of the organization, the one at the lower level is more likely to get short changed.

In a previous example (see Chapter 5), I described how a serious problem developed between psychiatry and psychology when the role of a ward psychologist, subordinated to the chief psychologist on the one hand and to the ward psychiatrist on the other, became the battleground in a heated struggle. That struggle highlighted two key questions: (a) What comes first, the care and treatment of the patient, or the education and training of the psychologist? (b) Can a psychologist serve two masters at one time—the chief of psychiatry and chief of psychology?

In that example, the chief of staff, in vigorous discussions with the chiefs of psychology and psychiatry, declared that the care of patients was the higher priority, and that on the ward, the psychologist would be subordinated to the psychiatrist. Yet, the psychologist could still remain under the wing of the department of psychology in matters of training, education, teaching, discipline, and other administrative relationships. This understanding led to a reduction of the problem and eventual peace and harmony between the two departments.

Multiple subordination may apply as well to persons in other disciplines—nursing, social work, rehabilitation, pastoral counseling, and so forth. Sometimes, a third element is added, namely, loyalty to an outside professional society that sets standards for patient care, ethical conduct, work, salary levels, and the like. Such societies dedicated to the welfare and advancement of their professions not infrequently pursue their interests through labor union conferences, negotiations, and contracts. The nursing profession has developed strong unions that negotiate periodically with management. In some states, new bargaining units fronting for professional or nonprofessional interests may be formed if at any time a sufficient number of employees prove that they have a common interest. These new bargaining units then claim the full loyalty of their members in any controversial issues involving management.

Multiple Subordination in Medical School Affiliations

When a hospital is affiliated with a medical school, a special form of multiple subordination appears. Many of the physicians in an affiliated hospital may enjoy coveted appointments on the faculty of the medical school. Indeed, in such affiliations, appointees may receive two salaries—one from the affiliated institution and one from the medical school. Individuals with academic stature appointed to high posts in the affiliating institutions further the university's program by contributing to research and teaching. They also help improve the quality of patient care in the affiliate and attract more competent professionals to their staffs. Complications can arise, however, when the physicians' loyalties become divided between the hospital, with its clinical mission, and the medical school with its special focus on education and research.

Case Illustration

Loyalty to Two Institutions

Hospital X is a county institution with a very heavy caseload. Staff is overworked and coverage is thin. The budget is tight; indeed, it has been cut repeatedly in recent years. Staff, therefore, suffers under the dual hardships of underfunding and the need to produce added revenue through more units of work. Nevertheless, hospital administration and medical school authorities do value their mutual agreements that grant the affiliated status to the hospital in exchange for space, use of clinical material, and support of training and research programs. The hospital acknowledges that in the long run its affiliated status helps it recruit more competent people and develop a better public image than nonaffiliated institutions. Benefits to patient care and treatment are almost always substantial.

The collaboration of a hospital and a medical school ought to be, and usually is, mutually enhancing. However, particularly in times of austerity, hospital authorities (in their drive to balance the budget) freeze or delay hiring, and when fiscal realities are really bad, employees are let go. Expenditures for services and equipment are carefully monitored. Telephone usage is restricted, travel curtailed, and consultant budgets severely pared.

To beef up revenues, management renews efforts to admit more patients, particularly patients who can pay. Third parties are scrutinized for every bit of reimbursement possible. New services with a potential for added income are introduced. At these stressful times, the professional staff works harder, and those faculty members striving to promote research find themselves enmeshed more and more in routine clinical services.

Caught in the dilemma of rising costs amid diminishing resources, hospital management pushes both faculty and trainees more and more into revenue-producing activities. Faculty reluctantly cuts down on teaching and research, while house officers resist treating more patients under conditions of diminished supervision and fewer didactic sessions. Sooner or later, the hospital may earn a reputation for using house officers as "slave labor." Applications drop, and the quality of applicants falls. The next step consists of anxious meetings between medical school deans, on the one hand, and hospital administrators and service chiefs on the other. Issues mainly concern (a) scrounging for new resources, and (b) faculty tolerance of deteriorating quality of education and patient care.

In summary, the one man–one boss concept disappeared a long time ago, leaving professionals with multiple loyalties and subordinations. The administrator must realize that there may be multiple tugs on his most talented professional employees. He feels also that new expectations have entered his life, flowing from the priorities and values of the medical school. As service chief appointments are made with the advice and counsel of the medical school—which may also supplement their salaries—and as house staff recruitment depends more and more upon the quality of training and supervision provided with the help of the medical school, the affiliated hospital administrator also becomes involved in a role conflict in which he, too, is doubly subordinated—once to the hospital's governing body, and again to the medical school (usually the dean's office).

UNCOVERING HIDDEN BELIEFS AND PRACTICES

ADO, or average daily occupancy, is one item of many that concern the administrator night and day. In almost all systems, it is necessary to keep ADO high. Particularly in the private sector, administrators know that full occupancy usually means robust health, whereas 70% occupancy may be close to the break-even point, and 50% occupancy means you may not see *that* particular administrator around for very long.

Case Illustration

The Sleuth Function of the Executive

ILLUSTRATION A: In a county hospital, the acute inpatient services were funded for an average daily occupancy of 63 beds. This was advance funding predicated on so-called adequate performance. Should ADO fall below 63, reduction of funds at the next budgetary go-around would be expected. This arrangement sometimes made the staff feel they were operating "under the gun."

Alas, in this particular hospital the average daily census over a number of months had been at the level of 57 beds. Each month, therefore, revenue from 180 "bed days" was lost. Multiply by $500 per day, and you have a monthly loss of around $90,000. On a 12-month basis, the staggering total would be over $1 million. Disaster loomed ahead.

In order to understand bed occupancy in this hospital, it was necessary to comprehend every detail of the process of counting and recording bed occupancy. The first controlling factor is the functioning of the six-bed emergency room

(ER) service, which in essence is the feeder for all the inpatient beds. If the ER has an adequate flow, the possibility of filling beds is good. If not, it becomes necessary to call the referring sources and tell them, "We need patients!" Fortunately, for this type of governmental hospital, serving mainly indigents, this practice was rarely necessary.

Why then, were the beds not being filled? Where was the slippage? In this illustration, I will point to only two types of slippage to illustrate how the administrator, in trying to correct flaws in the system, runs into unexpected, apparently small details of enormous importance.

In one inpatient ward of 33 beds, rooms on one side of the ward were designated for women; rooms on the other side for men. The reason given for this was to make it easier for the nurses to observe the comings and goings of both men and women, and to make sure that men and women did not end up in the same room, and certainly not in the same bed together. This practice, which initially was a seemingly harmless way of maintaining decorum in a mixed-sex ward, by degrees hardened into a proscription against admitting women to the men's side, and vice versa. Thus, sometimes when the physician in the emergency room called up to admit a male patient, he was told by the ward clerk or nurse assistant that no beds were available, although at that time rooms actually were empty on the women's side.

The point is that this practice had prevailed for many months, and although the necessity for keeping all beds filled was a well-advertised desideratum, no one had corrected it. Was it that keeping the sexes segregated had become too great a concern? Was it that this practice escaped solution because it meant fewer admissions and less work? At any rate, it had become so embedded that only an order from top administration could stop it. Here again one learns how subtle and entrenched resistances to change can become.

ILLUSTRATION B: A second example also illustrates the sleuth function of the executive. By probing into the admission process during the nighttime shifts (in fact, a sizable number of patients were admitted during the night), it was found that many patients worked up for admission *before* midnight actually were not officially assigned a bed until *after* midnight. In terms of ADO, the midnight census, it should be noted, was the most critical moment of the 24-hour day; it was the official point in time that determined reimbursement for beds filled. If a patient was officially admitted at 11:00 P.M., and he was counted in the midnight census, the hospital got credit for the whole previous day. If that 11:00 P.M. patient was not *officially* admitted until after midnight, the hospital lost credit for the previous day.

Many pre-midnight cases did not make the midnight count simply because of delays in processing information through the computer—delays due mainly to staff shortages. But the delays were extremely costly. In one month alone, 30 patient days had been lost due to these delays, at a cost of approximately $15,000! The problem was also one of definition. When should a patient be counted as an admission—when his workup was completed and a bed available, or when a group of workers was able to finish its recording and enter the data into their computers?

This problem was quickly corrected after the involved workers were brought together. Because the financial stakes were high, a general feeling of relief prevailed that such an important fiscal problem could be resolved in such a simple manner.

Comment

Many lessons can be drawn from these two illustrations. First, the administrator should never slacken his inquiries into how the system works. Second, learning experiences of this sort are endless; never does the administrator gain in his mind's eye a perfect picture of what goes on in his own institution. Third, his relentless inquiry is an object lesson to his staff to do likewise and to be prepared for his questions. Fourth, the unearthing of seemingly small details may become the key to major improvements. Fifth, the better the relationship with employees, who keep all systems going, the greater the ease of access to routinized practices that may be inimical to institutional goals.

SATISFACTION AND DISSATISFACTION

In the best hotels, management urges customers to rate their satisfaction or dissatisfaction with every aspect of service from check-in to checkout. Sometimes they ask for more mature reflections after the consumer has been away for some months. Polling of consumer and family satisfaction with mental hospital treatment has been increasingly accepted in recent years. It is, of course, essential for the survival of private for-profit institutions. Early 20th-century hospitals that housed most of the severely mentally ill patients in this country had very little to brag about; it was assumed that they were terrible places to be in.

For example, in the early 1940s at Boston Psychopathic Hospital (then Harvard's most important teaching and research facility), conditions were abominable.[35] Patients were admitted through an entrance in the back of the hospital, often accompanied by the police or by distraught relatives, and sometimes handcuffed or in straitjackets. Quickly shunted to the admission ward, they were then stripped of all clothing and possessions and put through a cleansing bath.

Then, clothed in hospital johnny and soft slippers—all "dangerous" accoutrements such as shoes, belts, rings, glasses having been removed—they were ushered into a ward of acute patients with little preparation for the sights and sounds of a bedlam environment. Of the 28 patients housed on that ward, most were sitting on wooden settees; some were wandering about. There was little communication among the patients, or between the patients and nurses or attendants. Many of the patients were in side rooms—in seclusion, in wet sheet packs, or in hot tubs. A few were in physical restraints, and a lucky few in occupational therapy elsewhere in the building. The doors to the ward were locked; only staff persons could unlock them.

In this climate, patients were tense, fearful, and bewildered, wondering what would happen to them. Were they safe? How long would they stay? Would they ever get out? When would they see their friends or relatives again? Soon the doctor would arrive. He would try to allay their anxieties while he obtained a history and did a physical exam, then hurriedly departed to his next duty.

As one wise clinician said, "We had learned more ways to keep patients sick than to get them well." Nevertheless, this was conventional psychiatric treatment of that day in a highly vaunted Harvard teaching hospital.

Happily, after 1943, under the superintendency of Dr. Harry C. Solomon, great strides were made in correcting these morbid conditions. Many new and advanced programs were developed so that in a space of 20 years, under a new name (Massachusetts Mental Health Center), that institution became one of the foremost university teaching/research centers in the world.

But the large state hospitals in our country lagged miserably.[36] The admitting units were especially bad. In 1971, I reported on the observations of a young Tufts medical student who interviewed patients shortly after admission to Boston State Hospital in order to ascertain their reactions to the process of admission. These patients, too, came in through a back door, a shabby rear entrance opposite a garbage pile and incinerator. Here they tarried three to four hours before seeing a doctor or attendant. When the admitting physician arrived, he examined the patient in a shabbily furnished room affording little privacy. As with Boston Psychopathic Hospital 30 years before, keys, jewelry, and money were taken away without explanation; then the patient was moved to the acute ward, where he met blank faces. There were no introductions, no tour or orientation to ward life. Staff attitudes reflected callous condescension, lack of personal interest, and an assumption that patients were either childish or incompetent. Year by year, the number of admissions increased without a concomitant increase in staff.

Appalled by the lack of humanism in one of the most important experiences in a patient's life, energetic measures were initiated to combat the routinization and impersonalization resulting from neglect and lack of humanistic quality control. It is not that the employees were inhumane, but that their innate humanity had to be rekindled from time to time. Apathy and neglect of patients is particularly likely to occur if management also overlooks employees' needs for attention, respect, and rewards, and fails to keep quality care of patients the shining ambition of all employees.

Case Illustration

The Chief Psychiatrist Becomes a Patient

At a VA hospital in 1973, as a new chief of psychiatry not yet known to employees, I presented myself for admission as a "depressed patient." The admission room was filled with patients of every description, noisy, no music, no television.

Apparently no one had thought of separating mental patients from the others. After a half-hour wait, my name was called by a clerk who obtained data for a punch card without even looking me in the eye. Then, when directions to the ward were given to me faster than I could absorb them, repetition was made in a tired, scolding voice. Alas, although I tried to follow the directions carefully, I wound up pacing long underground corridors until a kindly person sensed I needed help and took me by hand to the closed admission ward. Since my appearance on the admission ward had been delayed by my misadventure, the nurse gave me special attention, as might befit an older veteran who could have been rendered incompetent by a traumatic war experience. Altogether, although the first contacts left something to be desired, the admission ward was pleasant and the personnel were considerate. Certainly a big step above the treatment at admission.

In 1983, a study of 1,088 veterans from three war eras[37] was focused on the experiences of Hispanic veterans versus Anglo veterans with respect to their satisfaction with treatment received at several veterans' hospitals in Southern California. Although a majority of both groups felt that the treatment they received was satisfactory, 25% to 30% felt dissatisfied. Hispanics, by and large, were more dissatisfied than Anglos. They complained mostly about the attitudes of clerical and administrative personnel; there were numerous instances of long delays, cold and uncaring staff, red tape, and masses of paperwork before they could get care. They were frustrated by what they regarded as arbitrary evaluation processes for determining eligibility.

The impact was greater on Hispanics than on Anglos. The former felt there was definite racial discrimination against them; and because they had endured so much more poverty and racism in their backgrounds, they were less inclined than Anglos to fight the VA organization to obtain help. Further, the VA system was more alien to their values than to those of Anglo veterans. For Hispanic veterans, sensitivity to family values and manifestations of *personalismo* by caring personnel were very important. These were especially lacking in their initial contacts with lower-level clerical personnel, as indicated above, but once this barrier was negotiated, both Hispanics and Anglos found more respectful and dignified treatment from doctors and upper professional staff.

In general, however, there was clear reluctance of these veterans to use VA service unless their illnesses were severe and urgent, and other-than-VA services were financially unfeasible. Intensive interviews with these veterans revealed the depth of their feelings, illustrated by the following:

- "You go in at 7:30 in the morning and finally see a doctor at 1 in the afternoon—if you're lucky."[38]
- "Once I went there at 2 in the morning for a kidney stone problem. And I didn't get help until 9 in the morning. Then the treatment was hit-and-miss, so I went home and passed the stone myself. But the follow-up visits were fine."[39]

- "We were proud Mexicans. We fought in the war to prove that. But we were still Mexicans in the service, looked down upon. They always treated you as if you weren't smart enough."[40]
- "There is a difference in how minorities are treated. There is a condescension, a patronizing that is all too prevalent and too repetitive."[41]
- "The chief of cardiology; excellent. All the doctors who attended me; fine. . . . It seems to me it is the little ones who feel all-important."[42]
- "I know the VA. I've had to deal with it over the last 19 years. I've been given the runaround, been rejected, seen good doctors, seen too many piss-poor ones! Me and my wheelchair, we go here and there. We take a number and wait."[43]

Attitudes toward veteran care and treatment were also shaped to an extent by the war eras in which the veterans served. Older veterans who served in World War I were in general more accepting and more satisfied with VA care. They were more often poor and therefore necessarily turned to the VA for health care—thankful, often, that they did not have to depend on welfare. They tolerated the bureaucratic hassles and inefficiencies with greater equanimity. Vietnam veterans by contrast—younger, influenced by the critical, activistic spirit of the 1960s, and conscious of having served in an unpopular war—were least satisfied with VA medical/psychiatric services.

Another VA study of note[44] demonstrated that higher elopement rates were associated with lower personnel concern for patients, lower ward morale, and larger patient–staff discrepancies in perceived personal concern. When a lack of rapport existed between patient and staff (as indicated by discrepancy scores), patients were more often released before they were ready, and more reluctant to return to the hospital when they needed help.

Obviously, these studies are useful in documenting areas of inefficiency on which the VA can focus. Administrators are relying more and more on satisfaction/dissatisfaction studies not only to steer efforts to improve the life of patients, but also to increase their awareness of and cooperation with the therapeutic program. Very importantly, these studies reduce the anger and bitterness of patients and families that lead to grievances and lawsuits.

An interesting recent study by Grella and Grusky[45] of families of seriously ill mental patients reveals that interaction with a case manager specifically involving emotional support was the strongest factor associated with family satisfaction. The time spent by responsible professionals dealing with the families' emotional problems cannot be hurried, abrupt, or dominated by rejection. Lack of humane understanding, said one sage (Elvin Semrad), may be the most costly thing in the world.

Satisfaction/dissatisfaction surveys should be carried out as though they were full-fledged clinical evaluation research projects. The essential elements of a good satisfaction/dissatisfaction survey are as follows:[46]

1. The survey should be objective, that is, carried out by researchers who are not in the direct line of service and are not trying to please management.

2. The survey instrument should be short and administered face-to-face. Anything over 50 minutes strains the subject's attention span. Face-to-face interviews permit the best evaluation of the patient's comprehension of questions asked.
3. Both patients and significant others should be queried. Questions should be similar so that discrepancies between patient and family may be validated and analyzed.
4. A variety of ward staff members should also be included in the survey. Special survey instruments should be constructed to reflect satisfaction with their jobs, as well as satisfaction with the service given to patients.
5. Those creating survey questionnaires should utilize the sophisticated knowledge of experts in the construction of such instruments.
6. A broad range of aspects of care should be surveyed. For example, the following should be covered in the patient questionnaire: personal safety and ward security, the physical environment, information giving, the availability of treatment staff, staff humanism, perception of treatment, patient participation in treatment, auxiliary services and activities, cost of care, grievance procedures, discharge and aftercare planning, and other areas.
7. Determine how complainants have fared in the past, with whom their complaints were registered, and how they were received. How were their complaints acted upon, and with what result in terms of satisfaction/dissatisfaction?
8. Survey results should be conveyed to administration and fed back to all involved either as subjects of the survey or as formulators of corrective recommendations.
9. Resurvey at regular intervals.

SUMMARY AND COMMENTS

Human resource management today is more than hiring, firing, record keeping, and picnics.[47] It means maximizing productivity within a humane environment, opportunities for consultation and mediation, and recourse to grievance procedures. Administrators should be concerned with employees' health and welfare, their desire for advancement and need for fair compensation for work done. Evaluation of performance should be fair and just. In addition, in-service training, team building, and attention to morale are important.

Those conducting employment interviews must know about laws prohibiting unfair questions that may suggest discrimination related to sex, race, age, alien status, marital status, pregnancy status, and even conflicts with the law. Bias related to religious preference or physical or mental handicaps is also frowned upon unless the employer is prepared to demonstrate "undue hardship." Sexual harassment is a most sensitive area requiring watchfulness especially on the part of middle management. Sexual favors must not be sought by anyone on a quid pro quo basis, and the environment must not be a hostile one in terms of any unsolicited or unwelcome advances. Immediate counseling and referral to an appropriate personnel officer are indicated should infractions be suspected.

Human resource utilization depends more on community demands than on need. A high degree of flexibility in utilization of resources is a necessity. Reallocation of staff to specific target projects, redesigning of tasks, changes in composition of work teams, or phaseout of units regarded as unproductive are some of the methods that may be employed.

In one's concern for worker morale, special consideration should be given to middle management personnel. They have complex tasks involving mediation between upper management and workers in the front lines. Boundaries are not always clear, and since many middle managers are promoted upward from the front lines, conflicts in loyalties may be experienced. In any event, they must shift their concepts and values, and adopt new supervisory behaviors. Special training programs are indicated.

Another area of frustration for employees, highlighted by Bardwick[48] under the term *plateauing*, refers to the reduction of promotional opportunities in many organizations due to the sudden downturn in organizational expansions in recent years. This is particularly hard on dedicated, ambitious employees who have invested a considerable share of their adult years in an organization.

Other internal phenomena involving employees' behaviors that are recurring and troublesome include (a) end runs and reverse end runs, (b) closed dyads and broken dyads, (c) multiple subordinations, (d) hidden beliefs and practices, and (e) satisfactions/dissatisfactions of patients and staff and the challenge of evaluating same.

End runs refer to efforts of employees to bypass their superiors in order to reach higher officials in a hierarchy, usually for personal aggrandizement. It can be a most disconcerting event in an organization. Reverse end runs, which also involve definitive risks in terms of morale, occur when a higher official bypasses a lower official in order to explore what is going on at a still lower level.

Closed dyads refer to pairs of workers who tend to dissociate themselves from the larger group. They develop a special bond of understanding, often associated with a hostile or superior attitude and diminished communication outside the dyad. The *broken* dyad refers to a communication rift between two employees, a kind of feud in which little interaction occurs between the pair. Both closed and broken dyads are inimical to the natural flow of information necessary for optimum cooperation of workers in a system.

Multiple subordination refers to the familiar phenomenon in which more than one supervisor has responsibility for the time schedule and work of an employee; in turn, the employee reports to both of them. Often confusion arises in relation to boundaries of areas supervised, personality differences, and differing perceptions of authority over the person supervised. A special case of multiple subordination occurs in hospitals affiliated with medical schools, particularly where high-level professionals enjoy joint appointments and joint contributions to their salaries.

Hidden beliefs and practices, often without legitimate foundation and traced to antiquated rules and regulations, usually shape work to favor employee needs rather than organizational ends. They must be identified, exposed, and carefully excised from the living system.

Finally, the organization has great need for periodic surveys of the *satisfactions and dissatisfactions* of its clients, their relatives or significant others, and staff members. JCAHO surveys, patients' rights inspections, and the oversight actions of other regulatory and standard-setting bodies are worthwhile so far as they go, but they do not deal adequately with the more intimate experiences of the members of the hospital community.

Satisfaction/dissatisfaction surveys should be conducted on a face-to-face individual basis, and ideally should be carried out by an objective team skilled in research design and in questionnaire construction. A broad range of areas should be covered, including safety, physical environment, access to information, staff humanism, food, recreation, cost of care, patients' rights, discharge planning, and aftercare.

REFERENCES

1. Wolf JR: Human resource management. Psychiatr Annals 19:432–434, 1989
2. Equal Employment Opportunity Commission (EEOC) Guidelines on Discrimination Because of National Origin, Code of Federal Regulations, Title 29, Chapter XIV, Part 1606. EEOC Decision No. 71-969 (1970)
3. Equal Employment Opportunity Commission (EEOC), Title 7, Civil Rights Act of 1964, as amended. Authority transferred to EEOC by Federal Civil Rights Reorganization Plan of 1978.
4. *Johnson v. Pike Co.*, F. Supp. 490 (C.D. Calif. 1971); EEOC Decision No. 74-02 (1973)
5. *Phillips v. Martin Marietta Corp.*, 400 U.S. 542 (1971)
6. *Carter v. Gallagher*, 452 F. 2nd 315 (C.A. 1971)
7. *Gregory v. Litten*, 422 F. 2nd 631 (C.A. 1972)
8. *Carter v. Gallagher* supra
9. *Green v. Missouri Pacific R.R. Co.*, 523 F. 2nd 1290 (C.A. 8, 1975)
10. *Griggs v. Duke Power Co.*, 401 U.S. 424 (1971)
11. *Robinson v. Lorillard Corp.*, 444 F. 2nd 791 (C.A. 4 1971)
12. *U.S. v. St. Louis-San Francisco R.R. Co.*, 464 F. 2nd 301 (C.A. 8, 1972)
13. *Jones v. Lee Way Motor Freight, Inc.*, 431 F. 2nd 245 (C.A. 10, 1970)
14. Office of Affirmative Action Compliance: Harassment: Your Rights and Remedies. Los Angeles, County of Los Angeles, Office of Affirmative Action Compliance, Directive No. 4, March 9, 1989
15. Office of Affirmative Action Compliance: Harassment: Your Rights and Remedies. Los Angeles, County of Los Angeles, Office of Affirmative Action Compliance, Directive No. 4, March 9, 1989
16. Office of Affirmative Action Compliance: Harassment: Your Rights and Remedies. Los Angeles, County of Los Angeles, Office of Affirmative Action Compliance, Directive No. 4, March 9, 1989
17. Office of Affirmative Action Compliance: Harassment: Your Rights and Remedies. Los Angeles, County of Los Angeles, Office of Affirmative Action Compliance, Directive No. 4, March 9, 1989
18. Office of Affirmative Action Compliance: Guidelines for Preventing Sexual Harassment Com-

plaints. Los Angeles, Los Angeles County, Office of Affirmative Action Compliance (undated publications)

19. U.S. Civil Service Commission, Joe Ben Hudgens, Principal Deputy Counsel: Memorandum, June 16, 1981
20. Canales CJ (Personnel Officer, Los Angeles County–Olive View Medical Center, Sylmar, CA): Personal communication, September 1989
21. U.S. Consolidated Omnibus Budget Recommendation of 1985 (COBRA)
22. U.S. Immigration Reform Act, Section 89 of Tax Reform Act of 1986
23. Wolf JR: Human resource management. Psychiatr Annals 19:432–434, 1989
24. Bardwick JM: Plateauing. Hosp Forum 28:93, 95, 96, 98, 1985
25. Talbot JF: Middle managers in mental health: A study of management tasks. Admin and Policy in Ment Health 16:65–77, 1988
26. Ewalt PL: From clinician to manager, in White SL (ed): Middle Management in Mental Health. (New Directions for Mental Health Services, No. 8.) San Francisco, Jossey-Bass, 1980
27. Feldman S: Middle management muddle. Admin in Mental Health 8:3–11, 1980
28. Talbot JF: Middle managers in mental health: A study of management tasks. Admin and Policy in Ment Health 16:65–77, 1988
29. Greenblatt M: "End runs" and "reverse end runs": A note on organizational dynamics. Amer J Social Psychiatry 6:114–119, 1986
30. Kotin J, Sharaf MR: Management succession and administrative style. Psychiatry 30:237–248, 1967
31. Sharaf MR, Kotin J: Management succession revisited. Admin and Mental Health 60–62, Summer 1974
32. Schulberg B: What Makes Sammy Run? New York, Random House, 1941
33. Greenblatt M, Sharaf MR, Stone EM: Within the institution, Chapter 1 in Greenblatt M, Sharaf MR, Stone EM: Dynamics of Institutional Change: The Hospital in Transition. Pittsburgh, Pennsylvania, University of Pittsburgh Press, 1971, pp 13–14
34. 5 U.S.C. §2301(b) (9) (Supp.V.1981). Enacted as part of Civil Service Reform Act of 1978, Public Law No. 95-454, 92 Stat.111 codified as amended in scattered sections of 5, 10, 15, 28, 31, 38, 39, 42 U.S.C.
35. Greenblatt M, York RH, Brown EL: Eliminating major evils, Chapter 2 in Greenblatt M, York RH, Brown EL: From Custodial to Therapeutic Patient Care in Mental Hospitals: Explorations in Social Treatment. New York, Russell Sage Foundation, 1955
36. Greenblatt M, Sharaf MR, Stone EM: Research, Chapter 9 in Greenblatt M, Sharaf MR, Stone EM: Dynamics of Institutional Change: The Hospital in Transition. Pittsburgh, University of Pittsburgh Press, 1971, pp 232–234. Reprinted with permission
37. Becerra RM, Greenblatt M: Hispanics Seek Health Care: A Study of 1,088 Veterans of Three War Eras. Lanham, Maryland, University Press of America, 1983
38. Becerra RM, Greenblatt M: Hispanics Seek Health Care: A Study of 1,088 Veterans of Three War Eras. Lanham, Maryland, University Press of America, 1983, p 131
39. Becerra RM, Greenblatt M: Hispanics Seek Health Care: A Study of 1,088 Veterans of Three War Eras. Lanham, Maryland, University Press of America, 1983, p 131
40. Becerra RM, Greenblatt M: Hispanics Seek Health Care: A Study of 1,088 Veterans of Three War Eras. Lanham, Maryland, University Press of America, 1983, p 115
41. Becerra RM, Greenblatt M: Hispanics Seek Health Care: A Study of 1,088 Veterans of Three War Eras. Lanham, Maryland, University Press of America, 1983, p 123
42. Becerra RM, Greenblatt M: Hispanics Seek Health Care: A Study of 1,088 Veterans of Three War Eras. Lanham, Maryland, University Press of America, 1983, p 123
43. Becerra RM, Greenblatt M: Hispanics Seek Health Care: A Study of 1,088 Veterans of Three War Eras. Lanham, Maryland, University Press of America, 1983, p 126
44. Spiegel D, Younger JB: Ward climate and community stay of psychiatric patients. J Consult Clin Psychol 39:62–69, 1972
45. Grella CE, Grusky O: Families of the seriously mentally ill and their satisfaction with services. Hosp & Community Psychiatry 40:831–835, 1989
46. Norman ML, Greenblatt M, Essock-Vitale S: Satisfaction/Dissatisfaction Survey of Patients, Families, and Staff at Neuropsychiatric Institute, UCLA. Los Angeles, University of California, Los Angeles, Neuropsychiatric Institute & Hospital, 1983 (unpublished report)
47. Wolf JR: Human resource management. Psychiatr Annals 19:432–434, 1989
48. Bardwick JM: Plateauing. Hosp Forum 28:93, 95, 96, 98, 1985

Economics of Mental Health

FINANCING HEALTH CARE

Consider the recent explosive growth of the area of economics and mental health. In the late 1970s, when the Division of Biometry and Epidemiology of the National Institute of Mental Health began to develop the field,[1] there were then no well-recognized authorities, nor a significant bibliography; by 1987, a publication was forthcoming every two weeks. Doctoral training programs have now been initiated in several schools. Today we have an established body of knowledge, recognized specialists, and a flow of talented students and researchers. Let us consider herewith recent and current developments in this field.

The Deinstitutionalization Movement

Vast changes occurred in the mental health scene particularly after World War II. The lessons of that war hung heavily over policy makers for several years, ultimately finding expression in the report of the Joint Commission on Mental Illness and Health. The commission had attempted since 1955 to review and assess the whole mental health system in America; they reported their work in several notable volumes, the last of which, full of recommendations for the future, was called *Action for Mental Health* (1961).[2] *Action for Mental Health* said in so many words that the mental health system in America was, in effect, a nonsystem, a near disaster, and a discredit to a civilized nation. It recommended the phasing down of state and federal hospitals to a more manageable size, construction of small community mental health centers serving defined populations, an emphasis on ambulatory services and community care, mobilization of extramural resources to assist patients' retention in the community, training of large numbers of mental health professionals, and much greater utilization of paraprofessionals and volunteers.

The result was a great reduction of patients in large government hospitals, and considerable success in expanding community care. There was also greater attention to children, adolescents, substance abusers, and the elderly, and much more involvement of citizens in the total effort. This, in turn, was accompanied by *some* reduction in the stubborn stigma of mental illness, which had clung to its unfortunate victims for centuries. At the same time, the findings of psychopharmacological and psychobiological research strengthened the assumption that mental disease could be the result largely of genetic and neurophysiologic aberrations, and not faulty upbringing, laziness, or other characterological deficiencies.

Other Changes in the Mental Health Industry

It should be noted that these changes, commonly referred to as the deinstitutionalization of the mentally ill, were the basic elements of the largest organized effort to improve the plight of the mentally ill ever attempted in this nation. The movement was backed by the American Psychiatric Association, President Kennedy, the Congress, and literally dozens of professional and lay organizations. Particularly noteworthy was the emphasis on communitybased care, on planning services based on defined geographic areas and defined populations (catchment areas), and on participation of citizen groups in planning services and in membership on policy boards of hospitals and clinics. The need for many more trained professionals to treat the mentally ill was recognized, particularly in the core occupations—psychiatry, nursing, psychology, and social work—and many more government grants were awarded to facilitate training. Considerable emphasis also was directed to the need for increased research into the causes and treatment of mental illness, a recognition of the fact that our ignorance was profound, and that mental health as a developing science had lagged greatly behind medicine, surgery, and the other specialties.

The effects of these undertakings upon the economics of mental health were profound. At first, the federal government awarded grants to the states for construction of small, comprehensive community mental health centers. This was followed by grants for staffing of these centers. The agreements were as follows:

- The centers would offer at least five indispensable services: inpatient, outpatient, transitional, emergency care, and public education.
- Services would be offered to all individuals regardless of race, sex, ethnicity, color, or creed; a substantial amount of services would be offered to the poor and indigent.
- Funds allotted by the federal government would be for five years—full payment in the first year, gradually diminishing over the next four

years—with local jurisdictions taking over the funding after that. However, due to the difficulties of local jurisdictions in supporting the ventures, extensions of fiscal contracts for several more years were permitted.

- The size of the catchment areas to be served by the new, small comprehensive mental health centers would generally conform to a population of between 75,000 to 150,000 people, with exceptions based on special justifications. These new centers would be sited in, or close to, populated areas, unlike the old state mental hospitals.

The above concepts guided the development of a great new movement in American psychiatry. Never before had so much cooperation been developed between federal, state, and local levels on such a grand scale—all directed to reorganizing a national system of care that, on hard inspection, turned out to have been no system at all. As time went on, the concerted effort enlarged to include children's disorders, the elderly, alcoholism, and substance-abuse patients. Project support was also granted to mental hospitals for innovative demonstrations that would make the hospitals a better place to live for those longer-stay patients who could not be treated in the community or in the new community centers.

The federal expenditures for these programs were in the many, many millions of dollars. The states also loosened their purse strings and contributed even more, inasmuch as the comprehensive community mental health centers, after a period of time, had to be taken over by them or by other financial auspices. More than 750 comprehensive community mental health centers were established within two decades, thanks to the infusion of federal funds. After the federal funds disappeared, the vast majority managed to survive, although many experienced severe financial strains. Many, in order to continue, necessarily had to develop multiple sources of revenue: state and county governments, patient fees, third-party insurance, and private subscriptions.

The state and county mental hospitals, it should be mentioned, in several respects were greatly helped by the deinstitutionalization movement. The burdens of overcrowding were diminished by discharges of thousands of patients to community mental health care. For many hospitals, this meant a decided improvement in their staff-to-patient ratios. In addition, hospital improvement grants from the federal government stimulated innovative projects on patient care and greater attention in particular to chronic patients.

But, regrettably, in the 1970s the deinstitutionalization movement began to stall. Federal money ran out as the Congress faced other priorities; the rationale was that the federal effort had proved its point, and now it was time for other sectors to take over. Nixon as president was more interested in the fight against cancer, and certainly not in programs that had been identified with the Kennedys. As enthusiasm waned, important members of the psychiatric profession began to question what had truly been accomplished by this great movement. Certainly there had been a paucity of controlled studies to evaluate its impact on the health of communities or catchment areas. Fiscal austerity, political cutbacks, recession in the business world, and skepticism in the professional/scientific community began to assert their impact.

From the standpoint of economics of mental health, however, the deinstitutionalization movement was a unique event in history, characterized by direct large federal grants to the states to establish comprehensive community mental health centers and to enhance training and research. It stands in history as one of the greatest national efforts in modern times directed to a solution of the unyielding, stubborn problem of mental disease.

Supply and Demand

During the heyday of the movement, as vast sums of money were poured into improving care for the mentally ill, broad changes in both demand and supply occurred, led particularly by the private sector. As Feldman[3] has put it, demand rose not only as a result of decreased stigma and guilt, but also as a result of an almost explosive increase in advertising by the many new private sector hospitals.

> Such advertising . . . contributed to a 350% increase in adolescent admissions to private psychiatric hospitals in just four years. . . . On the supply side there has been a rapid growth in the number of psychiatric beds. In 1987 alone, these beds increased by nearly 30%, while beds for adolescents grew by about 1,600% . . . from 1983 to 1987. While general hospitals are in great financial difficulty, the psychiatric hospital business is booming. In fact, general hospital beds are being converted to psychiatric use at a record pace as hospitals discover that such beds are less expensive and that psychiatry . . . has far more attractive profit margins than medicine.[4]

Cost Escalation and Its Consequences

Mental health service had become an industry with vast potential, and insurance companies to a large extent financed a bull market that persisted over two decades. However, the prosperity curve, as has been pointed out above, began to weaken as costs escalated beyond inflation. The causes of the cost escalation were multiple:

- Advances in medical technology
- General economic inflation
- Increased public demand for health care
- Increase in the aging population
- Malpractice costs
- Fee-for-service systems
- Itemized billing

The magnitude of the increase in health care costs[5] is sharply illustrated by the following: In California, medical costs increased 200% in a 10-year period; in 1982, they were the largest single item in the California budget. In the United States as a whole, health care dollars increased 100% in 10 years (1974–1984), outrunning inflation by about 15% per year.[6]

As the growing costs of mental health care exceeded general inflation, several changes in public policy entered the picture. First was gradual attenuation of the concept that low-income persons must receive the same services as the privately insured, accompanied by emphasis on proving the cost-effectiveness of *all* treatment interventions. As a corollary, restrictions in services, cost cuts, and lowered quality of care were associated with a general decline in the influence of clinical personnel vis-à-vis administrative personnel in the formulation of health policy.

Progressively burdened by heavier taxes, the citizens in effect now joined a rebellion, expressed in California as Proposition 13 (1978) and the so-called Gann amendment to the state constitution (1979). Proposition 13 was passed overwhelmingly by voters threatened by rapid escalation of property taxes because of previously unheard-of inflation in property values. It cut taxes back to the preinflation period; but although it saved many taxpayers their homes, it reduced state revenues—and, as an inevitable corollary, state investment in health and welfare. The Gann amendment put a cap on spending such that government outlays could not exceed cost-of-living and population increases. A nationwide recession in the early 1980s, together with a $2 billion deficit that faced California in 1982 and followed in October 1987 by a stock market collapse, slowed California's support of welfare programs further.

On the national front, mention must be made of the enormous federal deficit that had accrued, including debt-servicing costs and trade deficits. These worries finally inspired the Gramm-Rudman-Hollings Act of 1985, which proposed neutralization of these deficits over a five-year period. The shock of implementation of the new laws was felt throughout the country. Although, fortunately, the stock market crash of 1987 did not lead to a major depression (as was feared), and the economy recovered quickly and remained strong, nevertheless the accumulated effects of all the above impacted tragically on systems of health and mental health care.

Measures to control runaway costs of patient care have been numerous. In California in 1983, in a bold and elaborate maneuver, responsibility for health care of medically indigent adults (MIAs)—who were formerly enrolled in cost-reimbursable plans in which choice of provider was largely left to the consumer—was transferred to the counties; but then the state paid the counties only 70% of expected costs of care. Insurance companies reduced benefits by reducing payments to providers, while beneficiaries were taxed by imposing more stringent eligibility requirements, higher deductibles, and higher copayments. Medi-Cal eliminated such benefits as hearing aids, prosthetic devices, and some drugs. Payments to physicians were reduced, and hospitalizations were restricted by requiring pretreatment authorization, current and retrospective utilization reviews, claims reviews, and conformity to quality assurance standards. Further, length of hospitalization was reduced by denial of payment for patients held beyond a specified number of days. In addition, by classifying diseases into diagnostic related groups and basing payments on averages of group costs, it was possible to save money by gradually depressing allowances for the diagnostic categories (see "Diagnostic Related Groups" later in this chapter).

In sum, changes in the social/political/economic scene impacted care and treatment in many ways. Care was denied to many. Quality of care suffered, and financing patterns changed from cost reimbursement *after* diagnosis and treatment to prospective financing. The historic autonomy that providers had enjoyed for generations gave way to third parties largely setting the conditions for medical/psychiatric services.

Effect on the Practitioner

Many practitioners have been distressed to see the economic motive so dominant in mental health care. They resent any intrusions into their practice that dilute the primacy of their personal relationship with patients. Chodoff,[7] in a penetrating analysis of the vicissitudes of psychotherapeutic practice, contrasts the kind of practice enjoyed by psychoanalysts and medical psychotherapists in Freud's time with what prevails in today's economic climate. Then, practice was individual, entrepreneurial, and unregulated.

> There was no requirement to make medical diagnosis, to define medical necessity, to establish criteria for "cure," or an end point of treatment; or to differentiate between the qualifications of physicians and other purveyors of psychotherapy. . . . This kind of individualistic therapeutic relationship continued for several decades after psychotherapy by psychiatrists took hold in the U.S., but it has been altered irrevocably.[8]

When insurance companies entered the field, federal employees could buy insurance from Blue Cross–Blue Shield that reimbursed 80% of fees for psychotherapy up to a lifetime limit of $50,000. Many a psychiatric resident was approved for psychoanalytic treatment during those days and subsequently turned toward psychoanalysis as a major career emphasis. After 1984, however, Blue Cross–Blue Shield limited mental health benefits to 70% in its high-option plan, with a maximum of 50 outpatient visits per year. Only the affluent could then afford intensive psychotherapy or psychoanalysis, and psychiatric residents' therapy was no longer supported.

Intrusion of insurance companies into the relationship has now made it necessary to formulate a specific diagnosis and to establish medical treatment as necessary and appropriate. Meantime, clinical psychologists have made great progress in establishing psychotherapeutic practices, achieving licensure in the 50 states and the District of Columbia. As they compete with psychiatrists, they add to a developing climate of cost consciousness. Now therapists must produce credible evidence of both clinical value and cost-effectiveness. As the pressure for cost-effectiveness discouraged long-term therapy, it drove many full-time private practitioners into part-time work in organized care settings. Thus, both independent office practice and the use of psychoanalytic techniques have declined.

Trends in Inpatient Psychiatric Care

As a result of the deinstitutionalization movement, there has been a very great reduction in state and county hospital beds. Transitional and community facilities and services have taken care of many of these patients, but unfortunately, community facilities have not expanded sufficiently to accommodate the large flow of patients out of the institutions. Thus, we have had an accumulation of discharged chronic mentally ill patients in the community, many of whom have added to the homeless population. The reasons why the deinstitutionalization movement stalled after a most dramatic and effective beginning are many and complex—partly political, partly economic, and partly due to waning interest of the public and even mental health professionals in community psychiatry. Adverse reports of disruptive, revolting, or aggressive behavior of chronic patients who had been released to the community made many citizens (and professionals, too) feel that the deinstitutionalization movement had gone too far.

Privatization*

In the late 1960s and through the 1970s, as noted earlier, *privatization* became big business. Dorwart and Schlesinger[11] have analyzed the causes of this phenomenon, which include:

- A large reservoir of unmet needs for psychiatric services, particularly among children, adolescents, substance abusers, and the elderly.
- Mandatory mental health insurance in many states.
- The increasing age of the American public, with a corresponding need for care for mental illness in the elderly.
- An increase in the number of mental health practitioners (psychiatrists, psychologists, and social workers).
- An increase in psychiatric services in acute care general hospitals.
- Lowered requirements for certificates of need for new construction in many states.
- Employers, recognizing loss of revenues due to absenteeism and diminished productivity from mental illness, drug abuse, and the like have encouraged the proliferation of employee assistance plans.
- Psychiatric illness has grown more socially acceptable as people become more psychologically aware, and as the psychiatric profession becomes remedicalized. In addition, the community is becoming educated to the

---

*The following sections borrow heavily from the work of Dorwart and Schlesinger,[9] as well as Dorwart, Epstein and Davidson.[10]

increasing effectiveness of treatment for a wide variety of psychological illnesses.

- As general hospitals encounter more and more trouble filling their beds, management shifts from medical to psychiatric beds, the latter usually being less costly and more in demand.
- State and county governments are trying to get out of the direct care business, with all its administrative headaches and high indirect costs. Instead, they are contracting out many services to the private sector. This works well in many cases; however, the private sector is not necessarily equipped to do a better job than the public sector for the same outlay of cash. Further, over time the private sector often becomes selective, accepting only less severe cases and those that are easier to treat.

Actually, mental health has been catching up to the private system model that has characterized the American health care system for decades. Both private investor-owned hospitals and private nonprofit general hospital units have led this trend. Separate units for children and increased services for patients with addictions have been characteristic. The units tend to locate in states with generous inpatient coverage under Medicaid or those with less stringent requirements for certificates of need.

The "new" economics resulting from these trends involves administrators in three areas of challenge (formulated by Dorwart and Schlesinger[12]):

1. *Proprietization;* that is, maximization of profits through the employment of marketing, advertising, and public relations techniques with the aim of increasing visibility and stimulating demand for services.
2. *Corporatization;* that is, the development of multihospital organizations that then allow for large-scale management systems and attending economies of scale.
3. *Competition* to reduce prices and costs, increase efficiency of utilization, and enhance responsiveness to changing community demands for service. Typically, private hospitals (especially for-profit ones) emphasize short-term treatment, the use of outpatient rather than inpatient sites, and adding new services and eliminating unprofitable services.

The implications for administrators in the new era have included not only a shift of focus from public to private organization, and expansion of services that are primarily profitable, but also aggressive cultivation of public agencies interested in contracting out services, and contracting with industry for services to employees.

Since the 1982 Supreme Court ruling that approved of professional advertising (so long as it was not false or misleading), the private sector has gone all out in this direction. Also, individual practitioners—formerly restrained from advertising by the American Medical Association on ethical grounds—may now respond to competition from the corporate sector by advertising their services. This presages a whole new view of private practice in the future.

Both positive and negative consequences of privatization are also discussed by Dorwart and Schlesinger.[13] Positive results of privatization include more services for the community, a reduction of the stigma of mental illness as a result of open and massive advertising, a marked increase in beds for children and adolescents, and an increase in treatment of eating disorders and substance-abuse cases. We can also expect that public knowledge about mental illness and its treatment will grow.

Negative results of privatization include increased emphasis of caregiving organizations on profit margin as opposed to humanitarian and quality concerns, reduced quality of care whenever overexpansion of beds in a highly competitive market occurs, and the phasing out of needed programs and services simply because profits cannot be achieved. According to some observers, the peak of competitiveness induced by the private systems will soon be passed, and many hospitals will not survive. This will result in loss of services to the community, loss of employment opportunities for health workers, and loss of investment capital.

The effect of privatization on the public sector has not yet been fully appreciated. It is fair to conclude that many of the public-sector "safety net" hospitals that have gone under in recent years have been casualties of the explosive growth of the private sector. Public hospitals have had trouble in recruitment and retention of professional workers because the private systems pay more. As an example, in California, board-certified psychiatrists who have given 10 years or more to county mental hospitals may now earn less in income than psychiatric residents just out of training who sign up with private for-profit outfits. The private system may provide the latter with an office to swell their income and to supply patients for the private institution that helps them. If young psychiatrists experience financial difficulties, the private facility may offer loans. Thus, the public-sector hospital ends up with less qualified professionals, while the private institution binds the better professionals to its service for the long term.

The implications of the privatization movement for training are also significant. Training for administration will most likely shift from schools of public health to schools of management. It will emphasize the bottom line and all the technologies and management systems necessary to meet the competition. Marketing strategies, public relations, and cost-effectiveness analyses will likely be the high priorities.

Since in the future many of our mental health professionals will be serving in the public sector, how will training programs accommodate these new careers? Will there be more concern with health care costs, maximization of bed occupancy, a preference for better treatment of patients with insurance coverage, more rapid client turnovers, treatment in ambulatory settings, and emphasis on innovative programs with greater profit return? Will the humanitarian tradition and ideals of medicine become dimmed over time?

Private For-Profit (PFP) versus Private Not-For-Profit (PNP) Hospitals[14,15]

As regards the difference between PFP and PNP institutions, it is expected that PFP will (a) be more aggressive in seeking insurance coverage; (b) be more likely to emphasize profit motive in competition with quality; (c) be more likely to limit access by ability to pay; (d) use ancillary services more and charge higher fees; (e) treat less seriously ill patients; (f) be less responsive to community needs; and (g) be subject to corporate taxes on profits. On the other hand, the PNP hospital will (a) have a more charity- and community-related mission; (b) emphasize professional values more; (c) treat sicker and more chronically ill patients; and (d) face increased costs related particularly to teaching and research. The PNP hospitals will be largely exempt from federal and state taxes. It is also hypothesized that as university hospitals (also PNP) experience an insufficiency of clinical material in specific discipline areas, they will rely more and more on clinical material in affiliated PNP hospitals (rather than PFP hospitals), as well as in state, county, and VA facilities.

When PFP institutions are making money, they may contribute to research and development with the ultimate aim of gaining an advantage in the marketplace over other competing PFP ventures. In recent years some academic/teaching university hospitals have sought joint ventures with PFP chains in the hope of gaining support for additional research staff, while assuring the PFP institution of high-quality academic talent to man the joint enterprises. Discoveries and innovations developed by the research staff that may be converted to clinical use and income generation are then jointly exploited by both the university and the PFP entity.

Development of Health Care Coverage*

In health care coverage, the United States has generally lagged behind other industrial nations. The first state workers' compensation plan appeared in 1910. Insurance to cover hospitalization was first developed by Blue Cross in 1930. Eight years later the California Medical Association started Blue Shield, a mechanism to reimburse physicians for services. In prepaid group practice programs introduced in the 1940s, Kaiser of California and the city government of New York (under Mayor LaGuardia) provided full medical and hospital insurance. These models led to today's health maintenance organizations, in which Kaiser is still a leading provider.

---

*This section follows exactly Roemer's summary of historic events in health care coverage.[16]

By 1957, two-thirds of Americans enjoyed health protection for hospital care, mostly through their place of work. This coverage, unfortunately, was lost upon retirement, when it was most needed. In 1965, Medicare and Medicaid were launched by the federal government, and private insurers came into the field with many new policies. In the late 1970s, bills were introduced into Congress for national health insurance, but none succeeded. The Congress deemed such a program too expensive; yet, in Canada, complete health insurance has been successful. By 1980, 75% of Americans enjoyed health insurance against major illnesses, and another 10% received coverage through Medicaid. But unfortunately, during the 1980s, benefits from many programs were curtailed, eligibility requirements were toughened, and copayments were raised.

Today, millions of Americans have no insurance, and millions more have inadequate coverage. The latest step forward, the Catastrophic Health Insurance Act of 1988—an amendment to the Medicare law—entitled elderly people to unlimited hospital care, based on a graduated tax on the elderly themselves. However, due to loud protests from many older citizens who claimed the law was discriminatory, this program was terminated.

Nevertheless, viewing the field historically, progress *has* been made. The large number of insurance plans aimed to provide health coverage to the American people today is testimony not only to a nation trying to bring health security up to the level of other advanced countries, but also to the ingenuity and imagination of the planners of these programs.

Blue Cross–Blue Shield[17,18]

Founded in 1929, Blue Cross–Blue Shield plans provide health insurance generally on a group cooperative basis. Roughly 85% of their membership is so enrolled, although individual coverage with less extensive benefits is possible. This form of nonfederal insurance is the one most extensively used today. In 1978, membership in Blue Cross had reached almost 73 million. It is estimated that more than 70 autonomous plans have developed since the introduction of Blue Cross–Blue Shield.

All Blue Cross plans offer some hospitalization coverage for mental conditions. The plans vary in the number of days of care provided, a common allowance being 30 days—considerably less than is allowed for medical illness. The coverage for physician services (Blue Shield) is largely limited to inpatient hospital care. Extension of Blue Cross–Blue Shield coverage is often provided by other insurance contracts, which usually pay 75% to 80% of charges after an initial deductible.

Many independent insurance companies are now in the field, having overcome their initial reluctance to take on mental health because of diagnostic vagaries, lack of adequate statistics to forecast risk, and the belief that mental care was often an indefinitely prolonged affair. However, since it has been shown that patients respond well to neuroleptic drugs and that hospital stays may be brief, it has become clear that costs can be contained. Further, utilization rates for mental disorders under Blue Cross–Blue Shield have been low compared to general health. As a result, the feasibility of including psychiatry in insurance plans has become increasingly obvious to the commercial sector.

Medicare and Medicaid

Passed in 1965, during the years of President Johnson's administration, Medicare and Medicaid were part of the War on Poverty legacy left by President Kennedy. Medicare and Medicaid then became part of the greatest social welfare program this nation had ever initiated for its people. The rich body of social legislation passed by the Congress in that period reflected both the nation's mourning of a departed leader and its desire to honor his memory by realizing his dreams. Medicare and Medicaid represent a historic turning point in the government's hopes to guarantee health services eventually to all the people.

> The Medicare program is a Federal health insurance program for people 65 or older. . . . It is run by the Health Care Financing Administration [HCFA] of the U.S. Department of Health and Human Services. Social Security Administration offices across the country take applications for Medicare and provide general information about the program.
> There are two parts to the Medicare program. *Hospital Insurance* (Part A) helps pay for inpatient hospital care, some inpatient care in a skilled nursing facility, home health care, and hospice care. *Medical Insurance* (Part B) helps pay for medically necessary doctors' services, outpatient hospital services, home health care, and a number of other medical services and supplies that are not covered by the hospital insurance part of Medicare.[19]

For both parts, either out-of-pocket payments are required (deductible or coinsurance) or additional coverage must be supplied through another insurance plan. "These out of pocket payments are set each year, according to formulas established by Congress."[20]

Psychiatric care represents only a small part of total Medicare expenditures for health (approximately 2.4% in 1981).[21] Part A provides a lifetime limit of 190 days for inpatient psychiatric care. Medicare Part B provides limited coverage for outpatient care and for pharmacotherapeutic visits after a fixed copayment. The initial psychiatric evaluation and medication follow-up office management visits are also covered.

The initial act required that hospitals develop utilization review plans and a medical staff committee to oversee and control utilization of services. A 1972 modification of the Social Security Act (Public Law 92-603) established Professional Standards Review Organizations (PSROs)—local nonprofit boards that (a) review concurrently all admissions, (b) evaluate medical care, and (c) collect data on medical practices and patient profiles. Local norms, standards, and criteria developed by hospital staffs are utilized as approved by area PSROs.[22,23]

Medicaid (Medi-Cal in California), essentially a program for indigents, covers charges for inpatient physician visits over a limited number of days (30 or less in most states). Payment for outpatient visits to psychiatrists, usually limited to 20 to 30 per year, are also covered, but unfortunately these reimbursements are set well below prevailing charges.

It should be noted that the Medicare and Medicaid legislation of 1965 tried to encourage a greater use of general hospital psychiatric units by providing a higher level of benefits for them than for public and private psychiatric hospitals. The latter were required to meet JCAHO standards of accreditation and were held to a lifetime limit of treatment not applicable to general hospital psychiatric units.[24]

In a polemical article, Wehrmacher[25] blames Medicare for many of the problems now besetting American medicine.

> Indisputable data now show that hospital costs have increased more rapidly than Medicare payments. . . . The economic viability of both urban and rural hospitals has been severely questioned. . . . More and more Americans are experiencing difficulty in gaining access to needed care, and because of the limitations of Medicare, an increasing number of experienced internists can no longer afford to absorb the financial loss of caring for Medicare patients.

Although Wehrmacher, an internist, attributes many evils to price control, administrators of health facilities—including mental health facilities—are likely to agree that the progressive constraints on payments under Medicare have imposed heavy burdens on patient services as well as hospital viability.

In addition to Blue Cross–Blue Shield, independent plans are numerous, including community, group, and individual prepaid plans; self-insured employer–employee union plans; and programs sponsored by private physicians.[26] The amount of protection varies greatly. Group plans include comprehensive coverage for basic benefits plus supplementary coverage, the latter often including nursing and drugs. The additional coverage usually requires significant initial deductibles. Individual plans usually provide less extensive coverage than group policies because individual subscribers are likely to require more services than groups, due to the factor of adverse selection.

Insurance companies may operate their own facilities and employ their own medical personnel, or they may contract with hospitals, physicians, or providers for services. The escalating costs of medical health care and the necessity to control runaway inflation have led to a number of plans that are being tested at the present time. These include payments based on diagnostic related groups (DRGs), health maintenance organizations (HMOs), preferred provider organizations (PPOs), and other managed care systems.

Prospective Payment Systems

Diagnostic Related Groups (DRGs).   Until 1982, Medicare paid for reasonable costs of necessary care, but unending double-digit inflation of hospital costs inspired Congress in 1983 to pass the Tax Equity and Fiscal Responsibility Act (TEFRA), which limited future payments to hospitals to an annual rate set by the secretary of health and human services. This in effect ended the era of cost-based reimbursements. Since then, truly revolutionary changes have occurred in the economics of health and mental health. The search for total control of runaway inflation was on, and numerous experiments have been tried to control health costs.

Understandably, the hospital industry was not pleased with the new law, which did not fully take account of differences in case types across hospitals, severity of illness, quality of care, or differences in case mix. Moreover, risk sharing with Medicare favored the federal government in that hospitals were liable for 75% of excessive costs, whereas they could keep only 50% of savings.

One way to control costs is to base payments on diagnosis, length of stay, severity of illness, or some formula taking into account multiple factors influencing cost. In the diagnostic related group (DRG) system, Medicare reimbursement reflects the cost of treating an average patient belonging to a specific DRG group. Thus, a hospital can project its revenue for a year by anticipating how many patients will be treated in each group. If hospital costs exceed total DRG payments, the hospital suffers a loss of revenue; on the other hand, if it manages to spend less than the DRG payments, it comes out with a surplus. This system, of course, moves the center of gravity from physician control of costs to payer control of costs. By setting the level of pay for a given diagnosis downward, the payer can effect economies of disbursements while forcing the hospitals to increase their efficiency of operation. It also tends to level quality of care to a predetermined average, to eliminate variability, and to encourage the institution to choose those diagnoses that yield higher rates wherever such a choice is possible. Other factors that must be figured into DRG-based costs include severity of the illness, its complications, previous history of illness, and psychosocial support systems. Training and research administrative costs would either have to be bypassed, or require additional allowances to be made, particularly in academic treatment centers.

Studies have shown that DRGs are not good predictors of costs of psychiatric services, although they may be applied with better results in medical and surgical diseases. For this reason, psychiatric hospitals and psychiatric units of general hospitals have been exempted from Medicare DRG prospective payments and continue to be paid mainly by retrospective methods, where calculations are made separately for each hospital based on base-year costs per discharge. In 1987, exemptions to DRGs in psychiatry applied to 460 psychiatric hospitals and 830 general hospital psychiatric units.

An important consideration recently underscored by the *New England Journal of Medicine*[27] pertains to the effect of the Medicare prospective payment system on the adoption of new technology. The focus of the article is on cochlear implants, which have been shown to be of significant value to patients suffering from hearing loss. According to estimates, 30% of those over 65 years of age and 50% of those over 85 have important hearing handicaps. As is well-known, hearing disabilities can increase the loneliness of older citizens, contribute to depression and disorientation, and greatly reduce quality of life.

Cochlear implants received FDA approval in 1984. President Reagan personally congratulated its inventor, and the press gave the approval high visibility. Implants had received the endorsement of the AMA in 1983, and of the American Academy of Otolaryngology—Head and Neck Surgery in 1985.

However, as a result of bureaucratic delays, DRG underpayments, and reluctance of Medicare to adopt device-specific DRG categories, three of five firms that developed cochlear implant devices for the United States have left the market, and no new firms have entered the market. "The prospective payment system has heightened the financial uncertainty of hospitals, predictably increasing their aversion to taking greater financial risks. . . . Evidence is accumulating that hospitals are not adopting new forms of technology because they anticipate ongoing losses."[28]

In summary, although still hotly debated,[29] the overhaul of the payment system for Medicare and Medicaid patients (1983)—with prices set by the government for nearly 500 different illnesses and treatments, stringent peer review procedures, ranking of hospital mortality rates, ranking of nursing homes, and so forth—has resulted in remarkable changes. Hospital stays have been shortened, outpatient treatment has been increased (from 19% of all surgery in 1981 to 40% in 1986), and home care has been encouraged (35% of American hospitals in 1988, as compared to 6.5% in 1976).[30]

However, 40% of the nation's 5,728 hospitals claim they now lose money when treating Medicare patients. Poor patients are quickly transferred to other institutions (a practice known as "dumping"), and many rural and inner city hospitals have been closed. At the same time, patients are asked to pay more in increased premiums and deductibles.

Health Maintenance Organizations (HMOs). Another way to keep costs down is through a prepayment plan (capitation fee) that admits a member to a so-called health maintenance organization that emphasizes prevention, health promotion, and use of outpatient services rather than hospitalization.

> During the last decade, growth in health maintenance organizations (HMOs) has resulted in a substantial increase in the number of people receiving prepaid mental health care. Proponents of prepaid plans . . . claim that they reduce the cost of mental health care by up to 50%, and provide adequate care for 90% of psychiatric problems.[31]

Federally mandated benefits include a minimum of 20 outpatient visits and 30 days of hospitalization. But contracts may exclude certain member groups—for example, the mentally retarded, or persons with organic psychosis or intractable personality disorders. Additional restrictions may include a requirement of "medical necessity," cost sharing, copayments and deductibles, mandatory periods between hospitalizations, and a lifetime ceiling on benefits. The use of gatekeepers, triage systems, and waiting lists are still other ways that utilization can be controlled.

The federal Health Maintenance Organization Act defines the basic health services the HMOs must provide. These include alcoholism, drug abuse, and mental illness care, but *parity with medical services is not required*. A typical HMO allows unlimited *medical* office visits and 365 acute care inpatient days with little or no copayment. This discrimination is hard to accept for several reasons. First, it has been shown that treatment for mental illness has an "offset" effect—that is, it reduces the demand for medical care, especially inpatient care.[32] Second, the separation of mental from medical disorders is arbitrary and unrealistic, since psychosomatic and somatopsychic illnesses are highly interrelated. Third, patients are encouraged under present conditions to present emotional complaints in the guise of physical ailments.[33]

Increasingly in the 1980s, HMOs are programs included under managed care. Large companies may have many HMO contracts, and they must monitor HMO costs; often HMOs begin by offering attractive rates, but rates may rise steeply once the provider system is established. Rates may rise with changes in community rates and higher administrative costs. Companies will find it necessary to obtain cost and utilization data in order to evaluate HMO effectiveness and to select the best HMO programs from among the many now competing in the field.[34]

The HMO industry has grown at a very rapid pace—since 1980, the enrollment has increased approximately 20% per annum. In 1986, there were 626 operational HMOs in the United States, with a total enrollment of about 26 million. In recent years a decided shift from not-for-profit to for-profit models has been noted, and concomitantly, a shift to use of individual practice association models rather than staff and group models of service providers (see below). More and more small HMO industries have been replaced by multistate networks of HMOs linked by common ownership and management.[35]

Three primary organizational models of HMOs have emerged:

1. The staff model, in which the HMO hires professionals to give services in an HMO's facility
2. The group model, in which the HMO contracts with a group of physicians to provide services to constituents (where two or more groups provide services, this is referred to as a network system)
3. The individual practice association (IPA) model, in which the HMO contracts with individual physicians to provide services that do not require the practitioner to alter his practice in other respects.

One expert in health care economics, Dennis Staton,[36] avers that HMOs resist providing mental health care, impose severe coverage limitations, and undertreat or ignore psychiatric symptomatology: "Chronically ill patients will continue to threaten all pre-paid systems and will be referred to the public sector."

Preferred Provider Organizations (PPOs). Patients who enroll as PPO members agree to select their physicians and hospitals from among those that have contracted with a corporation of insurance companies to provide services at lower cost. This, in effect, throws physicians and hospitals in competition with each other to attract clients—who are particularly important to hospitals if the inpatient census is close to, or below, the break-even point.

Employee Assistance Programs (EAPs).[37] Today's employee assistance programs grew out of the employee-counseling movement that began at the turn of the century. (The initial focus was on alcoholism.) Growth has been phenomenal in recent years, with approximately 2,000 EAPs established in the United States between 1972 and 1982; by 1984, the total number had increased to 8,000. More than half of the largest companies in the United States provide alcoholism services alone or in combination with clinical counseling on a variety of human troubles: conflicts among supervisors, peers, or subordinates; absenteeism; substance abuse; family discord; financial or legal problems; or undiagnosed psychiatric disorders.[38]

The Report of the American Psychiatric Association Committee on Occupational Psychiatry[39] indicates that 10% to 12% of the U.S. work force experiences serious personal problems, and an estimated 10 million workers suffer from alcohol abuse or dependency. The report cites a 52% improvement in attendance among employees who had sought help from EAP counselors. Health care costs decreased concomitantly.

Troubled employees come to the attention of EAP staff either self-referred or referred by management because of impaired work performance. The predominant services are (a) off-site counseling through a private provider, (b) short-term outpatient counseling, (c) employee assessment and referral, (d) on-site counseling, (e) inpatient hospitalization, and (f) long-term outpatient counseling. (These modalities are listed according to probable frequency of use in a variety of companies.) The EAP also functions as a liaison between employee and community, and between employee and management. EAPs often provide help not only to the employee but also to his family members; expenditures for children have grown more than expenditures for family.

The role for psychiatrists is a rich one. Psychiatrists serve as supervisors of nonpsychiatric helpers; as diagnosticians to distinguish psychiatric from nonpsychiatric illness; as educators, psychotherapists, medication supervisors, and general consultants. The psychiatrist is in a good position, also, to consult with middle and senior management about their interpersonal and organizational problems.

The *Wall Street Journal*[40] quotes a four-year study of mental health treatment at McDonnell Douglas Corporation. The conclusions underline the cost-benefit values of EAP, and assert that industry is demonstrating growing sophistication in comprehending the long-term values of comprehensive care. "Our approach is to provide whatever level of treatment is warranted by the assessment, rather than focus on short-term cost-containment objectives," said the McDonnell Douglas spokesman. A crucial component is the company's insistence that the whole family be included in treatment. Families of employees treated for chemical dependency *outside* of the EAP consumed an average of $8,400 more in medical services over four years than families who used EAP mental health treatment.

Other highlights of the study:

- Over four years, employees who used the EAP for chemical dependency treatment missed 44% fewer workdays, had 81% lower attrition, and filed $7,300 less in health-care claims than those who did not use the EAP.
- Forty percent of employees treated outside the EAP for alcoholism left the company within four years, compared with just 7.5% of those who used the EAP.
- Employees who sought mental health care through HMOs were four to five times more likely to quit or be fired within four years than those who used the EAP.

Managed Mental Health Care (Utilization Management)

Employers who pay for employee assistance plans, whatever their advantages, have nevertheless been stunned by the rapid escalation of costs of their benefit packages. Annual increases ranging from 15% to 30% for mental and nervous conditions have been reported.[41] Ten years ago, mental health benefits typically comprised 5% to 10% of total medical plan costs. Today, many large companies have seen this grow to 10% to 25% of total costs, and the mental health components are growing faster than medical costs in general.[42] Prudential, the largest insurance company in the world, covers 20 million Americans. Twelve years ago they developed a number of HMOs, eventually expanding to 30 cities and 1.8 million subscribers. Kaiser, the leader in the field, has 3 million people covered by HMOs.[43] Small wonder, therefore, that organizations with great investments in health care have turned to managed care, which claims to offer substantial savings without compromising quality of care.

A recent study (National Medical Audit) reviewed by Anderson[44] tells us that specialized management combined with preferred provider (PPO) services can reduce hospitalization of mental health/chemical-dependency cases by approximately one-half compared to nonspecialized review. There were no significant differences in quality of care as rated by reviewers (all board-certified psychiatrists). Inpatient utilization of services was reduced by an average of more than nine days per case, with a potential savings of $500 per day and an estimated savings of $4,500 per case. Mahoney estimates savings of 20% or more over traditional mental health care;[45] Feldman estimates savings as high as 40% or more in some programs.[46]

Managed care systems are dependent chiefly on two elements for effective results: the gatekeeper, and the provider organization. The gatekeeper is responsible for assessing patient needs, making a diagnosis, referring to an appropriate provider within the network, and monitoring progress. The provider network consists of the professionals needed to give quality treatment. Gatekeepers must consistently supervise and audit provider practice plans; in order to ensure control of the management system, they must also approve financial payments. Provider organizations offer discounts of 12% to 20% in return for gatekeeper referrals.[47]

Despite glowing accounts, managed care (utilization management) has been subjected to some harsh criticism. In a recent debate at the annual American Psychiatric Association convention, managed care was attacked as a "wild, unregulated, unbridled growth industry"[48] that operates on the basis of harassment and intrusion into the clinical treatment plan. Treatment goals, it was said, are tailored to fit economic definitions, and quality care is definitely not enhanced. Often, patients are treated in ambulatory care situations where active suicidal and homicidal tendencies should have dictated inpatient treatment. Sharfstein,[49] in particular, is critical of managed care, concluding that it is a threat to the patient–doctor relationship, to professional judgment, to the freedom to define a practice, and to ethical obligations to patients. Outcome research, said Doherty,[50] is urgently needed before taking any further premature leaps into managed care.

If managed care organizations are the "watchers" of patient treatment to ensure that money is spent wisely, some may ask, who will watch the watchers? The answer is suggested in the recent report by Sederer and St. Clair[51] in Massachusetts. New organizations have sprung up concerned with supervising and/or regulating the activities of managed care systems. For example, in Philadelphia, the Philadelphia Psychiatric Alliance is interested in monitoring managed systems, identifying poor systems and negotiating for better ones. The Physicians Association of New Haven County analyzes managed care contracts for prospective physician providers. The American Psychiatric Association has a task force on professional practice issues in managed care settings that develops guidelines for practice in staff model HMOs; it calls for government monitoring of marketing and advertising practices of managed care systems. The Massachusetts Psychiatric Society would develop criteria for certification of managed care systems, and would give approvals. It would also certify and monitor utilization review organizations: what services to allow, credentials and privileges granted the staff, and appeals mechanisms where denials of benefits are claimed.

Taking a historical view, we see that 50 years ago the psychiatrist and patient met together in a personal relationship dedicated toward helping the patient overcome his illness. The fees were fixed between them. If hospitalization was involved, the main pathway was through a state or county hospital (often remote from the patient's home) where admission was usually involuntary, the environment sterile and often frightening, illness chronic, and hospitalization prolonged. With the growth of the private sector and of psychiatric care in general hospitals, the situation was greatly relieved for those who could afford it. With the advent of Medicare and Medicaid, third parties stepped in both to assist in paying for the patient's treatment and to begin to monitor the type of treatment received.

More recently, as a result of continuing uncontrolled costs, a fourth element has emerged—namely, the managed care systems, which control admission to care, and all aspects of treatment on an individual basis. Managed care favors ambulatory care over hospitalization, pharmacotherapy over psychotherapy, and (where effective and financially feasible) alternative care such as day hospital, outpatient substance-abuse detoxification and rehabilitation.

Finally, a fifth element has become involved. Professional organizations, open to partnership with the state, are seeking to monitor managed care systems to make sure that the service they sell is not damaging to quality of care, or to the traditional values of humanitarian medicine.

Summary and Comments

Let me summarize what may appear to the reader as a very changing, confusing economic picture in mental health financing.

Historically, the deinstitutionalization movement must be regarded as one of the greatest events ever to affect mental health in this country. To a considerable extent, it was a post–World War II phenomenon that began in 1955 with extensive studies of the Joint Commission on Mental Illness and Health. Implementation was facilitated mainly in the 1960s and 1970s through the support of Presidents Kennedy and Johnson, the National Institute of Mental Health, the states, the American Psychiatric Association, and dozens of lay and professional organizations. In essence, the program called for rapid depopulation of state, county, and federal hospitals, shifting of treatment from intramural to extramural settings, construction and staffing of hundreds of small community mental health centers in populated areas, transitional and community facilities, community education, mobilization of citizen participation and support, and a very large expansion of training and research. Financing was mainly through federal grants for construction and staffing, plus state support, as well as additional support from public and private sources whenever it could be obtained.

The program was a success insofar as it reduced the population of governmental institutions greatly, expanded outpatient care, concentrated on the health of defined populations, and greatly increased citizen participation and involvement. The goals of expanded training of mental health professionals, research, and public education were to a large extent realized.

During this period, a veritable explosion occurred in private-sector involvement in mental health care and treatment, manifested by a great increase in private beds, many new services, and a concomitant increase in public demand for services. Health care costs—including costs for mental illness care—quickly ran out of control, fostering a very great effort both in the public and private sector to control escalation. The causes of the boom in health care and in runaway costs were numerous, including heavy advertising, great unmet needs for psychiatric services, inflation in the general economy, increased insurance coverage for mental illness, an aging population, adolescent turmoil, the drug culture, and (to an extent) the reduced stigma of mental illness in the public mind.

Health care coverage by the federal government and independent insurance companies became big business. One of the earliest and most important ventures in the private arena was Blue Cross and Blue Shield, and the most important in the public area was Medicare and Medicaid. Many private insurance carriers then quickly entered the field, bringing most working Americans under their protective umbrella.

The next most important approaches to controlling costs featured a shift in insurance philosophy from reimbursement of charges submitted by treating practitioners and facilities to prospective payment plans. These in effect solidified the control of third parties over clinical practice. The center of gravity shifted from physician control of costs and practice standards to payer control; the fiduciary relationship between doctor and patient was now severely impacted by a contractual economic relationship with an outside party. Understandably, this has been very hard for caregivers to swallow.

The names of the more prominent plans (now household words) are diagnostic related groups (DRGs), health maintenance organizations (HMOs), and employee assistance programs (EAPs). That these plans are effective in reducing costs is fairly well established. But whether they are too strongly dependent on the bottom line—and therefore not conducive to supporting quality care and treatment of the patient—is the question. Few will argue that the practice of medicine is now less gratifying to many practitioners than a generation ago.

The final instrument used by health carriers to effect a slowdown in cost escalation is managed care (utilization management), which monitors admission of patients to inpatient vis-à-vis ambulatory care, tries to reduce hospitalization time and use of costly procedures, and favors brief therapy over prolonged interpersonal relationships. Whether managed care is finally an unwanted intrusion into clinical care, a threat to the ethical obligations to the patient, a crippling camisole upon professional judgment, or an effective way out of economic chaos is now being hotly debated.

The economic picture has recently become further complicated by major fiscal deficiencies at the federal and state levels, the threatened business recession, increased costs of insurance coverage, and reduced payments to providers. The ramifications of these conditions have been corrosive, particularly in the mental health field. Many hospitals, both urban and rural, have gone out of business. Patients experience more difficulty gaining access to treatment. Many physicians cannot afford to treat Medicaid patients. Ethical/social dilemmas arise from pressure to serve lower-risk patients and to turn away chronic patients. And some physicians working for managed care systems, it is alleged, have been co-opted by accepting a risk-sharing partnership role with the company.

CONCEPTS AND TECHNIQUES USED IN BALANCING THE BUDGET

Because cuts in funding levels appear to be part of the administrator's life today, it is appropriate to review here methods used in balancing budgets. Before undertaking this task, let me point out that in the first years of austerity, the problem of balancing budgets was relatively easy and certainly less painful than subsequently. Administrators were asked to reduce budgets by a small amount—say, 5%—to "remove the fat." This supposedly would not affect the quality of services in any way. Many administrators went along with this charade, proclaiming publicly that service levels and efficiency would be maintained. At the next budget cut, however (perhaps another 5%), it was soon clear that service levels would have to be lowered, quantitatively or qualitatively. As a matter of fact, if service levels did not fall by this time, the administrator had probably been wasting resources.

The first decision facing management in the event of budget cuts is whether to cut by a given percentage across the board or to make selective reductions in services or programs. The latter, more often the choice, requires a reappraisal of priorities of present and future programs. To be considered are community needs and demands, the hospital mission as expressed in formal or informal documents, numbers and acuity of patients serviced, staff rights (e.g., seniority and expertise), labor contracts (including protective employment agreements), and political impacts. The unwavering goal, however, is to effect the savings mandated by those who control the budget.

Techniques to Effect Savings on Personnel

Since in most organizations personnel costs constitute the largest items of expenditures, usually 70% to 80% of the total budget, obviously any serious budget reduction sooner or later affects personnel. Medical personnel— that is, doctors—yield the largest savings of any category. Of late, nursing personnel have been in such short supply that the problem here is rather to recruit more nurses so that necessary programs can survive. In turn, this translates into funding nurse substitutes capable of carrying out duties that do not require highly specialized training, or signing up nurses from an outside registry where, unfortunately, per diem fees may be so high as to impose an unwanted drain upon the treasury.

Save by Reductions of Personnel

Savings through manipulation of personnel fall into the following categories:

1. No new hirings
2. Delays in hirings
3. Freeze hirings
4. Utilize personnel with lower-level training and expertise to carry out some of the functions of more expensive personnel
5. Reduce size of staff
6. Start "bumping"
7. Use part-time employees or consultants

No New Hirings. Plans for new programs or expansion and/or enrichment of old programs are abandoned; everything goes on hold. Exceptions may be made in some areas if the "holds" in other areas are sufficient to balance the budget.

Delays in Hirings. Replacements of personnel vacancies are possible, but only after a mandated period of delay. The delay may be long or short, depending on the importance of the job to be filled and the depth of budget cuts. With deep cuts, the hiatus may be prolonged; with superficial cuts, delays may be short. Management estimates the expected number of turnovers in a given period of time, and then figures out how much delay on the average, and in what personnel categories, will be needed to meet the deficit. Management must be aware that when the budget is tight, personnel tend to cling to their jobs, and vacancies tend to decrease in number. This is a tricky factor that has to be anticipated. It results, naturally, in extension of those vacancies that do arise to make up for the reduced turnovers.

To facilitate budget balancing by this device, administrators ask for justification for replacement of each vacant position; then, armed with this information, they make the final delay decision. At this point, therefore, program decisions are made not by clinical personnel but primarily by management with two factors in mind: the overall size of cuts to be made within a definitive time period, and the relative priorities and importance of programs as seen from the perspective of the institution as a whole.

Freeze in Hirings. In this case, each termination means in effect a loss of staff—a very unhappy event both for applicants hoping to be hired and for those who continue on the job, for the freeze puts a terrible load on remaining staff (particularly if attempts are made to keep units of service up). In austere times, indeed this is the goal: Reduce expenditures but keep revenue high. Under these conditions, morale falls, staff is overloaded, and patients receive less attention. Moreover, during special periods—days off for vacation, sick leave, family emergencies, educational leave, jury duty, and so on—services are seriously jeopardized, and staff coverage becomes dangerously thin. Staff educational activities, which give life blood to all institutions, particularly academically oriented institutions, are curtailed or neglected. When the freeze lifts, some personnel who have held on during the crisis decide they have had enough and leave.

Use Lower-Level Operatives.   As caregiving professionals are sacrificed to the maws of the budget crisis, pride in the proper care of patients gives way to erosion of professional standards and professional integrity. Ways to keep quality up by using less well-trained personnel to do jobs carried out by trained professionals are explored. Volunteers, for example, can help in such functions as escorting patients to other parts of the hospital for special tests, answering the phone, ward clerking, and supervising patients in a variety of activities where an additional reliable hand is needed. During the most severe period of a nursing shortage I witnessed, mature students from the university were recruited to assist nurses, and many of them did yeoman work. To be sure, they must be carefully instructed and monitored before they comprehend the subtleties of interpersonal work and can be trusted to use good judgment. Another device was to invite social-work students, already partially professionalized, to work with nurses on the ward. This was so successful that for a time the development of an intermediary specialty involving the skills of the two professions was contemplated.

Reduce Size of the Regular Labor Force.   This is the action that hurts the most. If a reduction in staff hits only one or a few departments, then openings may be sought for these personnel in other departments that are still allowed to hire. If not, openings may be sought in other hospitals or facilities belonging to the same administrative system. If this does not work, in some organizations "bumping" becomes the order of the day—a concession to seniority in which the senior employee in one area bumps a less senior employee in another area; after a chain of such events, the least tenured persons are pushed out of the system. In the view of many experts, bumping is a harsh and demoralizing process and should be used only as a last resort.

The bumping process tries to preserve workers' seniority rights, and as such has been justified by labor and management over the years. Unfortunately, it is founded on the principle that workers can be fitted into positions in different units like parts in an automobile factory. The facts are that the bumped person may not only lose status and income for which he has strived for years, but in addition, he loses his place within a human relations group that sustained his morale. With supportive friendships broken, loss of salary, and perhaps also longer travel time to get to the new job, the bumping process creates stresses all along the line.

Use Part-Time Employees and Consultants.   Devices of this sort aimed to reduce personnel expenditures include: reduce full-time people to part-time people; hire part-time people to replace full-timers when vacancies arise; reduce part-time people to even less time; and/or employ consultants to replace full-timers, or even part-timers, where this amounts to savings. The following comments are relevant to the use of these techniques:

- Reduction from full-time to part-time work in some systems cannot be accomplished without the incumbent's approval, except if the incumbent occupies his position as a temporary employee.
- Hiring part-time people to replace full-timers is often used successfully when the loss of a full-timer is too much for the program to bear and the part-timer makes the loss less traumatic, or where a good part-timer is able to carry out the most important functions of the full-timer with skill and dispatch.
- Employing part-time consultants to carry out tasks formerly carried out by regular employees has the (budgetary) virtues that the pay may be even less than that for part-timers, the consultant can be terminated more readily, and, in many systems, the consultant receives no perquisites. (Part-timers, too, may not receive perquisites if time spent is below a specified level.)

As an example of the last item above, in building up a psychopharmacology service in a county hospital where money was scarce and psychopharmacological expertise in short supply, part-time consultation was arranged with a psychopharmacologist of note from a nearby VA medical center where he was already employed at seven-eighths time. The plan was eminently successful. Not only did this distinguished teacher make rounds and provide specific bedside instruction for residents and staff, but he also made himself available by phone at all hours for specific advice and consultation.

Save through Reductions in Equipment, Supplies, and Telephone Charges

Although not as obviously as reductions in personnel, savings through reduction of equipment and supply costs can also affect staff morale and patient services greatly. One of the first economies concerns use of telephone by staff for personal calls; this requires special monitoring, with justification of all outside calls. However, imagine the frustrations of a social worker when told that outside calls must now be individually approved by management, or the chagrin of research personnel when the photocopy machine—afflicted by recurrent breakdowns—must be tolerated until the next budget year, when it may (or may not) be replaced by secondhand equipment. Repairs and maintenance activities are slowed down. Bathrooms and corridors are not assiduously cleaned; the environment is allowed to deteriorate. Travel allotments are cut, and—a final assault on dignity—professional personnel are ordered to sign in and out and to indicate time spent, hour by hour, on specific tasks. The savings may be significant, but the costs to morale and efficiency must always be kept in mind by administration.

Techniques Related to Increasing Revenue

The other side of the task of balancing the budget is increasing revenue. The following categories cover the most commonly used approaches:

1. Increase referrals
2. Speed up patient turnover
3. Increase and/or monitor charges
4. Itemize billing
5. Change the mix of patients
6. Develop and/or expand programs
7. Advertise
8. Start a fund-raising campaign

Increase Referrals

Oftentimes, referrals of new patients lag because referral sources either have lost touch or have been enticed elsewhere by more vigorous public relations and marketing programs. The following questions must be answered when intake suffers:

- Are referral sources gratefully acknowledged for the cases they do refer? Do they have clinical privileges, and do they feel welcome to visit their patients and participate in their treatment? Is there a financial gain to the referring persons in doing this? Are reports rendered to them at appropriate intervals? Is the patient referred back to them for further care? Is there a personal bond between referring physicians and the hospital physicians in charge?
- Are educational programs of value to the referral sources sponsored regularly by the institution? Are news bulletins and updates mailed regularly?
- Does the receiving hospital sponsor regular social events for the referring parties?
- Are open-house events sponsored by the hospital for referring physicians and other referring agencies?

Speed Up Turnover of Clients

Shorter inpatient hospitalization usually means increased intensity of patient care, higher reimbursements, and fewer days denied for payment by Medicare and other third-party payers.

Increase and/or Monitor Charges

In hospitals where rates can be set by management to reflect rising costs, this is a powerful tool for keeping revenue in line with expenditures. Rate setting becomes, then, a regular (usually annual) event. In addition, careful monitoring of eligibility of applicants for approval by Medicare or other payers is essential, for slippage here leads to losses and bad debts. Intensity of monitoring and follow-up of debtors is then titrated so as to yield greatest effectiveness in terms of revenue.

Itemize Billing

Itemized billing is generally superior as a revenue enhancer to all-inclusive rates. Itemized billing is a familiar process in private institutions (for-profit and not-for-profit), as well as in university hospitals that depend on third parties, but is not used as extensively in government hospitals, where all-inclusive per diem rates are generally the mode. Accounting procedures can be humongous tasks in maintaining itemized billing and probably are not cost-effective for many governmental hospitals.

Change the Mix of Patients

As third-party payers reduce rates through the use of diagnostic related groups (DRGs) or whatever other mechanisms, hospitals can no longer afford the burden of free humanitarian care. In teaching hospitals, costs of teaching staff and trainees are also heaped upon per diem rates of covered clients. Thus, on admission and throughout inpatient care, greater attention today is being paid to patient mix. In urban hospitals, the pressure to look after destitute homeless patients is great, and in some jurisdictions, pressure on hospitals is multiplied by county/state phaseouts of ambulatory care clinics. Insofar as care of indigents is not being handled by properly funded public systems of care, an unfair burden may be imposed upon nongovernmental systems.

Develop New Programs or Expand Old Ones

New programs and procedures of value to patients are emerging all the time. For example, laboratory tests to monitor neuroleptics arise as new drugs come upon the market. A device that identifies early motor signs of tardive dyskinesia may prove valuable as a diagnostic/preventive tool. Services for adolescent mentally ill and for substance-abuse cases are increasingly popular and constitute a major source of income. Hospice wards for dying patients, and now dedicated units for AIDS patients, are springing up in some places. Third-party reimbursement follows the trend, but with a variable lag as affordable rates are worked out for the public.

Advertise

Word of mouth is a great channel for spreading the good news about a high quality therapeutic institution; and maintenance of high quality care is a sine qua non for long term fiscal health. But reliance on word of mouth to augment referrals, although very important, may turn out to be a rather slow technique of market penetration. Today, hospitals must undertake vigorous short-term (as well as long-term) public relations/marketing programs to succeed in an increasingly competitive arena.

Public relations for these purposes may be divided into two types—internal and external. Internal public relations aims to utilize staff, trainees, patients, families, and volunteers (i.e., those already related to the internal functioning of the hospital) as ambassadors of goodwill. These individuals may number in the thousands, often increasing with the years. Their ambassadorial effectiveness depends primarily on their level of morale and satisfaction with their jobs, and secondarily on how their public relations potentialities are mobilized and organized. Obviously, employees of an institution with deteriorated internal relations are going to scare others away. Administrators concerned with internal relations should show interest, respect, and caring for these internal constituents. Staff, spouses, friends, and trainees are often the first to assist in development of volunteer services, gift shops, and beautification programs. Trainees, many of whom settle around the mother institution, become the referring personnel of tomorrow; patients and families may join community associations dedicated to enhancing the welfare of patients. There is a public relations gold mine here that is not sufficiently utilized in many institutions.

External advertising/public relations cannot develop in a planning vacuum. Immediate and long-term programs require careful thought and planning together with manpower identified specifically for these functions. The overall picture emphasizes image on the one hand, and specific attractive programs on the other.

Image making concentrates on developing goodwill and high reputation by projecting positive symbols characterizing the institution, glorifying professionals of high reputation or charismatic valence, or popularizing concepts and services that catch the imagination. For example, Stanford University, in its public relations, makes repeated use of its tower for immediate identification and recognition. Menninger Foundation exalts the Menninger name, and especially in the early days, a picture of intensive, psychoanalytically oriented therapy for their patients. Universities make the most of their research and educational advantages, building upon the fact that they are the promulgators of the latest knowledge and techniques and are particularly outstanding in the treatment of tertiary cases. Their remarkable DeBakeys, Shumways, and Cooleys become nexuses around which an aura of greatness is fostered.

Specific programs include the latest in drug treatment, alcoholism, adolescence, geriatrics, Alzheimer's and related disorders, brain imaging, smoking addiction, or whatever the imaginative public relations people can dream up. At another level, a speakers' bureau aimed to educate professionals and laypeople and to build bonds to the hospital is a good idea. In addition, church groups and citizen organizations that stir up interest in mental health, developmental disabilities, children's disorders, alcoholism, schizophrenia, affective disorders, battered children, runaway youth, and so forth are extraordinarily ripe for cultivation as friends and supporters of the institution.

Start a Fund-Raising Campaign

As conventional sources of support diminish or dry up, it becomes necessary to search for new sources of revenue. Multiplication of funding streams contributes to security; diversification is just as important in putting hospital and clinic programs on a sound footing as it is in developing a portfolio of stocks building toward the future. Increasingly, administrators in recent years have turned to the private sector to supplement whatever support they receive from governmental agencies (as in the case of state, county, and federal institutions) or third-party insurance, community groups, and private foundations (as in the case of corporate-based structures). The program should be worked out with an experienced development officer backed up by appropriate assistants. Start-up costs may be considerable, and planning will be both short- and long-term. Moreover, the efforts of the development officer must be coordinated with those of the individuals responsible for public relations and marketing, and many other individuals in the system may be called upon for support and cooperation. The naive notion that hiring a fund-raiser automatically increases contributions to the institution will soon be replaced by the reality that the development office functions mainly to elicit and organize the efforts of others.

A proper campaign first constructs a picture of what is needed by the institution for maintenance and development of current programs, and what is needed at the growing edge to ensure the institution's future. Capital projects, service programs, educational programs, and research and development needs are explored. How much is needed in each category, and how should those needs be formulated in the most attractive terms? What foundations, eleemosynary institutions, public and private potential donors, and constituents may be tapped? Potential donors must be researched in detail to establish their pattern of giving and areas of special interest and to formulate a plan of approach. Considerable sensitivity to and understanding of the potential donor's psychology and motivation is important. In particular, it should be understood that the development of a relationship of trust and confidence between development officers and the donor may be a long process. Thus, most campaigns take years to reach final goals. Feedback to constituents and the public as to progress in meeting those goals is necessary both during the campaign and thereafter—the latter to assure benefactors that their expectations are being met.

Contributions that come from bequests, the sale of land or property, or specialized arrangements with insurance companies require the expertise of lawyers and accountants. The experienced fund-raiser will tell the prospective donor that his contribution may be either *restricted* or *unrestricted*. Restricted contributions are designated for a particular program or project; the unrestricted contribution is disbursed at the discretion of the institution. The former type of giving is by far the most popular—often 90% of total giving. But the latter is extremely valuable because of the great need for financial flexibility in many enterprises where resource control is severely limited.

A further word about fund-raising is in order. As more and more health facilities of the nation depend on revenue raised from generous citizens, community organizations, foundations, friends, grateful patients or their family members, and staff members, they need the inspired collaboration of hospital administration, public relations personnel, and the professional staff. Several points should be noted:

1. To raise money one must *ask* people, associations, and foundations. Anyone who suffers a narcissistic wound if turned down by a potential donor is not fit for the job. The successful fund-raiser is enthusiastic because the program or project is worthy, and because the donor will gain much satisfaction from the joy of giving. But *ask* one must.
2. Fund-raising is easier if the potential donor believes that personnel in the institution are behind the project not only morally, but also with their own donations, however small they may be.
3. Donors become interested through the development of trusting, *personal* relationships over months or years.
4. Donors are interested in projects that have a deeply personal meaning for them.
5. Projects that honor a famous and beloved individual, or are aimed at the conquest of a specific disease, or relate to construction of a facility to house a worthy program are usually easier to fund than those that are general or merely conceptual.
6. Unrestricted funds, given for the use of management at its discretion, are hardest to come by but often most helpful to administrators tied by tight line-item budgetary rules.
7. In approaching grateful patients for donations, the administration should face the ethical question as to *when* and *how* an approach would be effective and justified. A patient suddenly relieved of heavy anxiety relative to a feared diagnosis of cancer should be allowed to settle down to a normal level before making a major financial commitment. He should not reflect later that the institution took advantage of his elation. The sophisticated institution will wait until the patient is discharged from care and a suitable interval has elapsed so as to permit mature reflection to modulate his generosity.

The interplay of political/economic forces, coping mechanisms, and survival strategies in the face of draconian cuts is dramatically illustrated in the following case.

Case Illustration

Draconian Cuts

It came to pass in California in 1989, as a result of population growth and subsequent greater demands upon the mental health service system (unfortunately coupled with a progressive depletion of resources), that a long-heralded crisis faced the state and counties, together with their local hospitals and clinics. The revenue picture had been very bad for years. It was not to be suspected from a glance at the total state budget, for in the year 1989, the budget was well over $40 billion, greater than that of all but a few *nations* of the world. The budget crisis for health and mental health arose from the fact that demands for many programs related to education, crime and safety, drugs, pollution, highway congestion, roads, gangs, and so forth were so strong that mental health—with low citizen and legislative support, poor public relations, and a poor image—could not get the attention it needed. Despite the size of the overall state budget, it yet was limited by special voter initiatives of 1978 and 1979 that greatly reduced revenue from domiciliary taxes and limited spending to population and cost-of-living increases. As "low men on the totem pole" with inadequate constituent support, fewer and fewer dollars trickled down to the poor mental patients.

In 1989, the word went out that many of the community clinics were scheduled for closure. It was estimated that this would release around 25,000 dependent patients onto the streets, or acute hospital services, or relatives and friends. Perhaps some patients with insurance coverage would find refuge in private care. The problem was further compounded by the fact that the state and county hospitals were also scheduled for draconian cuts, in addition to previous yearly curtailments.

At this point, advocacy lawyers got together to gain an injunction against closure of clinics on the basis that reductions in services would visit great hardship upon the population. An injunction was indeed granted by a superior court judge, and the clinics remained open. However, during the period of fearful anticipation of loss of services and loss of jobs, both staff and patients began to look elsewhere. At the same time, supervisors in the county of Los Angeles, at a loss for funds to keep clinics open and unable to raise additional money from the state, mounted an action for repeal of the original injunction with the state supreme court.

A critical incident occurred at this time in which a social worker at a somewhat denuded clinic (but one not necessarily targeted for total closure) was stabbed to death by a paranoid client overwrought by the tensions and uncertainties of a chaotic system. This happening received massive media attention and was used by the opponents of reductions in services as a warning of what would happen if seriously disturbed patients were abandoned by their therapists and thrust on their own. On the other hand, proponents of closure—those county officials responsible for implementing draconian cuts, come what may—used the incident to point out that the clinics were now in such disarray due to disaffected staff leaving for other jobs that the safety of remaining staff and patients could not be protected, and closure was the only alternative. Statements were made that patients could receive care in other county or state facilities. High-sounding words such as *consolidation* and *reorganization* were used, but in fact no replacement services were offered.

The most recent event in this sorry tale is that the supreme court of California has upheld the right of the county supervisors to close the clinics, although no satisfactory arrangements for care of deprived patients had been made.

This has shifted the scene of action to the state legislature, already hard-pressed by a multitude of petitioners for other causes. Thousands of patients, family members, and service providers descended upon Sacramento early in May 1989 to plead the cause and to try to stay the disaster. A conservative Republican governor used the plight of the mentally ill as a political bargaining chip with Democratic leaders to attain cuts in other areas. This battle between a Republic governor and Democratic leaders has been a very sorry scene, reflecting little credit on the ability of the citizens of California, our richest state, to look after their own.

However, a most recent burst of sunlight on the dismal scene has been the discovery of a tax windfall of between $1.9 and $2.5 billion. How the legislature will deal with this unexpected gift, how it will squirm out of the straitjacket of spending restraints, and whether enough will trickle down to rescue the county systems of health and mental health remains a mystery. Stay tuned.

This crisis in California illustrates the interplay of laws restricting the freedom of the legislature to raise taxes with political and judicial forces clamoring for better care for the mentally ill. In turn, social priorities concerning the place of the mentally ill in the esteem of the body politic are involved. In the end, the large legal-political-economic imperatives determine the fate of services to the mentally ill.

Risk Management[52]*

One constant and sometimes severe drain on the budget is the cost of settling claims of malpractice, neglect, lack of informed consent, and wrongful death, brought by aggrieved patients or relatives against the hospital or specific personnel. "The time, energy, anguish and money spent in preparation and defense, even if a suit is groundless, can shake the confidence and stability of the most skilled and sophisticated practitioner."[53]

The Malpractice Crisis

Malpractice insurance costs for the individual practitioner have sky-rocketed, particularly in the specialties of obstetrics/gynecology, general surgery, and orthopedics. (Some 60% of obstetricians, for example, have been sued at least once in their careers.) "The AMA reports that prior to 1981 an average of 3.2 claims per 100 physicians were made annually. Between 1981

---

*I am indebted to Carolyn Rhee, assistant administrator and risk manager at Los Angeles County–Olive View Medical Center, for sharing her knowledge of the program at the center.

and 1984 the rate increased to 8.2/100 and in 1985 it reached 10.1/100 physicians. . . . Not only have the number of suits increased, but judges and juries have increased the amounts awarded to successful claimants."[54]

In hospitals, staff physicians are generally protected by risk management departments whose work includes three elements: (a) *risk financing*, which investigates malpractice insurance coverage; (b) *malpractice claims management*, the processing of claims pending against the institution or its physicians or others; (c) a *risk management program* that identifies liability and endeavors to reduce risk by incident analysis, case study, and broad-based education.

Risk management systems vary. In the county of Los Angeles, individual hospitals have risk management departments that work with a professional risk management company whose lawyers advise on all potential cases, identify liability, prepare for litigation, represent the hospital and/or its personnel in court, and negotiate settlements. The professional management team, in the case of Los Angeles, is hired by the county department of health services. Claims against hospitals are paid by the individual hospitals. The total of payments for all facilities for a given year may be as high as $30 million. A typical hospital may pay approximately 1% to 2% of its overall budget in malpractice claims, but this percentage can vary widely on a year-by-year basis.

Patient satisfaction with the treatment received is all-important. A common cause of complaints is the anger and frustration that arise when patients feel they are handled impersonally or neglected. "No one listened to me," they say. Aside from hurt feelings, however, the fact is that malpractice claims are too often based on malpractice per se, for which the best defense is high-quality clinical care, including trust and free communication between doctor and patient.

In recent years, two major trends have contributed to the escalation of malpractice claims. The first relates to legislation and judicial decisions that have defined and broadened patients' rights—for example, judicial decisions on the right to treatment, the right to refuse treatment, and the duty to warn/protect (*Tarasoff*). Clarification of due process regarding admission, retention, and discharge; consent to treatment; and civil rights has expanded the liberties that patients enjoy and increased their voice in treatment. At the same time, it has limited the freedom of caregivers and made them more wary and responsible. The second factor relates to the growing sophistication of the public concerning medical and mental illness, and their rights to adequate and appropriate care. With the help of eager lawyers, the public has asserted these rights.

Patient–physician relationships are often central to the instigation of malpractice suits. An idea that has considerable currency is that financial compensation is due the patient if *anything* goes wrong, whether or not it results from physician error. Some patients feel there is always something that can be done to cure a condition; many are wary about physician recommendations and are ready to seek a second opinion.[55] Their suspiciousness of doctors' motivations is heightened by press reminders that some physicians are amoral or motivated only by the dollar sign. Finally, poor relationships between doctor and patient, lack of courtesy, hostile attitudes, and angry responses to questions or challenges to authority promote patient ire and may lead to litigation.

Risk Areas Warning List

The following areas have been identified by Kull[56] as the most common and costly areas of suits against psychiatrists:

1. Improper diagnosis and treatment
2. Wrongful commitment
3. Failure to secure an informed consent
4. Failure to assess, foresee, or prevent suicide
5. Failure to assess, foresee, or take precautions against homicide
6. Failure to assess, diagnose, and warn against tardive dyskinesia
7. Forced medication
8. Improper seclusion or restraint
9. Breach of confidentiality
10. Failure to warn and/or protect victims
11. Failure to provide reasonable aftercare and follow-up
12. Undue familiarity

The risk management department becomes alerted through incident reports provided by the medical staff. Risk management lawyers encourage staff members to report everything that has the slightest relevance, whether or not a claim is likely to result. Nurses are very good at reporting incidents; doctors are less conscientious. About 10% of incidents reported in one Los Angeles County hospital (Olive View Medical Center) become claims, and of these only one-third become lawsuits. Once claims are filed, lawyers and doctors work together, analyze records, and identify areas of vulnerability. It is very important that records be legible and that all abbreviations are interpretable readily from an approved list. Risk lawyers then coach defendants as to court procedures and practices. Wherever possible, defendants' names are deleted from claims so that no one person is liable. Finally, it should be noted that not all mistakes of personnel are covered by malpractice. For example, undue familiarity is outside the scope of malpractice and in all likelihood will not be defended by the designated risk management team.

Risk Reduction

Besides high-quality clinical staff and careful attention to patients' needs, fears, anxieties, and frustrations, what other measures may be taken to heighten awareness and reduce liability? Risk reduction is a function of the whole institution—management, physicians, and staff workers. The whole institution must be alerted to the potential heavy costs of lawsuits and unexpectedly large settlements.

A hospital medico-legal committee that reviews cases, keeps abreast of legal developments, and conducts grand rounds as well as teaching sessions for patients is a good idea. This group works directly with the hospital risk management department and assists in developing a data base that can track trends over time. The focus should be on major sources of critical incidents, and on those personnel and practices responsible for an excessive number of patient and family discontents.

Many states are alert to the need to address the malpractice crisis. Some states permit countersuits. Others reduce the time during which a person can bring suit (in effect, establishing a statute of limitations). More than 35 states have passed laws limiting malpractice awards and claims; a no-fault system has been suggested. Clarification of "standards of care" is desirable: Should it be based on a local standard or (as has been argued) on a national standard, given the free availability of the medical literature and modern media communication? Some states have abolished punitive damages altogether.[57]

Physician self-policing methods should be strengthened (e.g., more stringent peer review, and improved continuing education programs). Relicensing and recertification procedures should be expanded.

The malpractice crisis has changed the practice of medicine substantially. "Defensive medicine" has become the watchword. Patients and physicians both are more wary of each other. Physicians want to know which patients are inclined to sue, and patients want to check practitioners' lawsuit records. The cost of treatment goes up as more tests are ordered. Expenses for legal services escalate, while larger and larger settlements are ordered by the courts. It has been estimated that 12% to 25% of the increase in health care costs is attributable to malpractice fears and associated preventive maneuvers.[58]

Summary and Comments

Superseding most other considerations in administration is the necessity to balance the budget. Projections are made months and years ahead, and continuous monitoring of income against expenditures at regular, frequent intervals during the given year is necessary. The consequences of an unbalanced budget are serious. In some systems the administrator in charge is fined and/or subject to additional sanctions, including dismissal if the budget remains unbalanced. No system can long endure in debt without serious cutbacks in services, legal actions from creditors, loss of constituents, loss of reputation, bankruptcy, or organizational death. The consequences for patients and employees are shattering.

Techniques available to administration both to reduce expenditures and to augment revenues are discussed briefly in this chapter. The list is not exhaustive. In these austere times, balancing the budget requires the courage and toughness to resist the heartfelt entreaties of committed staff and needy patients. It also requires a great deal of thought, energy, and imagination to reorganize and make do with diminished resources.

The first decision facing management in the event of budget cuts is whether to cut across the board or to make selective reductions in services and programs. It is not an easy decision and requires considerable study and the wise weighing of many factors.

Savings through reduction of personnel is an early consideration, since personnel account for the majority of expenditures in most organizations. Mechanisms discussed in this chapter for accomplishing such savings include no new hirings, delay in hirings, freezing hirings, utilizing personnel with lower levels of training and expertise, reducing the total size of staff, and utilizing part-time employees or consultants. Further savings may be effected through reduction of equipment and supplies, or restrictions in use of such items as pharmaceuticals and telephone services.

Ways of increasing revenue are also vigorously explored when the budget ax falls. The following cover the most commonly used approaches: increased referrals to the facility from outside professionals or agencies, speeding up patient turnovers, increased charges and/or monitoring charges more closely, itemized billing, changing the mix of patients, development and/or expansion of programs, advertising, and starting a fund-raising campaign.

A fund-raising program of significant magnitude usually requires the advice and participation of expert personnel, together with the cooperation of public relations and marketing experts. Sensitivity toward and understanding of potential donors' psychology and motivations is important. Unrestricted funds are of exceptional value inasmuch as they increase administrative flexibility in the use of dollars.

In fund-raising, a specialty all its own, a rigorous program of solicitation should be projected, offering a variety of opportunities to excite the interest and imagination of prospective donors, emphasizing in particular programs and projects that may have personal meaning to the philanthropist. It is well to remember that a warm and trusting relationship with a prospective donor may take months or years to develop. Ethical problems in this field relate to when and how to ask for support from interested parties.

One possible severe drain on the budget is the cost of settling claims for malpractice, neglect, lack of informed consent, or wrongful death. Malpractice insurance costs have skyrocketed, particularly in the specialties of obstetrics/gynecology, general surgery, and orthopedics. Risk management departments help reduce claims and settlements by studying malpractice insurance coverage, the handling of claims, and by organizing a risk management program that includes case study and staff education. Patient–physician and patient–staff relationships are a key factor in the number of claims filed. Lack of courtesy and hostile-aggressive behavior must be avoided. The practice of defensive medicine as a preventive against liability suits is growing—a contemporary phenomenon that is understandable, but highly regrettable.

REFERENCES

1. McGuire TG: Growth of a field in policy research: The economics of mental health. Admin & Policy in Mental Health 17:165–175, 1990
2. Joint Commission on Mental Illness and Health: Action for Mental Health: Final Report. New York, Basic Books, 1961
3. Feldman S: Managed mental health: Ideas and issues. Paper presented at American College of Mental Health Administration, annual meeting, Santa Fe, New Mexico, April 1, 1989 (unpublished)
4. Feldman S: Managed mental health: Ideas and issues. Paper presented at American College of Mental Health Administration, annual meeting, Santa Fe, New Mexico, April 1, 1989 (unpublished)
5. RAND Corporation: Practices Governing Mental Health Policies. Santa Monica, California, RAND Corporation, 1984
6. England MJ: Emerging leadership in insurance in managed mental health. Presented at American Psychiatric Association, 142nd Annual Meeting, in symposium, Managed Mental Health: Problems and Prospects for Psychiatry, May 9, 1989, San Francisco, California
7. Chodoff P: Effects of the new economic climate on psychotherapeutic practice. Amer J Psychiatry 144:1293–1297, 1987
8. Chodoff P: Effects of the new economic climate on psychotherapeutic practice. Amer J Psychiatry 144:1293–1297, 1987
9. Dorwart RA, Schlesinger M: Privatization of psychiatric services. Amer J Psychiatry 145:543–553, 1988
10. Dorwart, RA, Epstein S, Davidson H: The shifting balance of public and private inpatient psychiatric services: Implications for administrators. Admin & Policy in Mental Health 16:4–13, 1988
11. Dorwart RA, Schlesinger M: Privatization of psychiatric services. Amer J Psychiatry 145:543–553, 1988
12. Dorwart RA, Schlesinger M: Privatization of psychiatric services. Amer J Psychiatry 145:543–553, 1988
13. Dorwart RA, Schlesinger M: Privatization of psychiatric services. Amer J Psychiatry 145:543–553, 1988
14. Dorwart RA, Schlesinger M: Privatization of psychiatric services. Amer J Psychiatry 145:543–553, 1988
15. Dorwart, RA, Epstein S, Davidson H: The shifting balance of public and private inpatient psychiatric services: Implications for administrators. Admin & Policy in Mental Health 16:4–13, 1988
16. Roemer MI: Development of health care coverage. UCLA Health Insights 7(5):2, 5, May 1989
17. English JT, McCarrick RG: The economics of psychiatry, in Kaplan HI, Sadock, BJ (eds): Comprehensive Textbook of Psychiatry, Fifth Edition. Baltimore, Maryland, Williams & Wilkins, 1989, pp 2074–2083
18. Brice RC: Financing of psychiatric services, in Talbott JA, Kaplan SR (eds): Psychiatric Administration. New York, Grune & Stratton, 1983, pp 357–366
19. U.S. Department of Health and Human Services, Health Care Financing Administration: The Medicare Handbook. Washington, D.C., U.S. Government Printing Office, Publication No. HCFA 19950, 1989, p 4
20. U.S. Department of Health and Human Services, Health Care Financing Administration: The Medicare Handbook. Washington, D.C., U.S. Government Printing Office, Publication No. HCFA 19950, 1989, p 4
21. Staton D: Mental health care economics and the future of psychiatric practice. Psychiatr Annals 19:421–427, 1989
22. Conklin TJ: Quality assurance, in Talbott JA, Kaplan SR (eds): Psychiatric Administration. New York, Grune & Stratton, 1983, pp 273–285
23. Greenblatt M: Discussion of Dr. Robert Gibson's paper entitled Peer review and PSRO, in Proceedings of Conference on The Crisis in Psychiatric Care and Insurance Coverage, sponsored by American Association for Social Psychiatry; Congressman James H. Scheur (D-N.Y.); and Human Service Group/American Health Services, Inc., Washington, D.C., June 11–12, 1976. Cambridge, Mass., Ballinger Books, 1978

24. Gibson RW, Levenson AI: Private psychiatric hospitals, in Talbott JA, Kaplan SR (eds): Psychiatric Administration. New York, Grune & Stratton, 1983, pp 89–101
25. Wehrmacher WH: Critical condition: American health care in jeopardy. Internal Med 9:81–85, 1988
26. English JT, McCarrick RG: The economics of psychiatry, in Kaplan HI, Sadock, BJ (eds): Comprehensive Textbook of Psychiatry, Fifth Edition. Baltimore, Maryland, Williams & Wilkins Co., 1989, pp 2074–2083
27. Kane NM, Manoukian PD: The effect of the Medicare prospective payment system on the adoption of new technology: The case of cochlear implants. NE J Med, 321:1378–1383, 1989
28. Kane NM, Manoukian PD: The effect of the Medicare prospective payment system on the adoption of new technology: The case of cochlear implants. NE J Med, 321:1378–1383, 1989
29. Kiesler CA, Morton TL: Prospective payment system for inpatient psychiatry. The advantages of controversy. Amer Psychologist 43:141–150, 1988
30. Malcolm AH: In health care policy, the latest word is fiscal. Living with the Reagan era's cost consciousness. New York Times, October 23, 1988, p E3
31. Altman L, Goldstein J: Impact of HMO model type on mental health service delivery: Variations in treatment and approaches. Admin in Mental Health 15:246–261, 1988
32. Goldman W: Mental health and substance abuse services in HMOs. Admin in Mental Health 15:189–199, 1988
33. Hornbrook MC: Mental health services in HMOs. An oxymoron? Admin in Mental Health 15:236–245, 1988
34. Wermert JF: Managing HMOs performance. Health Cost Management 5:11–19, 1988
35. Shandle M, Christianson JB: The organization of mental health care delivery in HMOs. Admin in Mental Health 15:201–225, 1988
36. Staton D: Mental health care economics and the future of psychiatric practice. Psychiatr Annals 19:421–427, 1989
37. Staton D: Mental health care economics and the future of psychiatric practice. Psychiatr Annals 19:421–427, 1989
38. American Psychiatric Assoc Committee on Occupational Psychiatry: Employee assistance programs and the role of the psychiatrists: Report of the Committee on Occupational Psychiatry. Amer J Psychiatry 146:690–694, 1989
39. American Psychiatric Assoc Committee on Occupational Psychiatry: Employee assistance programs and the role of the psychiatrists: Report of the Committee on Occupational Psychiatry. Amer J Psychiatry 146:6909–694, 1989
40. Winslow R: Spending to cut mental-health costs. Wall Street Journal, December 13, 1989
41. Mahoney JJ: How to manage managed mental health. National Underwriter, 91:52–53, 1987
42. Anderson DF: How effective is managed mental health care? Business & Health 7:34–35, 1989
43. England MJ: Emerging leadership in insurance in managed mental health. Presented at American Psychiatric Association, 142nd Annual Meeting, in symposium, Managed Mental Health: Problems and Prospects for Psychiatry, May 9, 1989, San Francisco, California
44. Anderson DF: How effective is managed mental health care? Business & Health 7:34–35, 1989
45. Mahoney JJ: How to manage managed mental health. National Underwriter, 91:52–53, 1987
46. Feldman S: Managed mental health: Ideas and issues. Paper presented at American College of Mental Health Administration, annual meeting, Santa FE, New Mexico, April 1, 1989 (unpublished)
47. Mahoney JJ: How to manage managed mental health. National Underwriter, 91:52–53, 1987
48. Harrington BS: Report on pros and cons of managed care aired in annual meeting debate. Psychiat News XXV(13):4, 24, 25, July 6, 1990
49. Harrington BS: Report on pros and cons of managed care aired in annual meeting debate. Psychiat News XXV(13):4, 24, 25, July 6, 1990
50. Harrington BS: Report on pros and cons of managed care aired in annual meeting debate. Psychiat News XXV(13):4, 24, 25, July 6, 1990
51. Sederer LI, St. Clair RL: Managed care and the Massachusetts experience. Amer J Psychiatry 196:1142–1148, 1989
52. Kull RK: Risk management: Avoiding the frontal malpractice assault. Carrier Foundation Letter, No. 140:1–4, February 1989
53. Kull RK: Risk management: Avoiding the frontal malpractice assault. Carrier Foundation Letter, NO. 140:1–4, February 1989

54. Stoline A, Weiner JP: The malpractice crisis, Chapter 12 in Stoline A. Weiner JP: The New Medical Marketplace: A Physician's Guide to the Health Care Revolution. Baltimore, Maryland: Johns Hopkins University Press, 1988, pp 143–155
55. Stoline A, Weiner JP: The malpractice crisis, Chapter 12 in Stoline A, Weiner JP: The New Medical Marketplace: A Physician's Guide to the Health Care Revolution. Baltimore, Maryland: Johns Hopkins University Press, 1988, pp 143–155
56. Kull RK: Risk management: Avoiding the frontal malpractice assault. Carrier Foundation Letter, No. 140:1–4, February 1989
57. Stoline A, Weiner JP: The malpractice crisis, Chapter 12 in Stoline A, Weiner JP: The New Medical Marketplace: A Physician's Guide to the Health Care Revolution. Baltimore, Maryland: Johns Hopkins University Press, 1988, pp 143–155
58. Stoline A, Weiner JP: The malpractice crisis, Chapter 12 in Stoline A, Weiner JP: The New Medical Marketplace: A Physician's Guide to the Health Care Revolution. Baltimore, Maryland: Johns Hopkins University Press, 1988, 143–155

8

Ethics of Administration

Ethics in medicine has become prominent in recent years as a result of the numerous social and technological changes in health practice, many of which are beyond the comprehension of the average citizen. In particular, medicine's increased ability to modify behavior and to prolong life has given rise to philosophical and ethical questions. A decline in political and professional authority after World War II[1] (including the authority of physicians), together with growing public concern about the behavior of persons who possess unusual power or expertise, has resulted in great media attention to situations of moral/ethical conflict.[2,3,4,5,6,7] Let us begin this odyssey with the patient.

On entering a general hospital, the patient is quickly stripped of dignity and autonomy.[8] Confined to a room and a bed, his civilian clothes are immediately removed. He must learn to manipulate hospital garb, with its inadequate coverage of the body. Nurses, orderlies, and physicians come and go as they do their work, often without knocking. Visiting hours are restricted; and in child care units, children are separated from their parents.

Hospitals have a right to refuse treatment to those who do not have the means. Socioeconomic level and type of insurance coverage to a large extent determine the quality and type of care received. With all this, a great deal of one's comfort and relief of apprehension depends primarily on the doctor, who is often very busy and may be overloaded with other patient responsibilities. Thus, dependency grows as confidence in the physician and the institution may be strained.

In psychiatry, more than in other branches of medicine, the law allows a declaration of incompetence, as well as involuntary detention and evaluation and even involuntary *treatment* of mentally ill patients. Such denial of normal human rights gives rise to public challenges to the power given to all physicians and especially to psychiatrists.[9]

Thus, there is little wonder that we are now greatly concerned with so many ethical and legal issues such as due process, informed consent, the right to adequate and appropriate treatment, the right to refuse treatment, the criteria for incompetence, equal access to treatment, equitable distribution of health resources, treatment under the least restrictive conditions, confidentiality, and conflict of interest in pursuing therapeutic goals.[10,11,12,13,14,15,16] We are also greatly concerned with research on human subjects and the withholding or withdrawal of life-sustaining measures.

In the past, physicians were less sensitive to the cost consequences of their clinical decisions than is the case today. They were responsible for the care of patients and for the conscience of the profession, while the payer was responsible for the financial burden. But times have changed greatly. Although the physician is still the guardian of medicine as a moral enterprise, he must now balance clinical acumen with conscience and cost; to make his task more difficult, this must be done under the scrutiny of powerful third parties. With all these changes, the physician's special place in society is still based on his unique knowledge and technical skill and the responsibilities invested in him by law. His primary responsibility in the midst of all these changes, however, is still to employ his unique knowledge and skills for the benefit of the patient, ethically and with the fullest use of his curative powers.[17]

HISTORY

The Hippocratic oath (see Appendix A toward the end of this chapter), promulgated in the 5th century B.C., is commonly regarded as the historical cornerstone guiding physicians' ethical conduct. Its tenets have been scrutinized for centuries, and although many believe the oath is out of date, its popularity as an historical landmark has endured. Under the influence of the Christian church, the Hippocratic oath enjoyed widespread use around the 10th century A.D. Many of its moral pronouncements are accepted unchanged today, such as its admonition to make the healing of the patient the primary concern of the physician, to refrain from doing harm, to respect confidentiality, and to treat patients within the limits of one's competence. It encourages a bond of trust between the patient, physician, and medical profession, and prohibits sexual relations with patients "both male and female persons, be they free or slaves."

The oath is clearly based on social values and relationships characteristic of those earlier times. Its prohibition against abortion, for example, is viewed differently today. Also, modern technology, with its advanced life support systems, has raised questions about the right to die and the physician's role in prolonging life where the quality of life has deteriorated. The Hippocratic guidelines are directed primarily to the conduct of the physician; they do not spell out the rights of patients, which, as is well-known, have been greatly elaborated in the last few decades. Further objections have been raised against an implied paternalism, for the oath treats the patient like a child or dependent member of a family.[18]

Finally, the oath, written in primitive times, makes no mention of group medicine or systems of delivery of care, nor does it touch upon the complexities of therapeutic organizations or the special ethical/moral problems besetting the administrator.

In the United States, the American Medical Association's Principles of Medical Ethics were first adopted in 1847, with the latest version coming forth in 1980. (See AMA Principles of Medical Ethics, Appendix B of this chapter.) The AMA principles broaden the physician's responsibilities to include not only the patient but also society and other health professionals. It expects physicians to respect the law and to expose those physicians who may be deficient in character and competence. It imposes an obligation to change the law where it is found contrary to the best interests of the patient. The physician must study and advance his scientific knowledge, share information with relevant others, and utilize the expertise of other professionals when indicated. Although the individual practitioner is free to choose whom he will serve, he must nevertheless "participate in activities contributing to an improved community."

In 1982, an unexpected surprise occurred when the Supreme Court allowed a lower court to bar the AMA from making any prohibitive references to advertisement and the soliciting of patients. This, in effect, shook the conceptual and ethical image of the profession of medicine severely, for up to this time numerous references had been made in successive revisions of the AMA code to the effect that advertising was incompatible with honorable standing in the profession. For a long time, advertising had been regarded as distinctly unprofessional and demeaning, as it tended to classify physicians with charlatans.

The Supreme Court decision emphasized the *trade* rather than the *professional* status of medicine, forcing physicians to compete as did other trades in the marketplace and thus to give the public the advantages of open competition among physicians and specialists. As indicated above, this was a serious blow to the self-image of the profession. In effect, the courts and the public viewed the medical profession as a self-serving organization intent on controlling supply and demand in the interest of maintaining high incomes. Self-regulation of medicine has therefore to an extent crossed over to market regulation, wherein the doctor is now the provider, the public is the consumer, and "product differentiation" by the public is the determinant of which provider will attract business.

In this instance, the law attempted to define what should be accepted as ethical behavior by the medical profession; however, the profession has been far from satisfied. The two motives—service to patients and economic gain—

that had always been in potential conflict were now rawly exposed in the highest court, with a shift in balance toward the economic side being the unhappy result.[19]

It should be noted that while this issue is still controversial insofar as the private practitioner is concerned, the private *institutions,* on the other hand—whether for-profit or not-for-profit—have been carrying on vigorous marketing activities for years. As third-party payments have been cut back and more corporate health facilities have come into the field, this competition has become exceptionally keen. Every day the public is bombarded by advertisements touting the merits of substance-abuse programs, adolescent services, or programs for elderly patients with dementia, with heavy emphasis on the quality of services offered.

In psychiatry, the AMA principles of ethics have been accepted with "annotations applicable to psychiatry." A special added draft for psychiatrists offered by Maurice Levine[20] in 1972 stresses the importance in psychiatric practice of self-observation and self-criticism. The psychiatrist must be aware of his own motivations and reactions in his treatment of the patient, and be prepared to seek additional supervision where countertransference feelings appear to prejudice the psychotherapeutic relationship.

Until 1970, medical ethics was largely the domain of the physician. Since that time, other professionals (in psychology, nursing, social work, and rehabilitation) have come into the field, and still other disciplines (theology, philosophy, law, behavioral science, and sociology) have become involved.[21] As Nisbet[22] has noted, there has been a decline of traditional social and moral authority in the West in the 20th century, and along with it a rise of hedonism and egalitarianism. Loss of trust and belief in the physician's moral integrity and loss of confidence in his dedication to humane values may be the results of this change in public attitude.

ETHICS AND THE LAW

Ethics and the law are intimately intertwined; however, they are not identical. Ethics deals with right versus wrong and with principles of desirable conduct, regardless of what the law says. Persons of high ethical principles do normally respect the law in their everyday life, though they may feel impelled to change the law to correspond to their ethical values. Some individuals feel so strongly about their ethical/moral beliefs that they choose drastic measures, even martyrdom, to assert their convictions. Great moral leaders like Martin Luther King, Jr., and Mahatma Gandhi have changed the course of nations by rallying masses around principles such as human rights and *satyagraha.*

The law may consecrate ethical principles through the decisions of courts or parliamentary bodies, but generally, the law becomes written after events have occurred that require rulings on matters of rights and justice. Ethics, on the other hand, exists as feelings and beliefs about right and wrong that exist long before acts are committed that demand legal intervention. Laws often appear absolute, but they are mostly arrived at through compromises among points of view—for the existence of the body of law depends on a majority willing to abide by it. Ethics reflects highly individualized beliefs not easily forced into compromise, as indeed there is often no practical necessity for it.

Although law and ethics often do coincide, there are instances when they do not.[23] An *ethical but illegal* situation may prevail, for example, when one thinks it appropriate to eliminate life supports for humanitarian reasons, even though the act is clearly illegal. At the institutional level, one may believe it is ethical to do something to drive competitors out of the market, although some of the tactics may be interpreted as illegal.

Legal but unethical situations can exist, as when a hospital administrator allows a physician of questionable competence to practice in an institution merely because the institution needs a higher census and more revenue. *Unethical and illegal* situations may arise when grossly discriminatory practices are allowed in a hospital, or when a public official is "bought off" in order to secure a certificate of need.

ETHICAL PRINCIPLES

Ethical principles have evolved in the hope of putting the complicated field of ethics in some reasonable order. The principles are numerous, just as the ethical quandaries met in life are numerous. It is difficult to arrange these principles in a hierarchy wherein a given principle is regarded as more important than others; the principles are not absolute. Much depends on the nuances of the specific life situations or clinical conditions that are being examined. These situations are best resolved when bright minds from various fields of thought and with varying perspectives seek consensus through argument and persuasion. However, in some ethical dilemmas, consensus appears impossible, and important controversies remain unresolved.

Ethical principles become immediately active as soon as one contemplates psychiatric intervention. The most important of these are the principles of beneficence, nonmaleficence, respect for persons, and justice.[24]

The principles of *beneficence* and its counterpart *nonmaleficence*[25] assert that the physician or mental health caregiver above all should do good and avoid harm. The Latin phrase *primum non nocere* (above all, do no harm) summarizes the concept very well. Only when that principle is satisfied should a physician intervene to relieve suffering and to assist nature in the healing process. Some believe that one of the physician's prime responsibilities is to prolong life, but this usually follows after efforts to relieve acute suffering.

Since many treatments carry risks and may produce side effects, the beneficence principle must often be modified by the *utilitarian* principle (i.e., the benefits must outweigh the risks). For example, when a patient presents with right lower quadrant pain, fever, and elevated white count, a diagnosis of acute appendicitis may lead to an operation, but the operation per se with the accompanying anesthesia is not without risk. If the diagnosis is correct, removal of the appendix leads to full recovery, but not before the patient (in the postoperative course) may temporarily experience more pain and discomfort than before surgery. Here the expected benefit outweighs the risks. Even in making the diagnosis, however, a risk is assumed that it may be wrong. Then all efforts and suffering have been in vain, and the treatment team has wasted time going in the wrong direction.

How then is the utilitarian principle different from the beneficence principle? There is indeed considerable overlap. The principle of utilitarianism basically says that the rightness or wrongness of an action is to be determined by the *consequences* of that action, and not by anything intrinsic in the act itself. These consequences usually have to do with "promoting happiness" or enhancing the "general welfare."

The principle of *respect for persons* presupposes that the physician has the welfare of the individual in mind as his highest priority at all times. It is close to, and overlaps with, the right to self-determination (autonomy). In psychiatry, as in other branches of medicine, we are interested in restoring function and maximizing competency. Since the patient's illness manifests itself in many areas of functioning, uncertainty arises as to which areas, functions, and competencies should become the prime targets. Should it be restoration of self-esteem; improved insight; relief of symptoms; return to job, family, and society; and/or a return to school and other educational endeavors?

The principle of *justice* applies in two contexts. One has to do with the availability of psychiatric attention and resources sufficient to give the patient his full opportunity to get well. The other is the proper distribution of therapeutic efforts and resources among a number of patients clamoring for attention when those resources are in limited supply. This latter problem impinges on issues of equitable access and other dilemmas that apply especially to ethics involved in the administration of systems of care.

Another principle that some regard as equal in importance to the principle of beneficence is the principle of *autonomy*.[26] It is founded on the right to self-determination. Operationally, in any medical intervention, this principle is honored by the process of gaining *informed consent*, which Redlich states is the cardinal principle governing doctor–patient relations and the fundamental ethical basis for *any* intervention.[27]

Informed Consent

Plaut[28] discusses the ethics of informed consent in a succinct, instructive paper. The relation between a physician and his patient is fiduciary, hence it imposes a duty of full disclosure. This principle has become all-important since the revelations of horrible Nazi experimentation on humans during

World War II. In the 1960s, the civil rights movement stimulated a reemphasis on individual autonomy. Watergate, too, contributed insofar as it resulted in a general loss of trust in authority.

What must be disclosed in informed consent?*[29]

1. The *nature* of the procedure. Here the question is how much detail must be disclosed.
2. The *purpose* of the intervention. Both diagnostic and therapeutic purposes must be served.
3. *Risks* of all procedures. Standards regarding details of disclosure vary from jurisdiction to jurisdiction; is it *full* disclosure of all risks, conformity with community practice standards, or standard fiduciary obligations under product liability law?
4. Disclosure of *benefits* poses few ethical problems. The physician must guard against exaggerating the potential benefits.
5. *Alternative treatments* must be discussed so that the patients can appreciate what is likely to happen if nothing is done, or if other options are pursued.

Plaut mentioned four exceptions that may be made to the above five requirements. The first is when an *emergency* dictates that procedures must be undertaken even if informed consent cannot be obtained from the patient or kin. The definition of emergency is up to the physician and should be carefully explicated in the record. The second is when a *waiver* may be allowed, as in the case in which the patient specifically requests not to be informed. In this instance, the physician must be assured that the patient is competent to choose a waiver. The physician's ethical decision here is to balance the values of the patient's autonomy against his right to health.

Incompetence of a patient to give consent constitutes a third exception. This difficult decision hinges on the patient's understanding of his illness, his situation, and its gravity; the degree of his insight into the impairment of his own judgment; and the role of his physician and other caretakers. Judicial involvement is often necessary to make the final decision in many of these cases.

Finally, *therapeutic privilege*, in which the physician in effect substitutes his judgment for that of the patient in the interest of his health, is an ethically vexing question.

Plaut points out that in fully informed consent the patient should understand that confidentiality can be broken by (a) the physician, based on his duty to warn anyone whose life is threatened by the patient (per the *Tarasoff* ruling, discussed later); (b) the courts, which may subpoena records (as when the patient is in an automobile accident); and (c) the hospital, based on the fact that records are open to the gaze of employees and review organizations.

*Strictly speaking, it is not "consent" that must be informed, but the *patient* who must make a decision regarding consent.

Whether the physician should discuss the cost of care with a sick patient and how much his treatment plan should be affected by the bottom line are difficult questions to resolve. Budget shortfalls often determine the number of patients an institution can treat, the nature of the treatment, the length of hospitalization, and the adequacy of aftercare. It would be highly unethical to select a more expensive treatment over a less expensive one where the latter would be perfectly adequate. And it would be equally unethical to extend the hospital stay of a patient who can pay over one who cannot pay. Yet these practices may occur, dictated often by the necessity for institutional survival. It is important also to note that when a physician is employed by a hospital, or is a participant in its financial support, he must resist as far as possible letting financial considerations affect his clinical judgment.

Finally, Gutheil et al.,[30] suggest that obtaining informed consent need not be a mere formality, but instead can be a focal point for the formation of a therapeutic alliance: "The patient becomes a coexperimenter rather than [a] passive object of experimentation." The alliance is strengthened by the mutual acceptance of problems and uncertainties involved in the practice of medicine.

The principle of autonomy is also linked to the principle of *privacy*, which is greatly respected everywhere as a basic human right. Privacy means personal control of access to one's body or mind; in law, it is linked to freedom from intrusion by the state or a third person. If competent, an individual must be free to make his own decisions. If incompetent, decisions may be made by the court or by a guardian or conservator appointed by the court. (Considerable writings in law define conditions under which an individual may be regarded as incompetent and thus deprived of freedom.) The principles of *confidentiality* and *privilege* arise as corollaries to the notion of privacy. In confidentiality, communications from the patient to the physician are held in trust and may not be released abroad without the patient's consent. It is elemental in holding onto the patient's trust, so he may be free to divulge what is troubling him and thereby make healing possible. *Privilege* refers to the right of persons acting on behalf of the patient in a judicial or quasi-judicial setting to withhold confidential information entrusted to them.

Finally, to complete the list of primary ethical principles, there is the principle of *concern for the general welfare*. This broadens the range of ethical considerations enormously, for it not only touches on the question of equitable access, but also on the allocation of resources in short supply and the decision in critical times as to who shall survive. Much has been said in recent years to the effect that all patients should have a right to adequate and appropriate treatment, but we see instead an increasing reduction of treatment benefits to many individuals in the population.[31]

Concern for the general welfare has also been the basis for laws to prevent the spread of infectious disease, as well as laws that require reporting of gunshot wounds, child and elderly abuse, and fraudulent practice by colleagues. Emphasizing the point also is the *Tarasoff* decision in California, in which the court ruled that psychotherapists have a duty to take reasonable steps to protect a third party when a patient has made threats in a psychotherapeutic setting.

However difficult it is to define ethical principles, it is even more difficult to apply them in practice. What is more, since they are often in conflict with one another, the very best judgment is necessary to serve the welfare of patients caught in complicated situations. For example, in *Tarasoff*, the ethical goal is to protect the third party, but without damage to the therapeutic relationship. In the case of depressed individuals who are competent, the principle of beneficence urges treatment of the patient, but a patient's refusal of treatment may be honored in keeping with the principle of autonomy and self-determination. In still another context, the laudable principle of concern for the general welfare runs aground upon the hard reality of discrimination against those who cannot pay.

THE RIGHTS OF PATIENTS

The long struggle for the rights of the mentally ill has been characterized by progressive inclusion of ethical principles into major judicial actions or into law through legislative initiatives. In a few short decades, the rights of patients have come strongly to the fore; the courts and the legislature have assumed responsibility in a sphere that formerly was primarily the realm of the physician. At the same time as patients' rights have been enunciated, the rights of professional caregivers to treat patients according to the best dictates of their profession have been eroded. While a great deal of attention has been paid to patient rights, and properly so, rather little has been said about the rights of physicians and other professionals who treat them—or, for that matter, to the rights of administrators who set the climate, govern the organization, and take much of the blame when things go wrong.

In this section, I will deal with the evolution of patient rights within a combined ethical, legal, and judicial context and also try to spell out a framework for a balance among the rights, privileges, and obligations of three parties—patients, caregivers, and managers.

Early actions on rights were attempts to atone for society's neglect of its mentally ill criminal offenders.[32] In the *Baxstrom* (1961) case in New York[33] the subject (a nondangerous person) was incarcerated in Dannemora, a New York institution for the mentally ill offender, long after penalty for the crime would normally have been served—merely because he was mentally ill. After a court trial, Baxstrom was eventually transferred to a civil institution for the mentally ill; he was followed by 900 other psychiatric offenders in the same category. Although there was much concern that mentally ill patients coming from institutions of such fearsome reputation as Dannemora would wreak havoc in civil facilities, these patients behaved as well as noncriminal mental cases, and eventually many were able to be discharged to the community.[34,35]

Massachusetts followed suit in 1967 after examination of 750 criminally insane individuals incarcerated in Bridgewater State Hospital. The results were similar to the experience in New York.[36,37]

In 1966, Judge Bazelon in the District of Columbia, in deciding about a man named Rouse—who had been imprisoned in a mental facility four times longer than any sentence could have been imposed for his crime of carrying a weapon without a license—ruled that since the man was not getting adequate treatment, he must be released. Thus, the judge declared that a mentally ill person being held against his will is entitled to *adequate and appropriate* treatment; lacking this, the institution has no right to retain him. This ruling became a landmark decision in relation to the right to freedom of involuntary patients.[38] Again in 1966 (*Lake v. Cameron*),[39] Judge Bazelon ruled that a person may not be confined for treatment if other, less restrictive, nonhospital facilities can be found. This became the doctrine of "the least restrictive alternative." A series of decisions in similar mental illness cases focused on how far the courts should go in establishing standards for adequate and appropriate treatment for prisoners who are involuntarily detained.[40,41,42,43,44]

The next steps in the rights of patients were taken not in relation to criminally incarcerated mentally ill persons as in the above, but in relation to *civil* commitment cases. The most famous occurred in Alabama in *Wyatt v. Stickney* (1971),[45] in which Judge Johnson of the federal district court found that care and treatment in the Alabama hospitals, both for the mentally ill and for the retarded, were inadequate by any standards. After much expert testimony, he declared the right to treatment to be a constitutional right and outlined standards in three fundamental areas: (a) humane psychological and physical environment, (b) qualified staff in sufficient numbers to administer adequate treatment, and (c) an individualized treatment plan. Despite the objections of Governor George Wallace at the time that the federal government was obtruding into the affairs of the state, and that Alabama did not have the resources to meet the standards set by the judge, Johnson insisted that the state must raise the funds to treat the patients properly or abandon its program altogether. He suggested the sale of state lands as one approach to raising money. Eventually, he appointed a master to ensure proper treatment for patients confined against their will.*

Wyatt (1971) in Alabama was soon followed by *Donaldson v. O'Connor* (1972) in Florida.[47] In *Donaldson* the court (the Fifth Circuit Court of Appeals) fined the superintendent and his assistant for retaining the plaintiff in Chatahoochee State Hospital for 15 years although he had received no treat-

---

*It is important to note that Stonewall Stickney, the first commissioner of Alabama, who took office in 1968, had initiated a series of reforms in Alabama's system. "In the waning days of Governor Brewer's administration, before Wallace took over," the Alabama institutions were integrated. A team approach was inaugurated, organized discharge planning was instituted, and families were encouraged to care for patients at home (p 130).[46]

ment. On appeal, the U.S. Supreme Court upheld the decision, declaring that the state may not constitutionally confine in a custodial institution a non-dangerous person capable of surviving on the outside with the help of friends or relatives. The high court added the concept of dangerousness as a standard for commitment but, notably, skirted the issue of a constitutional right to treatment (which the lower court had averred).

Since *Wyatt*, state after state has expanded the rights of patients. A new echelon of lawyers specializing in mental health law has emerged, and forensic psychiatry has received great new impetus as a specialty within clinical psychiatry and in the education of mental health professionals. Mechanisms for patient advocacy—for example, notably, the human rights board set up by Judge Johnson—and many other citizen groups, independently organized or instigated by legislative initiatives in the various states, have come to pass. Now, periodic patient-rights advocacy inspections of mental hospitals are required procedures in many states.

Johnson's treatment of the Alabama case is not only notable for his formulation of criteria in establishing adequate and appropriate treatment—and in his insistence on state responsibility to increase the resources designated for the mentally ill—but also for his great patience in allowing step-by-step progress toward his goals and in monitoring that progress directly from his office. The Alabama project has taken many years; staff had to be instructed in new attitudes and methods in patient care, new staff had to be recruited, and political reaction from conservative elements had to be dealt with.

The range of rights that flowed from *Wyatt* and from enlightened actions in other states has been very broad indeed.[48] Briefly summarized, these include the rights to privacy; to manage personal affairs; to marry or divorce; to register and vote; to hold professional, occupational, and vehicular licenses; to make a will; to take regular exercise; to enjoy religious worship; and to communicate with family, friends, doctor and/or lawyer, and the administrator of the mental health system responsible for the patient. The right to protection from harm was asserted in the *Willowbrook* case.[49] The right to treatment in the least restrictive alternative, as noted above, was asserted by Judge Bazelon (*Lake v. Cameron*, 1966).[50]

The right to receive compensation for work done in institutions was declared by Judge A. E. Robinson in District of Columbia federal court "as long as the institution derives any consequential economic benefit." This ended the practice of "institutional peonage," in which psychiatric facilities employed patients who for years would help run departments and services of hospitals, without compensation. Not infrequently in those days, if patients were good workers and the institution was short of employees, the patient's treatment program would take second place to the hospital's need for hands.

The above rights have been achieved on behalf of mentally ill adults through the efforts of men on the bench like Johnson, the efforts of the Civil Liberties Union, and enlightened initiatives in various states introduced by progressive legislators. Landmark achievements on behalf of the mentally retarded and children suffering from emotional disorders occurred in Pennsylvania (1971),[51] where the right to appropriate education was secured for retarded children.

Thus, in recent years important *ethical* concepts have been identified and incorporated into the judicial/legal annals of the federal government and the states. Where rights are to be withheld, the patient is entitled to a hearing by qualified representatives of the court and can be represented by counsel. Withholding of rights depends on a finding that the mentally ill patient is incompetent (except in cases of emergency), that the treatment is necessary to prevent danger to self or others, and that without treatment deterioration in the patient's condition would be expected (see the *Riese* case).[52]

Whereas a substantial body of law has developed concerning the right to treatment, a seemingly contradictory *right to refuse treatment* under certain conditions has also arisen.[53] Not only did *Wyatt* allow psychotic patients who were not adjudged incompetent to refuse electrotherapy and lobotomy, but so does California law (1971 Cal. Welfare and Institutional Code, Sec. 5325 (F) West Supp.).[54] *Winters v. Miller* (1971)[55] permitted mental patients to refuse medication on religious grounds. Recent California law restricts medication use on patients who refuse unless an emergency exists, or the patient is incompetent and a court approves the use of pharmacological agents.[56]

On the face of it, the right of psychotic, committed patients to refuse treatment is a triumph of the ethical principles of autonomy and self-determination. However, this right runs into complications and has been the subject of much controversy. If an acutely suicidal, but voluntary, patient refuses to give permission for electroconvulsive treatment, his life may be endangered by the delays involved in placing him on involuntary status and gaining court permission for treatment. Before that, around-the-clock suicide precautions, heavy doses of medication, or physical restraints might be necessary. Still another problem: A psychotic patient who intimidates other patients on the ward but refuses any therapeutic interventions may create a climate of apprehension, as well as command a virtual monopoly of staff time. These are situations that a staff fears; they lower morale and reduce therapeutic efficiency and effectiveness.

THE BALANCE OF RIGHTS, PRIVILEGES, AND RESPONSIBILITIES[57]

We have reached the point where we must think in terms not only of the rights of patients, but also of the balancing of rights, privileges, and responsibilities of three interdependent parties—the patient, therapeutic staff, and administration. The rights of patients cannot go so far as to cripple staff personnel's ability to carry out their professional roles effectively and with reasonable morale and freedom from fear. The rights of patients cannot go so far as to cripple management's ability to sustain morale, retain able employees, or recruit new employees under conditions (which, unfortunately, prevail too often) of low wages and shortages of trained staff. This leads to the concept of another right—that of *management,* through the coordinated efforts of all, to render the best possible service to constituents, to keep staff risks low and morale high, and to reduce the burden of complaints, litigations, and settlements that may jeopardize survival of the organization.

Patient Responsibilities

To balance the numerous rights that patients now possess, the following expectations should be considered as part of *their* responsibilities: They must not act aggressively toward others or destroy property, and they may be expected to do a number of ward chores, participate in ward society, cooperate in treatment, become free of chemical dependencies, utilize hospital services fully, become increasingly self-sufficient and able to leave the hospital, and become self-supporting and productive citizens.

Employees

Employees have many rights that they have gained through the years, either via civil service or labor contracts. Through grievance procedures or contact with labor representatives, they can obtain corrective action. More severe measures open to them, but not encouraged by management, are work slowdowns, mass sick calls, work stoppages, or strikes.

Gibson[58] in 1976 outlined a number of rights for medical staff that seem quite appropriate today. He included:

1. The right of staff to have sufficient resources to provide adequate health care [Budgetary shortfalls have challenged our concept of adequate care for the mentally ill. Shorter hospitalizations, reliance on pharmaceuticals, and inadequate aftercare have become more serious in recent years. It behooves mental health professionals to continue to press for quality care for all the mentally ill and for the resources needed to provide it.]
2. The right to participate in the allocation of resources and the setting of priorities
3. The right of staff to be accountable for clinical matters to the highest governing authority
4. The right of staff to the free and complete exercise of clinical judgment and skill
5. The right to have clinical practice reviewed by peers
6. The right of staff to practice without excessive and unnecessary regulations

Thus, in the main, the rights of patients and the rights of staff are *not* in conflict; together, patients and staff share a common goal—adequate health care for the mentally ill. To this I would add that here, too, management is vitally involved.

Workers' responsibilities are to keep foremost in their scale of values the lives and welfare of patients, and the necessity to cooperate with management in policies and programs and with all the members of the treatment team. They must conduct themselves ethically, avoiding conflicts of interest. They should strive to increase their skills in the art of caring for patients, to further the good name of the institution in the community, and to become ambassadors of goodwill on behalf of the mentally ill.

Management

Management has both the right and responsibility to conduct the business of its institution within the law, to admit qualified individuals for the best treatment it can supply, to be free and nondiscriminatory in the use of resources, to conduct business with dignity, honesty, and probity, and to represent the institution before the public. Management is expected to develop and maintain ties with outside agencies, institutions, and professional societies. Management also has the right and responsibility to declare emergencies when the institution is beset by strikes or physical catastrophes such as fires and earthquakes, to issue proper orders to staff, and to call upon emergency services in the community. Management must never cede any rights or privileges to labor that would make it difficult or impossible to provide services at satisfactory professional and ethical levels.

ETHICAL CHALLENGES FOR THE ADMINISTRATOR[59]

The practice of medicine is by its very nature an ethical enterprise. Insofar as the physician possesses unique skills, and the patient in sickness entrusts his body and mind to the physician, ethics is involved in every nuance of the doctor–patient relationship. The ethical concerns of the administrator, however, go beyond the individual one-to-one relationship to include relationships among many groups within the institution, as well as between the institution and outside individuals, agencies, societies, and institutions. Insofar as the administrator mediates between these elements, and/or apportions time and resources among them, he is engaged (so to speak) in a higher ethic, one that requires constant study, judgment, balance, conference with experts, and also critical self-examination. It is the ethical responsibility of the administrator to integrate to the best of his ability the many constituencies, agencies, and concerns in a complex, changing world.

Since the institution usually cannot serve all constituents ideally,[60] the administrator always feels a sense of inadequacy with respect to the underlying mandate of society to help secure "life, liberty, and the pursuit of happiness" for all. Scarce resources and compromises with optimal care are realities of life. As Kane[61] has so eloquently pointed out, society has thrust administrators into situations of discrimination against the poor and the near poor. It is a form of social Darwinism that leaves conscientious individuals in a state of perpetual unrest. This dilemma gives rise to still another ethical quandary: To what extent should the individual undertake social/political action to try to remedy a sorry state of affairs, and what should be the nature of that action—the writing of letters of petition (at the mild end), or civil disobedience (at the extreme)?

Inasmuch as the administrator is given power, he has an ethical responsibility to use that power wisely. He must recognize what *forms* of power are available for his use and understand their legal and moral boundaries. Russell,[62] Raven,[63,64,65] Galbraith,[66] McLelland,[67] and others[68,69] have developed taxonomies of power that would be useful for the administrator to know (see "Taxonomy of Power" in Chapter 11). The exercise of power with due respect for justice, autonomy, and respect for people is the great challenge. Power is exercised in the setting of policies for admission and treatment of patients, in standards of behavior for patients and staff, and in the hiring and firing of employees. Social power is exercised insofar as the administrator is usually the social leader of the organization; his comportment is a standard for others to follow. Among the difficult policy decisions the administrator may often make are those that relate to targeting of resources toward acute versus chronic patients, or elderly versus young patients;[70,71] the relative emphasis on research or education versus clinical services; and clinical/philosophical decisions as to the relative importance of somatic, pharmacologic, psychologic, or socially rehabilitative modalities of treatment.

In pursuit of the cost-containment objective, the question is how far to trade off quality care for cost—whether it is better to provide service of lower quality to the many, or service of higher quality to the few.[72,73] Finally, the supreme question: At what point in a deteriorating environment is it unethical to continue in the role as administrator as opposed to phasing out a program, or simply leaving the scene?

ETHICAL CONCERNS IN SPECIAL CLINICAL AREAS

Issues in Inpatient Practice[74,75]

The trend in recent years has been in the direction of "narrowing the criteria for involuntary hospitalization, strengthening the presumption of patient competence to make treatment decisions, and circumscribing the freedom of attending psychiatrists."[76] In some jurisdictions, the court itself rules on the competence of each case. As stated earlier, ethical considerations require that professionals be alert to the consequences of treatment delays on the welfare of other patients, families, and staff.

A moral obligation of the inpatient psychiatrist is to keep the patient's welfare primary in the midst of a number of influences from other quarters—the state, the courts, the insurance carriers, and regulatory and bureaucratic agencies. The intervention of the courts in recent decades unfortunately has fostered an adversarial climate of diminished trust, pitting the patient against the doctor and the institution. Likewise, the necessity to meet regulatory standards should not force an assumption that quality of care is equivalent to conformity to regulatory requirements. Nor should it be assumed that informed consent necessarily implies that the patient understands fully the nature of his illness, the significance of treatment proposed in relation to other possibilities, or that he is competent to make a wise choice among several treatment options. Specification of criteria for competence and presentation before the courts may be necessary where patient and psychiatrist disagree. Yet, we should never lose sight of the fact that patient wishes and choices are an all-important ingredient in trying to work out an optimal collaboration between the patient and his therapists.

Emergency Psychiatry[77]

In any emergency department, the patient has a right to appropriate and *timely* professional attention; however, the more acute the nature of his illness, the greater the necessity to make quick decisions. Concerns about the protection of patient and staff against violence make emergency care a highly vulnerable area. Specialized professional training and experience are very important in emergency services as compared to inpatient settings, where calm deliberation is more often possible. Precautions must be taken to remove harmful objects, weapons, and contraband; at times, restraints may be required. Sophisticated knowledge and use of medication are important. Information from the referring physician or agency and contact with responsible kin are essential when it is necessary to start treatment at once.

As with inpatients, confidentiality must be respected, as well as the patient's right to refuse treatment unless an emergency exists and the patient is judged incompetent. Breaches of confidentiality may occur when venereal disease is diagnosed, other infectious disease is present, or a gunshot wound is obvious. *Tarasoff* must be invoked to protect a threatened third party, and minors need parental consent unless they are legally emancipated.

Community Psychiatry[78,79]

Faced often with inadequate resources, the community psychiatrist must nevertheless solve stressful problems that present both clinical and ethical challenges, such as the dangerous patient who needs hospitalization but for whom no public beds are available, or the schizophrenic patient who can benefit from psychotherapy but whose treatment would require that professionals be pulled from other areas of demand. Here, as elsewhere, sensitive ethical/moral/clinical judgments must be made in relation to priorities where resources are low.

The community psychiatrist is also faced with multiple constituencies, including police, politicians, minority groups, public agencies, hospitals, and other referring sources. An important question is the form and type of community participation in the affairs of the facility that should be encouraged. What kind of community board, with what representation, and with what responsibilities or powers in governance should be favored? What community needs should be placed in highest priority?

Mental Health Data Systems[80]

Ethics and laws regarding privacy, confidentiality, and privilege apply whether records are paper charts or electronic files. Privacy is jeopardized as a function of the number of people involved in the patient's treatment. Single-location automated systems are more secure than multiple-location systems exposed at more sites, with more terminals involved and more people having access. If multilocation systems are linked to criminal justice systems or to welfare systems, risk of information exposure is increased. This risk must be balanced against the advantages of a larger data base, which provides ease in monitoring and following up patients through several systems and affords the ability to keep track of drug usage, duplicate resource utilization, and missed appointments.

AIDS[81,82,83,84,85,86,87]

AIDS (acquired immune deficiency syndrome) was first described in 1981; the virus that causes it (HIV) was identified in 1983. HIV infection, detected by serological tests, is spread primarily through intimate sexual contact and exchange of fluids. Particularly vulnerable are homosexuals, intravenous drug users, and hemophiliacs (through transfusions of contaminated blood). By 1989, 115,000 clinical cases were reported by the Centers for Disease Control. Perhaps 1.5 million people in the United States are now infected with the virus (HIV positive), and maybe 5 to 10 million people worldwide. The time elapsing from discovery of positive serology to death is estimated at eight to nine years, whereas time from active clinical outbreak to death is estimated at less than 18 months. It is estimated that approximately 60% of cases with positive tests will eventually develop evidence of dementia.

Clinically, the AIDS virus produced its pathology by destroying the T_4 helper cells essential to maintaining immunological competence. The initial infection may be a mild self-limiting illness, but within weeks or months HIV positivity may develop, progressing eventually to fatal infection, carcinoma, and neurological disease.

Although AIDS is feared by the public and by professionals, an ethical obligation exists to provide access to medical treatment and an unbiased decision regarding the commencement and termination of treatment. Whereas the physician in the community does not have a duty to accept every patient referred to him, if a treatment relationship *has* been established and a physician learns the patient is HIV positive, termination of treatment for that reason alone makes the doctor legally liable for abandonment. Such refusal would be seen as ethically wrong and discriminatory, according to the AMA Principles of Medical Ethics. Refusal to treat could result in emotional distress, loss of income, pain and suffering, and the ultimate acceleration of the disease process.

Apart from the moral obligation to treat, the physician also has a moral obligation to inform the patient fully as to the meaning of the tests, the modes of transmission of the virus, risk behaviors, the protection afforded by confidentiality, and the availability of additional counseling. He also has responsibility for postcounseling, for example, the meaning and limitation of test results, the necessity to inform sex partners and drug-using contacts, availability of state services, and availability of additional counseling for psychosocial problems.

Ethically, in the case of HIV positivity and/or signs of ARC (AIDS-related complex) or AIDS, should the physician notify the spouse, other sex partners, and the public health authorities? Despite the moral obligation of the physician, under normal conditions, to hold confidences secret, in this case is disclosure warranted to protect others? AIDS is reportable in every state, although seropositivity is not. It is best if the patient cooperates, but what if he refuses? In that instance, the physician may opt for civil commitment, but civil commitment may not be used simply to interrupt the transmission of venereal disease. It may, however, be used if the patient is mentally ill and in need of treatment, and it may necessitate involuntary commitment if the patient is dangerous to self or others, or is gravely disabled.

In California, disclosure of HIV positivity to the spouse is included in the consent for the test; disclosure to third parties or the Department of Public Health is not allowed without additional written consent from the patient. However, ARC or AIDS is reportable to the health department without written consent.

The legal obligations of the physician vary from state to state. In California, the *Tarasoff* decision in effect obligates the therapist to take reasonable steps to protect a third party whose life is threatened by a patient in therapy. However, in the case of HIV positivity, the question arises whether the court rulings in *Tarasoff* apply.

Staff reactions to AIDS patients vary. Many are fearful, or do not understand the basic facts about transmission. Counseling with staff is therefore a necessity, and strict precautions regarding safe handling of body fluids should be observed, not only for AIDS patients but for *all* patients.

AIDS and Public Policy

Although testing for HIV infection is by and large voluntary, as is notification of sexual partners, reports of transmission of AIDS from patients to health care providers, and vice versa, have motivated calls for the routine screening of both parties.[88] In addition, as a result of the growing numbers of infants who contract AIDS from their mothers perinatally, routine screening of pregnant mothers and newborns has been strongly urged. Pregnant mothers are already tested for syphilis and hepatitis B, and the screening of newborns for phenylketonuria and other congenital conditions is standard.[89] Since AMA delegates (1990) called for HIV infection to be classified as a sexually transmitted disease, the pressure to have AIDS and HIV brought under control through statutory provisions has been growing.

Concerning the reporting of names of HIV-infected persons to public health departments, a sharp debate has ensued, with much opposition coming from those emphasizing privacy and confidentiality. Yet recently, four medical societies in New York state have demanded that HIV infection be made a reportable condition in order to improve the prospects of early clinical intervention. Public health officials note that despite a long-established rule to notify partners in the control of venereal disease, notification of sexual and needle-sharing partners at risk for AIDS has been the exception rather than the rule. However, since 1988 the Centers for Disease Control have made partner notification a condition for the granting of funds from its HIV prevention program. Recognition of the clinician's heavy responsibility in these matters has finally led to a number of states passing legislation that permit disclosure to persons at risk. Some states have used the authority of quarantine to influence individuals who persist in unsafe sex practices, and 20 states have enacted statutes permitting prosecution of persons whose behavior poses a risk of HIV transmission.

In a provocative *New England Journal of Medicine* article,[90] Bayer concludes that the most important factor accounting for the changes in public policy ("An End to HIV Exceptionalism") has been the therapeutic advances in the management of HIV opportunistic infection, and the hope of slowing the course of HIV progression by early identification of those infected.

Bayer asks what the guidelines should be apropos health care *providers* who are HIV seropositive. This problem has alarmed the health care community since the discovery that several patients of HIV-infected professionals have also turned up with positive serology. Brennan, in another provocative article,[91] though disinclined on a cost/benefit basis to screen all health care workers routinely, does recommend that HIV-positive providers warn their patients; further, he suggests that hospitals offer such individuals alternative jobs. He also urges hospitals to explore ways and means to insure providers against the expenses associated with occupational transmission of AIDS.

THERAPIST–PATIENT SEXUAL CONTACT

Barton and Barton (1984)[92] reported on 273 ethical complaints received by the American Psychiatric Association during a 30-year period (1950–1980). In 63 of these cases, the physician was judged guilty by the national ethics committee of the APA; 102 were judged not guilty, and 108 either were under investigation or had no action taken. Classification of complaints was consistent with the various categories of the AMA code of ethics.

In sum, ethical complaints increased greatly in the last decade, attributed in part to greater APA district branch awareness and to explicit instructions to district branches to report such complaints. Other factors of wider social significance are presumed to be the general increase in alertness of the American public to the misbehavior of public figures (ever since the Watergate scandals) and the decline in recent decades in the public's esteem of authority per se. The public in general is today better informed about medical practice, more sophisticated, and more critical than ever before.

Complaints received by the ethics committee particularly emphasized improper conduct (including sexual misconduct), failure to safeguard the public, failure to carry out duties to patients, violations of confidentiality, improper billing for services, and/or excessive fees. Of these, the most troublesome and alarming from the ethical viewpoint is improper sexual contact with patients. Violation of professional trust and responsibility, potential damage to patients, and tarnishing of the public image of psychiatry are the major concerns. Under civil law, a therapist who engages in such activity during treatment may be liable for malpractice.

Definition of Sexual Intimacy

"Sexual intimacy can be defined as touching, fondling, kissing or erotic acts including intercourse between a patient and a therapist. . . . The crucial factor . . . must be the context in which they appear."[93] In Minnesota law, touching a patient's intimate parts or allowing a patient to touch a therapist for the purpose of satisfying sexual or aggressive impulses is a legal offense. The law specifies "intimate parts" as including the genital areas, groin, inner thigh, buttocks, and breasts (regardless of whether clothing covers the area).[94] In Massachusetts law,[95] sexual contact means "the touching of an intimate part of another person"; this definition includes sexual intercourse, sodomy, and oral copulation.

Prevalence of Sexual Intimacies between Therapist and Patient

According to prevalence data based on self-reports obtained from questionnaires, sexual contacts between therapists and clients are of sufficient frequency to be taken seriously by all professions engaged in the treatment of patients. In an anonymous questionnaire sent to a random sample of psychiatrists, obstetricians-gynecologists, surgeons, internists, and general practitioners, Kardener et al.[96] and Schoener et al.[97] reported that 5% to 13% of respondents indicated they had engaged in erotic behavior with patients. Involvement of male physicians and therapists with female patients was considerably more common than involvement of female physicians and therapists with male patients. Many who had sex contacts with patients had done so repeatedly.

A national survey of the American Psychological Association (1977),[98] which yielded a 70% return of inquiries, found that 5.5% of males and 0.6% of females had engaged in sexual intercourse with patients. In addition, 2.6% of male therapists and 0.3% of female therapists had intercourse with patients within three months *after* therapy terminated. Allowing for error in data of this kind, insurance estimates have suggested that one in five psychotherapists might be intimate with one or more patients! Pope et al.[99] report that 1 out of every 10 malpractice suits handled through the American Psychological Association insurance trust involves allegations of sexual misconduct.

Sexual contacts between therapists and clients are not limited to physicians and psychologists, but have also been reported in the therapeutic relationships of the clergy, allied professionals, and paraprofessionals.

Another significant sidelight is that in a national survey of psychiatric *residents*, 4.9% of 548 respondents indicated that they had been sexually involved with psychiatric educators, and 0.9% indicated they had been involved with patients.[100] Data from women members of the American Psychological Association (clinical division) indicated that 23% of recent doctorate recipients had been sexually involved with their instructors.[101] Involvement during graduate education was statistically related to later sexual involvement with patients. An expanded training curriculum to include specific education on sexual exploitation was strongly recommended. Strongly held also was the view that to function in today's new ethical climate, clinicians require formal education in moral science.[102]

Views on Therapist–Patient Sexual Intimacies

For years, Semrad taught his psychiatric residents at Harvard, "As soon as you touch the patient, therapy is finished" (quoted by his students). The overwhelming opinion (98%) of professionals in this field is that sexual intimacies between therapist and patient are inappropriate, unethical, and harmful.[103,104] Some claim that this practice may be on the rise, and many fear that the esteem of the professions may suffer irreparable damage if it continues. Although many condemn the practice, only a fraction of clinicians who have knowledge of such activities have bothered to report them. Ethical and legal pressures to do so, however, have been mounting.

Despite the antagonism of the vast majority of professionals toward sexual intimacies with patients, the opinions of professionals are not unanimous.

A small group maintains that it may be therapeutic in some cases, even justifiable clinically and legally if the patient gives consent. Some prefer to believe that if treatment is discontinued, or if sexual contact begins only *after* the termination of therapy, a sexual relationship is acceptable.[105] The question has arisen as to how long after termination of therapy a therapist and patient who have become romantically entangled during therapy should wait before consummating their relationship. In response to this question, some have said that sexual relations between a therapist and patient are *never* justified. Attorneys defending therapists have attempted to introduce as evidence that the patients were seductive or were overtaken by psychotic confusion between fantasy and reality.[106]

Effects on Patients

In a study of 318 psychologists who had treated 559 patients reporting sexual involvement with previous therapists, 90% of the therapists' patients indicated they had suffered ill effects. The adverse reactions included increased depression, loss of motivation, impaired social adjustment, emotional disturbance, suicidal feelings or attempts, and increased drug or alcohol use. Eleven percent were hospitalized, and 1% committed suicide.[107] In a psychoanalytically oriented paper, the catalogue of negative effects included ambivalence and mistrust, patients' doubts as to their own sense of reality, fixation of childhood traumata, increased bondage to the offending therapist, exacerbation of preexisting problems concerning intimacy with men, and increased burdens of guilt and shame. Not the least of the negative consequences was the abrupt termination of the relationship, leaving the patient confused and abandoned.[108,109] Indeed, once sexual activity began, therapy ended immediately for one-third of the patients (usually initiated by the patient). This often left the patient with an added load of distress—still in need of treatment, but in a quandary as to whether to turn for help again to another psychotherapist.

Legal Aspects

In 1970, Masters and Johnson,[110] in their study on human sexual inadequacy noted "frequent" histories of therapists' seduction of patients. Physicians of every discipline were involved, as well as behaviorists, theologians, and legal advisors. The highest frequency involved male therapists with female patients, the latter often married to inadequate husbands. Masters and Johnson point out that in a psychotherapeutic relationship, the patient is always in a vulnerable position. Even if orgastic potency is achieved in sex with the therapist, there is no assurance of the ability to transfer such success to a rejected (or rejecting) husband. They suggest that this kind of exploitation of power and position by the therapist be considered grounds for a charge of rape.

Stone, in 1976, took issue with this pronouncement, suggesting that "unless new criminal statutes are enacted, criminal charges of rape or related sexual offenses against psychotherapists who exploit their patients are a remote possibility at best" (p 1139).[111] However, there is evidence that in the ensuing years both the professions and state licensing authorities have been paying more attention to the problem.

In 1985 and 1986, the Minnesota legislature criminalized sexual contact by a therapist with a current or emotionally dependent former patient, established sexual exploitation by a therapist as a statutory cause of action, and required that all licensed health professionals report to the board of medical examiners any physician who engaged in sex or sexually suggestive contact with patients.[112,113] A task force developed a statewide program to educate mental health providers and consumers on problems of therapist sexual abuse.

In 1986, Wisconsin made therapist sexual misconduct a felony, and in 1988 therapists were required to report sexual exploitation revealed in treatment.[114] California, Florida, Illinois, and Maine have followed the leads of Wisconsin and Minnesota. Lymberis[115] believes that by the year 2000, every state will pass some type of legislation to curb sex exploitation related to psychotherapy treatment.

Possible Solutions

A wide range of suggestions has been advanced to ameliorate or halt the practice of sex exploitation within the context of psychotherapy. It is understood that any actions taken to curb sexual transgressions should logically apply to all who are engaged in a therapeutic relationship.

First, it would seem important to introduce education on moral behavior in undergraduate and graduate curricula. Evidently, only a small minority of trainees are exposed to the facts of therapist–patient exploitation: its prevalence, tragic effect on both parties, and possible dire consequences. In the case of the therapist, ethical, social, professional, and legal sequelae can be drastic; in the case of the client, confusion, depression, and disorganization can be severe. An important element in training would be to alert the professional to his statutory duties (as expressed in specific jurisdictions) to notify authorities if and when a colleague is suspected of unethical practice. In some instances, as when a significant danger of harm to another individual is threatened, the *Tarasoff* doctrine may be invoked, although it may involve a breach of confidentiality.[116]

Since the professional's misconduct may be linked to unresolved neurotic conflicts and/or character difficulties, it behooves the individual to seek help when he senses that his professional restraint and control are threatened in a relationship. It then behooves the role models, teachers, and supervisors of students and trainees to discuss this problem area fully and to encourage early searches for help.

As for the patient, our concern here is paramount, for the primary ethical principle guiding the treating professions is "First, do no harm." Since the time of Hippocrates, it has been forbidden to take sexual advantage of a patient. It would be well also if we understood better what clinical factors predispose the *patient* to sexual victimization. Kluft[117] suggests that the majority are severely symptomatic, the victims of incest or other previous abuse. He posits a constellation of four factors that make these patients vulnerable: severe symptoms, "idiosyncratic" dynamics, atypical socialization, and cognitive difficulties. Gutheil[118] points out that patients with borderline personality are particularly inclined to sexual acting-out.

In the city of Minneapolis, efforts are made to bring the patient and therapist together in a face-to-face meeting with an impartial mediator presiding, and with support persons chosen by each of the participants.[119] In response to urgent requests for help, a posttherapy support group was established at the UCLA Psychology Clinic to provide group and individual therapy to those who had been sexually involved with their therapists.[120]

Finally, it behooves professional organizations and societies to assume responsibility to educate their members, alert their ethics committees, and notify state licensing boards of all disciplinary actions. The publication of the names of members suspended or expelled for sexual violations must also be considered.[121]

THE BIOETHICS SERVICE*

Ethics committees were introduced to the medical world as a result of the 1976 New Jersey Supreme Court decision approving the cessation of Karen Ann Quinlan's life supports. In 1983, the Indiana court, in the Baby Doe case, refused to intervene in a physician's and hospital's decision to forgo treatment of a handicapped newborn. The argument was that the benefit of treatment was not worth the emotional and financial costs. In response to such cases, the Department of Health and Human Services published guidelines encouraging hospitals to develop ethics committees. It is estimated that about one-half of all hospitals now have such committees, the majority set up within the past five years.[122]

Bioethics services are based on ethical consultations and recommendations derived from discussions with personnel appointed to a hospital bioethics committee. Individuals initiating a request for consultation, and others who can contribute information and expertise, are included in such discussions. The committee, appointed by the chief of staff or hospital director, is broad ranged (in California it is based on recommendations of the council of

---

*I am indebted to Alan Steinberg, Ph.D., formerly chairman of the ethics committee of the Department of Veterans Affairs Medical Center, Sepulveda, California, for sharing his extensive knowledge and experience.

the state medical association), including members from a variety of backgrounds such as law, the ministry, medicine, nursing, psychiatry, dietetics, research, and philosophy, as well as laypersons. Committee members are on rotational call and can be contacted at any time. The petitioner fills out a consultation request that is placed in the patient's permanent record.

It should be said that before the ethics committee is ready for its role, education of its members is essential. Experts are brought in to lecture and discuss ethics in its manifold dimensions for months before operations begin. Subjects such as the relationship between ethics and the law, organ transplants, dialysis, resuscitation, withholding of treatment, informed consent, and problems of scarce resources are studied. Education of the hospital staff is also a function of the committee; this has been effective in raising staff levels of awareness of ethical problems, improving communication with families, and possibly reducing threats of litigation. As consultants to medical and nursing staff, patients, and families, the committee helps sort out legal, religious, ethical, and medical issues. On a regular basis, the committee reviews and upgrades policy on such matters as criteria for death, supportive care for the terminally ill, cardiopulmonary resuscitation, and withdrawal of life supports.

Most of the problems confronting the committee are from the medical and surgical side of the hospital; only about 10% stem from psychiatry. Problems arising from ethical dilemmas in medical and surgical intensive care, coronary care units, and dialysis comprise about 60% to 70% of the total. DNR ("do not resuscitate") orders generate problems mainly in medical/surgical departments.

Some problems familiar in the field of psychiatry include ethicality of research; validity of consent procedures in schizophrenic, manic-depressive, and Alzheimer's diseases; judgment and decision-making competence of severely ill patients; informed consent; duty to warn (*Tarasoff*); and involuntary commitment. An incompatibility of drugs noted in a physician's prescription may alert the pharmacy to contact the ethics committee. The rehabilitation department faces problems of distribution of protheses and artificial limbs, particularly when these are in short supply. Dietetics will be concerned if the patient is not receiving enough nutrition to sustain life.

Strategic meetings convened to attack such problems must include members of the ethics committee, the patient's primary care provider, and as many other knowledgeable and involved parties as it is possible to bring together. At a subsequent meeting, it may be appropriate to include the patient and family members. After precise delineation of the problem as it appears in the clinical setting, vital questions concern hospital policy, federal and state laws, ethical values, and possible conflicts among these. Much discussion and argumentation may ensue, with different perspectives presented and clarified. Often the lawyer's testimony alone, or a review of house rules, can lead to consensus; however, unanimity is not demanded. A final report with recommendations and possible options for action is usually based on majority rule.

Committee members come from various persuasions and with varying strengths of conviction as to right and wrong. However, a common ground of agreement tends to take shape with repeated discussions. This common ground includes emphasis on the quality of the patient's life, care burdens and costs of sustaining life, significance of advances in technology, and costs versus benefits in a world of finite resources.

Mention should be made of the assignment of durable powers of attorney for health care. This allows the individual to select a proxy decision maker to make decisions about health care in the event the patient becomes incompetent. The attorney, in fact, carries out the patient's will as to what type of treatment to permit in the terminal phase. It is, in effect, legal advanced death care planning. Many people are now filling out the durable power of attorney form when making their wills, and some when entering the hospital.

Finally, ethics committees may someday have a decisionary or disciplinary role in enforcing policy respecting the allocation of scarce resources in matters of life and death. The role of committee members, therefore, can never be considered superficial or casual; it is profoundly involved with the most important of human values.

Case Illustration

Ethical Vicissitudes of an Emergency Service*

The Los Angeles County mental health system has been progressively underfunded year after year. Although the population of Los Angeles has increased, available funds for mental health have diminished. Massive sudden shifts of funds have followed such social catastrophes as the Watts riots, when monies were diverted from the state to the county to establish the Martin Luther King, Jr., General Hospital, the Drew Postgraduate Center, and a new psychiatric institute. Although the pressure for treatment of acute emergency cases has increased, the available state and private facilities to which the county's acute care hospitals can refer patients for continued care has diminished. This disastrous situation had grown to the point where the several county hospital chiefs of psychiatry in 1987 formulated a white paper, entitled "Declaration of Conscience,"[124] that called attention to the sorry state of affairs and urged county commissioners and the government in Sacramento to take immediate corrective action. The Declaration of Conscience proclaimed that three conditions were unacceptable and getting worse:

1. Patients in acute need were being turned away from overcrowded emergency service facilities.
2. Those who gained admission to emergency services were often forced to sleep on mattresses on the floor, or on wooden benches, making treatment difficult and causing great distress to caregiving personnel. The danger

*Case example was presented at the American Psychiatric Association annual meeting, in the symposium "Ethical Issues and Changing Health Care Economics," May 8, 1989, San Francisco, and published in *Administration and Policy in Mental Health*.[123]

of assault and injury to treating personnel by disturbed patients was stressed.

3. Due to serious reductions in referral beds at the county hospitals, as well as at the state hospitals and private facilities under contract, many patients overstayed their time in the emergency room or were discharged prematurely without adequate arrangements for continued care. Too often, they were discharged onto the streets.

Excerpts from the Declaration of Conscience called attention to the following:

. . . the ENORMITY OF EXISTING PROBLEMS AND THE UNACCEPTABILITY OF CONDITIONS in Los Angeles County psychiatric emergency and inpatient settings (p 1).[125]
. . . overcrowding . . . sick people are sleeping on mattresses on the floor . . . no beds (p 2).[126]
. . . we need 660 more acute and subacute psychiatric beds to care for our sickest patients, as recommended by the Department of Mental Health (p 4).[127]
. . . the system so demeans the patients and their families that they become bitter and resistant to efforts to help them (p 5).[128]

The declaration received excellent support from mental health associations, medical and psychiatric organizations, and other professional groups, as well as extensive coverage in the press. The state department of mental health presented a plan for $300 million to restore the mental health system to sanity; significant moral support was also offered by county supervisors. Unfortunately, the large amounts of money needed to cure the situation could only be supplied by the government in Sacramento. There, the legislature's vote for a very small augmentation of funds was red-penciled by the Governor.

Two years passed. Then a second Declaration of Conscience[129] came forth, this time pleading on behalf of the needs of the whole state. The situation had deteriorated even further. Closures of community clinics and reduction in services in the hospitals had been ordered. This section declaration announced:

San Diego County refuses admission to 9 out of 10 persons seeking hospitalization for acute mental illness due to lack of beds. (San Diego has sued the state for its lack of access to state hospital treatment [and for inequity in state support].)
Placer County turns away 3 out of 4 . . .
Rural northern California counties . . . no longer offer outpatient therapy other than medication.
San Francisco has stopped providing hospitalization on a voluntary basis.
Twenty thousand persons are losing their outpatient treatment as Los Angeles shuts down 8 outpatient clinics and reduces services at the remaining clinic sites.[130]

As Bruce Bronzan*[131] put it, of 8 million residents in Los Angeles County, 1.2 million are in need of mental health care, of which almost half suffer from major mental disorders. The county mental health system is only able to assist 90,000,

*Assemblyman Bronzan is a champion of the rights of the mentally ill in California.

and if the new proposals to scale back what is already a horrendously inadequate system are approved, 20,000 more people will go without needed treatment.

The governor, however, threatened a 40% reduction in local mental health funding (i.e., $229 million) if the legislature did not agree to cut:

- Welfare cost-of-living allowances
- In-home supportive services for the elderly and disabled
- State family planning (to be eliminated entirely)

How could this sorry state of affairs come to pass in the richest state in the union? The causes are multiple and complicated. Executive and legislative support had been meager for years, and public passivity contributed greatly to the low priorities for mental health. The Gann amendment of 1979, which limited the amount of state government budget increases to population growth and to inflation, throttled many worthy enterprises, and Proposition 13 seriously limited revenues obtained from taxes on residential and commercial property. Thus, even if more funds were to materialize suddenly, governing bodies would be unable to use them. Robbing Peter to pay Paul, therefore, became the major game in California.

What are the implications for the mental health administrator? He is beset on all sides with assaults on his ethical conscience. First, he is galled by having to bow to the hard realities of fiscal predominance over humanitarian concerns. (There has been a gradual and steady shift of power from clinicians to the framers of the budget.) Physicians resent the fact that medical input has had less and less influence, and that too often decisions on health, life, and death hinge on the judgment of fiscal authorities.

Violations of ethical principles and the American code of fair play are numerous:

1. Access to health care in our hospitals and clinics is not equitable. When the emergency room is overloaded, priority is given to police cases, which constitute approximately 40% of admissions. Where choice is possible, preference is given to suicidal, homicidal, or dangerously aggressive patients or to cases complicated by medical disease. Thus, many people (probably equally deserving) may be turned away.

2. Successful arrangements for transfer to continuing treatment are far easier for those covered by third-party payments, but for those patients without insurance coverage, the sad reality often is that nobody wants them. What is seriously demeaning to professional staff is that they have been made the instruments for this discrimination.

3. When the emergency care holding area is overcrowded, beds are available only to those who require special attention; the rest sleep on the floor. Vital decisions are in the hands of overburdened staff, who do not have opportunities for ethical consultation or reflection.

4. Staff in the psychiatric emergency unit are exposed to far greater risks

of injury from violent patients than in any other part of the hospital. This imbalance has resulted in repeated attempts to obtain extra compensation—so-called hazard pay—but to no avail.

5. At times, emergency patients must be held beyond the three-day period allowed by law, simply because there is no place to send them. Thus, a faulty system imposes an additional burden on personnel through no fault of their own.
6. If medical or surgical disease complicates the acute mental picture, the possibilities of referral outside for continuing care are greatly reduced. Thus, the more complicated the cases, the greater the chances of discrimination against them.
7. Since professional integrity is often seriously compromised by these conditions, the ethical choice is: What is the level at which one must rebel, or move out of this career to another type of livelihood?
8. Finally, should we continue to teach new generations of students in inferior facilities where ethical standards and professional ideals are constantly undermined?

Two further problems may be mentioned, also typical of ethical dilemmas faced by the administrator. One is the duty owed the public vis-à-vis the duty owed the therapeutic organization to which one belongs. It is similar in some ways to the stress felt by every citizen in deciding between his public and private role. For example, as the level of care for patients declines, when is it his duty to inform the public, and how does he do it? If four patients in a row commit suicide, how is this to be communicated? It will scare the public and give rise to numerous investigations, accusations, and maybe litigations; heads may fall, including that of the administrator.

A second ethical problem that arises pertains to the degree and kind of social/political action an administrator ought to engage in. The Declaration of Conscience illustrates this very well. The heads of psychiatric programs of Los Angeles County, in a collective political action, formulated a white paper exposing the faults in the mental health services system and distributed thousands of the documents to legislators, the media, and medical and lay organizations. None of this activity was subordinated to the control of the various hospital directors, to whom the psychiatric chiefs were normally responsible. Although hospital directors knew what the psychiatry chiefs were doing, the psychopolitical action took on a life of its own. Hospital directors *could* have objected on the grounds that they might be embarrassed, and that normal channels were circumvented, but fortunately none did—hoping, it was surmised, that some good might come of it.

Yet, to the signators of the declaration, it was an unusual action, which might be interpreted by some as an end run or as whistle-blowing by disgruntled employees. In truth, to set the record straight, the hospital directors whose institutions were once again exposed for inadequate services had for years been trying in many ways to correct the inadequacies.

ETHICS OF RESEARCH

> When Hippocrates suspended upside down his first group of patients who were suffering from intractable leg pain, and thus established the differential diagnosis between what is now known as ruptured intervertebral disc on the one hand, and fatal cancer on the other, he performed the first experiment of its kind, yet no one questioned his legal right to perform it.[132]

Since that time, over 2,000 years, many generations of physician-scientists have carried on studies using humans without being questioned as to their legality. It was assumed that the codes of ethics of physicians and scientists guaranteed greater safeguards than legal injunctions. However, the experiments during World War II, initiated and supported by the National Socialist (Nazi) government of Germany, changed all that. These criminal experiments were not motivated by efforts to improve services to patients but by the political goals of a totalitarian government—in other words, the genocide of non-German populations. They were performed in concentration camps on victims who had no say. From this horrible experience arose the postwar Nürnberg (or Nuremberg) Code, which became "the basic principles which must be observed to satisfy moral, ethical, and legal concepts with regard to medical experiments."[133]

The principles of the Nürnberg Code are contained in these 10 rules:

1. Enlightened voluntary consent, in the absence of duress, coercion, or deceit, and with full disclosure of hazards and inconveniences
2. Humanitarian purpose, unachievable by other means
3. Sound basis on all other sources of knowledge, including animal experimentation
4. Avoidance of all unnecessary physical and mental suffering and/or injury
5. Absence of a priori reason to believe that death or disabling injury will occur
6. Risk proportional to humanitarian importance of problem
7. Proper preparation for adequate protection against even remote possibilities of injury, disability, or death
8. Experimenter is scientifically qualified, possessing the highest degree of skill, and exercising the highest degree of care
9. Option for discontinuance always available to subject on request
10. Discontinuance mandatory whenever experimenter discerns danger of injury, disability, or death of subject

In the decades since World War II, a veritable explosion of scientific research has occurred; thus, the Nürnberg principles have assumed great importance in guiding the use of humans in experimentation. Time has also produced additional clarification and acceptance of what is meant by enlightened informed consent: elucidation of the nature and purpose of the experiment, the benefits and risks, and the expected course of the disease if investigations are *not* carried out. Of special concern has been the use of retarded children, the elderly, and persons suffering from incurable disease, or classes of individuals who are disfranchised (such as prisoners). With regard to the latter class, courts have doubted whether consent can ever be voluntary where choices are limited or are influenced by the desire of subjects to gain favor with those who control their lives.

The postwar years also brought considerable refinement in the technology of experimentation. This applied particularly to experimental designs in which double-blind and placebo controls were used and where sophisticated statistical analyses were applied. Evaluation of subject status also improved greatly through the development of assessment scales that measured overt behavior as well as subjective attitudes and expectations. Ethical questions arose in some experiments as to the justifications for excluding patients from drug trials where the experimental drug had the possibility of benefiting the individual. These became passionate issues in regard to diseases such as AIDS, where experimental drugs might reduce suffering greatly and even postpone death. A further ethical problem arose as to whether and when to interrupt a research program in which early results promised benefits. In such a case some individuals might be helped, but the premature closure of the study could sacrifice vital information that might be useful to a larger population.

A landmark study by Beecher[134] published in the prestigious *New England Journal of Medicine* (1966) called attention to the fact that many patients were used in experiments where the risks had never been satisfactorily explained to them, and "further hundreds [of patients] have not known that they were subjects of an experiment although grave consequences have been suffered as a direct result." Documented by examples from leading medical schools, university hospitals, private hospitals, government military departments, governmental institutes (the National Institutes of Health [NIH]), and VA hospitals, these charges had great impact at a time when funds available for research were growing by leaps and bounds, and when many new investigators were entering the field of medicine each year.

Beecher states that of 100 human studies published consecutively in 1964 in an excellent journal, 12 seemed to be unethical. He was particularly concerned that informed consent was not mentioned in the majority of examples he compiled. His "Example No. 17" is worth mentioning as a blatant violation of humane principles: "Live cancer cells were injected into 22 human subjects as part of a study of immunity to cancer. According to a recent review, the subjects (hospitalized patients) were 'merely told they would be receiving "some cells" . . . the word cancer was entirely omitted.' "

Articles like Beecher's led a growing concern about the legal and ethical vulnerability of scientists. A national effort included NIH's requirement for human subject protection committees to preapprove investigations supported by government funds. The need for the subject (or his legal guardian) to understand the meaning of informed consent was also stressed, and scientific journals were encouraged to consider whether they should publish any data obtained unethically.

Finally, the use of animals for medical experimentation has for years drawn the fire of antivivisectionists (now animal-rights activists). The two main questions that characterize the animal-rights debates are: (a) Is the subjugation of one species to the purpose of another ethical? (b) Are the experiments on animals carried out with utmost humane regard for the pain and suffering of the animals?

ETHICS IN TRAINING

Compared to 50 years ago, the medical graduate of today has had to make many new accommodations. Then, women in medicine were conspicuous for their rarity. Of those who graduated, the essential avenues open were pediatrics, obstetrics, psychiatry, and research; the demanding surgical specialties were regarded as not appropriate for the "weaker" sex.

Today, the male graduate is learning to accept the female medic as an equal. Women are in many fields, and female students now have members of their own sex to look up to. New standards of fairness, sharing, and collaboration among professionals of both sexes are being accepted. Female medical students today are gradually approaching equality in numbers to male students all over the country.

Medical students of 50 years ago rarely married during their student days, and many were in debt at graduation. Today, marriage and children are much more common. However, many graduates still have a burden of debt to repay. After many sacrifices and long years devoted to mastering a specialty, the altruistic aspects of medicine are taking a back seat to practical considerations—more reason, therefore, to emphasize in the training years ethical principles in the practice of medicine. Chief amongst these, Redlich and Pope[135] emphasize (a) do no harm, (b) do not exploit, (c) obtain informed consent, (d) treat patients with respect and dignity, (e) practice with competence, and (f) practice within the framework of social equity and justice.

Michels[136] raises the question whether voluntary informed consent should be obtained from the patient prior to his participation in the education of residents.

The education of the doctor is a process to which large public and private resources have been committed over and above the tuition paid by the individual student. Previous generations of practitioners, teachers, and researchers have made the field what it is today; hence, it may be argued that the new physician therefore owes a debt of service to the community and to the next generation. This debt may be discharged through teaching, research, mentorship, and taking special pains to encourage the dedication of young physicians to the humanitarian ideals of medicine.

SUMMARY AND COMMENTS

The Hippocratic oath, promulgated in the fifth century B.C., is the foundation of ethics in the practice of medicine. Its admonition was to make the healing of the patient the primary concern of the physician, who must refrain from doing harm, respect confidentiality, treat patients within the limits of personal competence, and refrain from sexual relations with patients. The American Medical Association's principles, first adopted in 1847, emphasized the physician's responsibility not only to patients but also to society, other professionals, and the law. In psychiatry, the AMA principles have been modified to include the need for self-observation and self-criticism.

Ethical considerations in practice, teaching, and research have received more and more attention in recent years. Concern with these principles becomes acute when psychiatric intervention is contemplated. Principles such as *beneficence, maleficence, utilitarianism, respect, justice,* and *equitable access*—as well as *autonomy, privacy, confidentiality, privileged communication,* and *concern for the general welfare*—must all be defined, understood, and applied appropriately in practice. Their application may be very difficult, however, for both wisdom and refined judgment are required when principles may be in conflict with each other. Probably the cardinal element governing doctor–patient relationships, and fundamental to any intervention, is the principle of informed consent.

In the long struggle for the rights of patients, many ethical principles have been embodied in the law. Early rights were defined in relation to mentally ill offenders, for whom the doctrines of adequate and appropriate treatment, least restrictive alternatives, and rights to freedom for involuntary patients were enunciated by the courts. The concept of dangerousness as a criterion for commitment has also been a fundamental advance.

After the famous Alabama case *Wyatt v. Stickney,* the rights of patients were greatly enlarged to include the rights to marry, divorce, manage personal affairs, register and vote, and communicate with family (or friends, lawyer, or religious adviser), among others. Rights to appropriate education and protection from harm were declared early in relation to confined retarded persons. The right to compensation for work done arose in the quest to end the practice of institutional peonage. The right to due process and to refuse treatment are further expansions of patients' liberties. It soon became obvious that rights of patients should be developed in balance with the rights and responsibilities of treatment and administrative personnel—both interested in maximizing the patient's potential for recovery. This is clearly a major area for future development.

Ethical concerns may be different for different arenas of psychiatric practice (e.g., inpatient, emergency, or community), and special problems arise in the handling of information systems. Two recent areas of special interest include AIDS cases and cases of therapist–patient sexual contacts. The recent introduction of bioethics committees in many, if not most, hospitals in the nation is in part a response to scarce resources and medicine's remarkable ability to prolong life. Who shall survive is often the question.

Attention to ethical/moral issues in research has been accentuated by the discovery of bizarre inhumane experiments carried out during World War II by the National Socialist (Nazi) government of Germany. This gave rise to the Nürnberg Code and a reemphasis on enlightened informed consent. It is of universal importance that humane principles in the treatment of patients and in the conduct of research be emphasized in all training programs.

APPENDIX A—OATH OF HIPPOCRATES[137]

I swear by Apollo Physician and Asclepius and Hygieia and Panaceia and all the gods and goddesses, making them my witnesses, that I will fulfill according to my ability and judgment this oath and this covenant:

To hold him who has taught me this art as equal to my parents and to live my life in partnership with him, and if he is in need of money to give him a share of mine, and to regard his offspring as equal to my brothers in male lineage and to teach them this art—if they desire to learn it—without fee and covenant; to give a share of precepts and oral instruction and all the other learning to my sons and to the sons of him who has instructed me and to pupils who have signed the covenant and have taken an oath according to the medical law, but to no one else.

I will apply dietetic measure for the benefit of the sick according to my ability and judgment; I will keep them from harm and injustice.

I will neither give a deadly drug to anybody if asked for it, nor will I make a suggestion to this effect. Similarly I will not give to a woman an abortive remedy. In purity and holiness I will guard my life and my art.

I will not use the knife, not even of sufferers from the stone, but will withdraw in favor of such men as are engaged in this work.

Whatever houses I may visit, I will come for the benefit of the sick, remaining free of all intentional injustice, of all mischief, and in particular of sexual relations with both female and male persons, be they free or slaves.

What I may see or hear in the course of the treatment or even outside of the treatment in regard to the life of men, which on no account one must spread abroad, I will keep to myself, holding such things shameful to be spoken about.

If I fulfill this oath and do not violate it, may it be granted to me to enjoy life and art, being honored with fame among all men for all time to come; if I transgress it and swear falsely, may the opposite of all this be my lot.

APPENDIX B—AMERICAN MEDICAL ASSOCIATION PRINCIPLES OF MEDICAL ETHICS*[138]

Preamble: The medical profession has long subscribed to a body of ethical statements developed primarily for the benefit of the patient. As a member of this profession, a physician must recognize responsibility not only to patients, but also to society, to other health professionals, and to self. The following Principles adopted by the American Medical Association are not laws, but standards of conduct which define the essentials of honorable behavior for the physician.

I. A physician shall be dedicated to providing competent medical service with compassion and respect for human dignity.

II. A physician shall deal honestly with patients and colleagues, and strive to expose those physicians deficient in character or competence, or who engage in fraud or deception.

III. A physician shall respect the law and also recognize a responsibility to seek changes in those requirements which are contrary to the best interests of the patient.

IV. A physician shall respect the right of patients, of colleagues, and of other health professionals, and shall safeguard patient confidences within the constraints of the law.

V. A physician shall continue to study, apply and advance scientific knowledge, make relevant information available to patients, colleagues, and the public, obtain consultation, and use the talents of other health professionals when indicated.

VI. A physician shall, in the provision of appropriate patient care, except in emergencies, be free to choose whom to serve, with whom to associate, and the environment in which to provide medical services.

VII. A physician shall recognize a responsibility to participate in activities contributing to an improved community.

(adopted July 22, 1980)

REFERENCES

1. Nisbet R: The Twilight of Authority. New York, Oxford University Press, 1975
2. Redlich F, Mollica RF: Overview: Ethical issues in contemporary psychiatry. Amer J Psychiatry 133:125–136, 1976
3. Callahan D: Shattuck lecture: Contemporary biomedical ethics. NE J Med 302:1228–1233, 1980
4. Redlich F, Pope, K: Editorial: Ethics of mental health training. J Nerv Ment Dis 168:709–714, 1980

5. Annas GJ: The hospital: A human rights wasteland. Civil Liberties Review I:9–29, Fall 1974
6. Jonsen AR, Siegler M, Winslade WJ: Clinical Ethics. New York, Macmillan, 1982
7. Fink PJ: (Presidential address) On being ethical in an unethical world. Amer J Psychiatry 146:1097–1104, 1989
8. Annas GJ: The hospital: A human rights wasteland. Civil Liberties Review I:9–29, 1974
9. Galbraith JF: The Anatomy of Power. Boston, Houghton Mifflin, 1983
10. *Rouse v. Cameron*, 373F 2d 481 (D.C. Cir. 1966)
11. Callahan, D: Setting Limits: Medical Goals in an Aging Society. New York, Simon & Schuster, 1987
12. *Wyatt v. Stickney*, 325 F Supp. 781,784 (M.D. Ala. 1971)
13. *Winters v. Miller*, 446 F 2d 65 (2nd Cir. 1971)
14. Lake v. Cameron, 364 F 2d 657 (D.C. Cir. 1966)
15. Jones LR, Parlour RR (eds.): Wyatt v. Stickney: Retrospect and prospect. New York, Grune & Stratton, 1981
16. Sider, RC: Ethical issues in inpatient practice. Psychiatr Med 4:445–454, 1986
17. Stoline A, Weiner JP: The physician as ethicist, Chapter 9 in Stoline A, Weiner JP: The New Medical Marketplace. Baltimore, Maryland, Johns Hopkins University Press, 1988, pp 111–116
18. Dyer AR: The Hippocratic tradition in medicine and psychiatry, in Dyer AR: Ethics and Psychiatry: Toward Professional Definition. Washington, DC, American Psychiatric Press, 1988, pp 29–41
19. Dyer AR: The place of ethics in the definition of a profession, in Dyer AR: Ethics and Psychiatry: Toward Professional Definition. Washington, DC, American Psychiatric Press, 1988, pp 15–28
20. Levine M: Psychiatry and Ethics. New York, George Braziller, 1972, pp 323–341; quoted by AR Dyer in: The Hippocratic tradition in medicine and psychiatry, in Dyer AR: Ethics and Psychiatry: Toward Professional Definition. Washington, DC, American Psychiatric Press, 1988
21. Redlich R, Mollica RF: Overview: Ethical issues in contemporary psychiatry. Amer J Psychiatry 133:125–136, 1976
22. Nisbet R: Twilight of Authority. New York, Oxford University Press, 1975
23. Oglesby DK: Ethics and hospital administration. Hosp Health Service Admin 30:29–43, 1985
24. Winslade WJ: Ethics in psychiatry, in Kaplan HI, Sadock BJ (eds): Comprehensive Textbook of Psychiatry, ed 5. Baltimore, Maryland, Williams & Wilkins, 1989, pp 2124–2131
25. Wettstein RM: Ethics and involuntary treatment. Admin Ment Health 15:110–119, 1987
26. Reece RD: The new medical ethics and mental health administration. Psychiat Annals 19:428–431, 1989
27. Redlich F, Mollica RF: Overview: Ethical issues in contemporary psychiatry. Amer J Psychiatry 133:125–136, 1976
28. Plaut EA: The ethics of informed consent: An overview. Psychiat J Univ Ottawa 14:435–438, 1989
29. Boyarsky S: Informed consent—current concepts. Legal Aspects of Medical Practice 16:3–5, 10–11, 1988
30. Gutheil TG, Bursztajn H, Brodsky A: Sounding board. Malpractice prevention through the sharing of uncertainty: Informed consent and the therapeutic alliance. NE J Med 311:49–51, 1984
31. Kane T: Opinion—Systematic discrimination: A strategy for survival. Admin and Policy in Mental Health 16:179–182, 1989
32. Greenblatt J: Class-action suits and the rights of patients, Chapter 6 in Greenblatt M: Psychopolitics. New York, Grune & Stratton, 1978, pp 73–99
33. *Baxstrom v. Herold*, 383 US 107 00 (1966)
34. Steadman HJ, Halfon A: The Baxstrom patients: Backgrounds and outcomes. Sem in Psychiatry 3:376–385, 1971
35. Steadman HJ: Follow-up on Baxstrom patients returned to hospitals for the criminally insane. Amer J Psychiatry 130:317, 1973
36. Flaschner FN (Special Assistant Attorney General): Interim Report to the Honorable Elliot L. Richardson, Attorney General (Massachusetts), May 19, 1967
37. Flaschner FN (Special Assistant Attorney General): Progress Report to the Honorable Elliot L. Richardson, Attorney General (Massachusetts) re Bridgewater Release Project, October 29, 1968

38. *Rouse v. Cameron*, 373 F 2d 451 (DC Cir 1966)
39. *Lake v. Cameron*, 364 F 2d 657 (DC Cir 1966)
40. *Nason v. Superintendent of Bridgewater State Hospital*, 233 NE 2d 908 (Mass 1968)
41. *Tribby v. Cameron*, 397 F 2d 104 (DC Cir 1967)
42. *Covington v. Cameron*, 419 F 2d 617 (DC Cir 1969)
43. *Dixon v. Commonwealth of Pennsylvania*, 325 F Supp 966 (MD Pa 1971)
44. *McCray v. Maryland*, 4363 (Cir Ct Montg Co Md, filed November 11, 1971)
45. *Wyatt v. Stickney*, 325 F Supp 781, 784 (MD Ala 1971)
46. Greenblatt M: Wyatt v. Stickney: A study in psychopolitics, in Jones LR, Parlour RR (eds): Wyatt v. Stickney: Retrospect and Prospect. New York, Grune & Stratton 1981, pp 129–139
47. *Donaldson v. O'Connor*, Civil Action No. 1693 (ND Fla, decided November 28, 1972)
48. *Wyatt v. Stickney*, 325 F Supp 781, 784 (MD Ala 1971)
49. *New York State Association for Retarded Children, Inc., et al., v. Rockefeller*, 357 F Supp 752 (ED NY 1973)
50. *Lake v. Cameron*, 364 F 2d 657 (DC Cir 1966)
51. *Pennsylvania Association for Retarded Children v. Commonwealth of Pennsylvania*, 334 F Supp 1257 (ED Pa 1971)
52. *Riese v. St. Mary's Hospital and Medical Center*, 196 Cal.App.3d 1388, 243 Cal.Rptr. 241 (1987, Modified 1988)
53. Michaels R: The right to refuse treatment. Hosp Community Psychiatry 32:251–255, 1981
54. Stone AA: Mental Health and Law: A System in Transition. See Chapter 6, The right to refuse treatment, pp 97–108, particularly p 99. Rockville, Maryland, NIMH Crime & Delinquency Issues, US Dept of Health, Education, and Welfare, US Public Health Service, Alcohol, Drug and Mental Health Administration, 1976
55. *Winters vs Miller*, 446 F 2d 65 (2d Cir 1971)
56. *Riese v. St. Mary's Hospital and Medical Center*, 196 Cal.App.3d 1388, 243 Cal.Rptr. 241 (1987, Modified 1988)
57. Greenblatt M: Psychopolitics. New York, Grune & Stratton, 1978. See The subtle balance between rights, privileges, and responsibilities, pp 90–95, in Chapter 6, Class-action suits and the rights of patients
58. Gibson RW: The rights of staff in the treatment of the mentally ill. Hosp & Community Psychiatry 27:855–859, 1976
59. Greenblatt M: Ethics of administration: The California crisis. Admin and Policy in Mental Health 17:177–183, 1990
60. [No byline]: Income, sex, and race are factors in who gets kidney transplants: Study report. AHA News 25:2, Issue no. 4, January 23, 1989
61. Kane T: Opinion—Systematic discrimination: A strategy for survival. Admin and Policy in Mental Health 16:179–182, 1989
62. Russell B: Power. The Role of Man's Will to Power in the World's Economic and Political Affairs. New York, WW Norton, 1938
63. Raven BH: A taxonomy of power in human relations. Psychiatr Annals 16:633–636, 1986
64. French JRP Jr, Raven BH: The basis of social power, in Cartwright P (ed): Studies in Social Power. Ann Arbor, Michigan, Institute for Social Research, 1959, pp 150–167
65. Raven BH: Social influence and power, in Steiner ID, Fishbein M (eds): Current Studies in Social Psychology. New York, Holt, Rinehart & Winston, 1965, pp 372–382
66. Galbraith JK: The Anatomy of Power. Boston, Houghton Mifflin, 1983
67. McLelland DC: Power, The Inner Experience. New York, Halsted Press, John Wiley & Sons, Irvington Publishers, 1975
68. Greenblatt M: The use and abuse of power in the administration of systems. Psychiatr Annals 16:650–652, 1986
69. Greenblatt M: Psychopolitics and the search for power: The meaning of power, Chapter 13 in Psychopolitics. New York, Grune & Stratton, 1978, pp 210–226
70. Callahan D: Shattuck lecture: Contemporary biomedical ethics. NE J Med 302:1228–1233, 1980
71. Callahan D: Setting Limits: Medical Goals in an Aging Society. New York, Simon & Schuster, 1987
72. Rinella V: Ethical issues and psychiatric cost containment strategies. Intl J Law Psychiatry, 9:125–136, 1986
73. American Psychiatric Association, Ethics Committee: The New Mental Health Economics and the Impact on the Ethics of Psychiatric Practice: A Report of the Hastings Center

Conference on Psychiatric Ethics and New Economics. Ethics Newsletter (American Psychiatric Association, Washington, DC) IV:1–7, April/May 1988

74. Sider RC: Ethical issues in inpatient practice. Psychiatr Med 4:445–454, 1986
75. Wettstein RM: Ethics and involuntary treatment. Admin in Ment Health 15:110–119, 1987
76. Sider RC: Ethical issues in inpatient practice. Psychiatr Med 4:445–454, 1986
77. Julavits WF: Legal issues in emergency psychiatry. Psychiatric Clinics of North America, 6:335–345, 1983
78. Moffic HS: Ethical dilemmas for community psychiatrists. An administrative example. Community Psychiatrist (Publication of American Association of Community Psychiatrists) 3:8–9, 1988
79. Perlman B: Ethical concerns in community mental health. Amer J Community Psychol 5:45–57, 1977
80. Walken GH, Lyon M: Ethical issues in computerized mental health data systems. Hosp Community Psychiatry 7:11–16, 1986
81. Eth S: Ethical treatment of patients with AIDS. Psychiatr Annals 18:571–576, 1988
82. Dyer AR: AIDS, ethics and psychiatry. Psychiatr Annals 18:577–581, 1988
83. Bisbing SB: Psychiatric patients and AIDS. Psychiatr Annals 18:582–586, 1988
84. Ginsburg HM: HIV related diseases and the future of the delivery of psychiatric care. Psychiatr Annals 18:563–570, 1988
85. Zonona H, Norko M, Stier D: The AIDS patients and the psychiatric unit: Ethical and legal issues. Psychiatr Annals 18:587–592, 1988
86. Yarnell EK, Battin MP: AIDS, psychiatry, and euthanasia. Psychiatr Annals 18:598–603, 1988
87. Tanay E: Psychiatric reflections: AIDS and education. Psychiatr Annals 18:594–597, 1988
88. Angell M: A dual approach to the AIDS epidemic. NE J Med 324:1498–1500, 1991
89. Bayer R: Public health policy and the AIDS epidemic. An end to HIV exceptionalism. NE J Med 324:1500–1504, 1991
90. Bayer R: Public health policy and the AIDS epidemic. An end to HIV exceptionalism. NE J Med 324:1500–1504, 1991
91. Brennan TA: Transmission of the human immunodeficiency virus in the health care setting. Time for action. NE J Med 324:1504–1509, 1991
92. Barton WE, Barton GM: A study of ethical complaints, Chapter 5 in Barton WE, Barton GM: Ethics and Law in Mental Health Administration. New York, International Universities Press, 1984, pp 91, 104–110
93. Zalen SL: Sexualization of therapeutic relationships: The dual vulnerability of patient and therapist. Psychotherapy 22:178–185, Summer 1985
94. Gartrell N, Herman JL, Olarte S, Feldstein M, Localio R: Management and rehabilitation of sexually exploitive therapist. Hosp & Community Psychiatry 39:1070–1074, 1988
95. Massachusetts Senate Bill 1406. Chapter 1474. An Act to Add Section 43.43 to the Civil Code Relating to Psychotherapy; and Senate Bill 1277. Chapter 1448. An Act to Add Sections 337 and 728 to the Business and Professional Code, Relating to Psychotherapists
96. Kardener SH, Fuller M, Mensh IN: A survey of physicians' attitudes and practices regarding erotic and nonerotic contacts with patients. Amer J Psychiatry 130:1077–1081, 1973
97. Schoener G, Milgrom JH, Gonsiorek J: Sexual exploitation of clients by therapists. Women & Therapy 3:63–69, 1984
98. Holroyd JC, Brodsky AM: Psychologists' attitudes and practices regarding erotic and nonerotic physical contact with patients. Amer Psychologist 32:843–849, 1977
99. Pope KS, Keith-Spiegel P, Tabachnick BG: Sexual attraction to clients: The human therapist and the (sometimes) inhuman training system. Amer Psychologist 41:147–158, 1986
100. Gartrell N, Herman J, Olarte S, Localio R, Feldstein M: Psychiatric residents' sexual contact with educators and patients: Results of a national survey. Amer J Psychiatry 156:690–694, 1988
101. Pope KS, Keith-Spiegel P, Tabachnick BG: Sexual attraction to clients: The human therapist and the (sometimes) inhuman training system. Amer Psychologist 41:147–158, 1986
102. Pellegrino ED: (Editorial) Medical ethics, education, and the physician's image. JAMA 235:1043–1044, 1976
103. Herman JL, Gartrell N, Olarte S, Feldstein M, Localio R: Psychiatrist–patient sexual contacts: Results of a national survey. II. Psychiatrists' attitudes. Amer J Psychiatry 144:164–169, 1987
104. Pope KS, Bouhoutsos JC: Sexual intimacy between therapists and patients. New York, Praeger, 1986

105. Herman JL, Gartrell N, Olarte S, Feldstein M, Localio R: Psychiatrist–patient sexual contacts: Results of a national survey. II. Psychiatrists' attitudes. Amer J Psychiatry 144:164–169, 1987

106. Brown LS: Harmful effects of posttermination sexual and romantic relationships between therapists and their former clients. Psychotherapy 25:249–255, 1988

107. Bouhoutsos J, Holroyd J, Lerman H, Forer BR, Greenberg M: Sexual intimacy between psychotherapists and patients. Professional Psychol: Research & Practice 14:185–196, 1983

108. Apfel RJ, Simon B: Patient–therapist sexual contact. Psychodynamic perspectives on the causes and results. Psychother Psychosom 43:57–62, 1985

109. Apfel RJ, Simon B: Patient-therapist sexual contact. II. Problems of subsequent psychotherapy. Psychother Psychosom 43:63–68, 1985

110. Masters WH, Johnson VE: Treatment failures, Chapter 15 in Masters WH, Johnson VE: Human Sexual Inadequacy. Boston, Little, Brown, 1970, pp 388–391

111. Stone AA: The legal implications of sexual activity between psychiatrist and patient. Amer J Psychiatry 133:1138–1141, 1976, p 1139

112. Gartrell N, Herman JL, Olarte S, Feldstein M, Localio R: Management and rehabilitation of sexually exploitive therapists. Hosp & Community Psychiatry 39:1070–1074, 1988

113. Gartrell N, Herman JL, Olarte S, Feldstein M, Localio R, Schoener G: Sexual abuse of patients by therapists. Strategies for offender management and rehabilitation, in Miller RD (ed): Legal Implications of Hospital Policies and Practices. New Directions in Mental Health Services, No. 41. San Francisco, Jossey-Bass, 1989, pp 55–66

114. Bemmann KC, Goodwin J: New laws about sexual misconduct by therapists: Knowledge and attitudes among Wisconsin psychiatrists. Wisconsin Med J 88:11–16, 1989

115. Lymberis M: Predicts all states will act to curb patient–therapist sex. Clinical Psychiatric News 18:1 and 19, 1990

116. Eth S, Leong GB: Therapist sexual misconduct and the duty to protect, in Beck JC (ed): Confidentiality vs. the Duty to Protect: Foreseeable Harm in the Practice of Psychiatry. Washington, DC, American Psychiatric Press, 1990, pp 107–120

117. Kluft RP: Treating the patient who has been sexually exploited by a previous therapist. Psychiatric Clinics of North America 12:483–500, 1989

118. Gutheil TG: Borderline personality disorder, boundary violations, and patient–therapist sex: Medico-legal pitfalls. Amer J Psychiatry 146:597–602, 1989

119. Bouhoutsos JC, Brodsky A: Mediation in therapist–client sex: A model. Psychotherapy 22:189–193, 1985

120. Sonne J, Meyer CB, Borys D, Marshall V: Clients' reactions to sexual intimacy in therapy. Amer J Orthopsychiatry 55:183–189, 1985

121. Gartrell N, Herman J, Olarte S, Feldstein M, Localio R: Reporting practices of psychiatrists who know of sexual misconduct by colleagues. Amer J Orthopsychiatry 52:287–295, 1987

122. Abraham L: Ethics committee weighs life and death decisions. Amer Med News [no volume number]:3, 19–20, February 10, 1989

123. Greenblatt M: Ethics of administration: The California crisis. Admin & Policy in Ment Health 17:177–183, 1990

124. Greenblatt M, Sloane RB, Miller MH, Thomas CS, Titus ED (signatories): Declaration of Conscience, October 9, 1987, Los Angeles. Also published in Southern California Psychiatric Society Newsletter 35:4–6, 1987

125. Greenblatt M, Sloane RB, Miller MH, Thomas CS, Titus ED (signatories): Declaration of Conscience, October 9, 1987, Los Angeles, p 1. Also published in Southern California Psychiatric Society Newsletter 35:4–6, 1987

126. Greenblatt M, Sloane RB, Miller MH, Thomas CS, Titus ED (signatories): Declaration of Conscience, October 9, 1987, Los Angeles, p 2. Also published in Southern California Psychiatric Society Newsletter 35:4–6, 1987

127. Greenblatt M, Sloane RB, Miller MH, Thomas CS, Titus ED (signatories): Declaration of Conscience, October 9, 1987, Los Angeles, p 4. Also published in Southern California Psychiatric Society Newsletter 35:4–6, 1987

128. Greenblatt M, Sloane RB, Miller MH, Thomas CS, Titus ED (signatories): Declaration of Conscience, October 9, 1987, Los Angeles, p 5. Also published in Southern California Psychiatric Society Newsletter 35:4–6, 1987

129. California Psychiatric Association, together with Chiefs of Psychiatry of California Medical Schools: A Declaration of Conscience to All Californians. March 1989

130. California Psychiatric Association, together with Chiefs of Psychiatry of California Medical Schools: A Declaration of Conscience to All Californians. March 1989
131. Bronzan B (D) Chair, Assembly Health Committee, California State Legislature: Letter to the Editor. Los Angeles Times, Metro Section, part 2, p 6, March 24, 1989
132. Alexander L: Limitations of experimentation in human beings with special reference to psychiatric patients. Dis Nerv Sys, Monograph Supplement 27:61–65, 1966
133. Alexander L: Limitations of experimentation in human beings with special reference to psychiatric patients. Dis Nerv Sys, Monograph Supplement 27:61–65, 1966
134. Beecher HK: Ethics and clinical research. NE J Med 274:1354–1360, 1966
135. Redlich F, Pope KE: (Editorial) Ethics of mental health training. J Nerv Ment Dis 168:709–714, 1980
136. Tardiff K: Michels discusses ethical concerns in AAP keynote. Bull Assoc Acad Psychiatry 17:1, 24–25, 1989
137. Oath of Hippocrates, in Temkin O, Temkin CL (eds): Ancient Medicine: Selected Papers of Ludwig Edelstein. Baltimore, Johns Hopkins University Press, 1967
138. American Medical Association: Principles of Medical Ethics. Chicago, American Medical Association, 1980

9

Education and Research

EDUCATION OF THE ADMINISTRATOR

In a field that is extraordinarily complicated and at the same time desperately lacking in critical research (not only on administration per se, but also on the training of administrators), what are the fundamental *questions* related to the training of administrators—and where do we stand on these questions today?

Who Is to Be Trained?

In earlier years,[1,2,3,4,5] arguments as to who should lead centered around the relative desirability of M.D.s versus formally trained mental health administrators as heads of therapeutic institutions. At that time, almost all administrators of mental health facilities, including county and state departments of mental health, were physicians. Indeed, Walter E. Barton (medical director of the APA, 1963–1974) and the American Psychiatric Association took the position that psychiatrists were best suited to lead because of their clinical training and deep understanding of human needs.

However, this was before the great increase in the number and diversity of services following World War II, and before the great deinstitutionalization movement. It was also before the unhappy austerity era, when budgetary deficits and cuts in services became almost regular events. It was before the flowering of third-party payment systems, prospective reimbursements, managed care, private and corporate expansions of mental health services, and the intrusions of judicial and legislative decisions into psychiatric practice. It was before the heyday of surveillance by standard-setting organizations and patient-rights agencies.

Together, the above developments have made administration so complicated and its technical mastery so remote from the curricula taught in medical
schools that, in fact, psychiatrists almost disappeared from many administrative positions: as commissioners of mental health,[6] superintendents of
mental hospitals, directors of community mental health centers—even as
executives in private institutions and corporate chains.

The new leaders have come from many directions—some from nonmedical health specialties, some from public health administrative training
programs, and some from law, welfare, and rehabilitation. And flags that
unfurl today are as likely to read "cost-effectiveness" as "high-quality
treatment."

What Is the Nature of the Job?

Today, administrative training resembles medical training in some respects. When the physician receives his M.D. degree, he has a basic education that fits him for general practice, but not for specialties such as
neurosurgery, psychiatry, or anesthesiology. In like manner, administrators
today practice in a variety of organizations and contexts, each with its unique
history, rules and regulations, value orientations, and goals. Specialization is
overtaking generalized training. Today, we are eager to find individuals with
the relevant knowledge and experience to head up such programs as chemical
dependency, child and adolescent psychiatry, geriatrics, or community
psychiatry.

The demands of a given administrative position in an organization also
vary with the goals of the organization and its resources, pattern of governance, and relationships with other institutions in the community at large. In
a for-profit system, public relations, marketing, and development (fund-raising) may become the areas in which an executive must prove himself. In a
university setting, the search for the most creative and productive scientists
or academic department heads, together with the resources to maximize their
creative potential, may become the concern of the day. An activistic ethnic
community will shape the agenda of an organization and its leaders in one
direction; on the other hand, a genteel, well-heeled, sedate community of
senior citizens will shape quite another agenda for the institution it supports.

The Training Program

In view of the diversity of roles and functions in today's administrative
jobs, training *programs*, too, vary. Training is necessarily divided into didactic
instruction and field experience. When to begin training, and whether this
training should be given to everyone in a training program or simply those
with special interest or career tracks, are primary questions. The Psychiatric
Residency Review Committee has expressed itself as recommending *some*
training in administration for everyone, and the American Association of

Directors of Psychiatric Residency Training has in recent years recognized the importance of administration training in its curricula. A recent survey of training directors[7] informs us that there is a definite trend toward starting education in administration in the advanced years of residency. Several writers also advocate enrollment in formal courses in health administration such as are offered in public health schools, and/or further work toward an advanced degree in administration.

Experiential Training

What should be the form and substance of the experiential component of training, where should it be sited, and how long should it last? It is obviously reasonable to make the experience as relevant as possible to the realities of the leadership challenge to be faced. As for the site of experiences, in the residency years it would seem reasonable first to exploit the residents' ward experiences, for the ward as a small community indeed presents a rich microcosm of opportunities to learn about administration. Supervision of the ward chief by an experienced administrator would be highly desirable. The teaching strategy would then center around "cases" of system dysfunction that have led to significant deviation from desired institutional goals and purposes. The etiology, diagnosis, remedial actions, and eventual outcomes of interventions in such cases then round out an approach to the living system, which in many ways is analogous to medicine's traditional approach to the individual patient (see "The Social System Clinician View" in Chapter 3).

One teaching technique used successfully with psychiatric residents is called "desk rounds." With students gathered around his desk, the administrator picks up mail, reports, and memos almost at random, explaining the problem, background, and approaches applied to the handling of the issues presented. The students immediately gain insight into the diversity of challenges the executive faces and the reasoning and actions directed to resolution of the problems. Both formal and informal aspects of the system come into bold relief, as well as outside conditions and forces controlling the final decision. The executive's job to look after the *total* system becomes clearer with each example. His definition of problems, assessment of their positive or negative impact on the system, and his delegation of functions along with guidelines as to implementation give the student an inside view of the command functions of the executive.

Backgrounds, Talents, and Skills

In several studies of promising young psychiatrists[8] and of high-level administrators (commissioners and other "illustrious" executives),[9,10,11,12] the following impressions stand out:

- In their formative years, many of the subjects had already asserted their leadership potentialities in Boy Scouts, high school, and college activities.[13] They were recognized by their peers as having that extra something that stamped them as leaders. It is likely that in these early years, basic leadership talents were honed and quickened by natural experiences—and early lessons learned in these contexts influenced their style and effectiveness in later years.

- Many future leaders were influenced by senior figures—mentors— whom they admired and decided to emulate.[14] These senior figures were often themselves successful administrators. In recent years, social scientists have made much of the phenomenon of modeling. It is a two-way affair, featuring on the one hand strong idealization of a leader by a younger person, and on the other hand a warm, nurturing relationship initiated by the mentor. One writer[15] has asked whether *anyone* has succeeded in business without having some unselfish sponsor or mentor.
- In their later years, many of these subjects achieved high-level positions in federal, state, and county mental health programs. By and large, they did not learn their work from formal sources; they learned by doing.

These observations raise questions as to whether leadership is primarily based on biological endowment, enhanced in early years by opportunities to develop potentialities, or developed through formal training programs. In this respect, Livingston,[16] in his provocative article, "Myth of the Well-Educated Manager," throws out the following challenge: "Men who get to the top in management have developed skills not taught in formal management education programs." He states categorically that there is a "lack of correlation between scholastic standing and success in business," and that problem-finding and problem-solving skills must be developed through direct personal experience on the job. Much further research is certainly indicated on (a) the relationship between early leadership potentialities and future career patterns, (b) the importance of mentorship in the development of interests and careers in mental health administration, and (c) the relationship between formal training and subsequent performance as administrators.

Grusky, Thompson, and Tillipman[17] discuss the relative values of clinical versus administrative backgrounds for mental health care administrators. Both points of view are clearly needed. The clinician aspiring to be an administrator has a lot to learn about social systems, budgets, law, building construction, and maintenance. Contrariwise, the administrator aspiring to be an executive in a clinical care system has a lot to learn about patient pathology, systems of care, and about the values and ideals of medical/psychiatric practitioners.

Although the talents needed for leadership must rest to a great extent on innate endowment, most would probably agree that they can also be shaped and honed by education and experience. One proponent of this view[18] divides the universe of skills needed by an executive into technical, human, and conceptual skills (see Chapter 12). Katz states that these skills can be learned through case study and role-playing of complex management situations. Nichols and Stevens,[19] too, stress the importance of developing the skill of *listening* to other people (Chapter 12). With good attention and practice, more of the substance of a conversation can be later recalled. One can also become more aware of the multiple messages a conversation carries—some overt, some covert.

Role as a Conceptual Approach in Training

Role theory supplies yet another approach to the enigma of training for leadership. In addition to managerial functions that keep the organization going on a day-to-day basis, we see the good executive naturally assuming a variety of other roles: judicial, social, paternal, or avuncular roles; roles as community leader; and roles as teacher, scholar, and researcher. Each role is appropriate to a given time, place, and situation. (See Chapter 12 for discussion of multiple roles.)

Although these are not necessarily stressed in formal didactic or experiential components of a curriculum, the complete executive ought to be able to function comfortably in all of these roles.

Health Factors: Physical and Mental Impairment

Common sense dictates that the administrator who is in a job vital to the health and welfare of many people should exercise every precaution necessary to protect his own physical and mental health. Therefore, in preparation for high responsibility, the administrator should pay attention to achieving a balanced life, with proper alternation of work, rest, and play; good nutrition and hygiene; early medical attention to signs and symptoms of illness; and the development of a stable family life, which is important to peace of mind.[20] Recent publications[21,22,23] emphasize the high cost of illness and disability both to the leader and to the organization he represents. In this connection, it is well to consider possible ways of reducing administrative stress, as suggested in Chapter 12.

Educational Programs and Opportunities

Contemporary wisdom holds that education can be very helpful in preparing for leadership roles.[24,25] Educational modalities include classroom exercises, mentoring, and on-the-job experiences. Today, formal educational opportunities in mental health care administration are highly diversified; increasingly, the attempt is to fit the training curriculum to the job. For example, medical directors in state hospitals particularly require persistence and sustained energy in the face of delayed personal gratification and institutional resistance to change. In these settings, charisma and vision are important combatants against staff demoralization. Sophistication in the workings of local and state politics is often a necessary skill. A systems orientation may provide some insurance against vulnerability to mundane in-house demands, and creative use of resources in short supply is often a necessary skill. Optimal preparation for such roles therefore might include mentoring, fellowship experience in public psychiatric administration, a political "internship," emphasis on health care economics, and administrative experience in parallel systems. On the other hand, training for chief of psychiatry in a general hospital might emphasize clinical competence and alignment with medical staff values more than alignment with conventional administrative or executive functions.

In view of changing community needs and not-infrequent budget instability, preparation for a top-level administrative job today must be broad. For example, knowledge of risk management, community values and lifestyles, marketing mechanisms, and hospital finance and the development of skills in management of rapid change are particularly important. Conflict resolution skills are increasingly significant in acute general hospitals, where psychiatric services must be integrated into a multidiscipline environment. The reactions of ancillary service personnel to psychiatric patients may require considerable attention. Other possible sources of conflict in such an environment include competition among physicians of various disciplines, physician–nurse tensions, in-house medical staff prerogatives versus those of private practitioners, and intrusions of third-party payers into management decisions (see Chapter 5).

Some fundamental questions in contemplating the ideal educational curriculum for mental health care administrators are: What should be the nature of a mental health care delivery system in a good society? Are there some characteristics that all mental health care administrators should have in common? And is there a model curriculum that could fit most (if not all) needs? There are no pat answers to these questions; however, a wide variety of educational standards and curricula do exist at the present time, of which the following are good examples.

To assume the lead in the identification and certification of specialized knowledge and ability in the field, in 1953 the American Psychiatric Association founded the Committee on Certification of Mental Health Administrators—now called the Committee on Certification in Administrative Psychiatry.[26,27] The Association of Mental Health Administrators (AMHA), under the auspices of the American College of Healthcare Executives (ACHE), and the American College of Physician Executives (ACPE), under the auspices of the American Board of Medical Management, also offer certification examinations. Continuing education programs in mental health care administration are offered by selected professional associations. For general education, the American Psychiatric Association encourages the presentation of administrative topics at its annual meeting, as does the American Association of Directors of Psychiatric Residency Training (AADPRT).

Several national professional associations specifically address the administration of mental health services, and education is a major component of their mission. These include the American College of Mental Health Administration (ACMHA), a multidisciplinary association that stresses the importance of clinical training in preparation for administrative roles, and the aforementioned AMHA.

Some continuing education programs have been targeted primarily for clinicians. The department of psychiatry at Wright State University School of Medicine sponsored a successful series of nine annual courses of five days' duration dedicated to administration of mental health systems. In 1989, Dartmouth Medical College offered a well-received special program called "Blueprint for the 1990s." Courses at other schools of medicine—Albert Einstein College of Medicine, Cornell University Medical Center, University of Maryland College of Medicine, University of North Carolina at Chapel Hill, and Emory University—were offered for a time but have been discontinued (often through loss or demise of an inspirational leader).

With regard to continuing medical education for multispecialty positions, the ACPE presents annually a series of physicians-in-management seminars, a management development program for chiefs of service and department chairmen, and a program for chief residents. Harvard School of Public Health offers an intensive program for chiefs of clinical services, and Harvard Medical School conducts an annual program on leadership for physician executives. Annual programs at the Physicians Leadership Institute—cosponsored by Arizona State University, the Western Network of Education and Health Administration, and the ACPE—offer continuing education and certification credit.

Degree programs are becoming more popular among physicians, psychologists, social workers, and psychiatric nurses. Nationally, there has been a surge of interest in programs offering a master's degree in business and administration, examples of which include the master's program in administrative medicine (M.S.) at the University of Wisconsin-Madison,[28] which was designed exclusively for physicians; the Sloan master's of science in management program (M.S.) at Stanford University; the Sloan Program in Health Services Administration (M.P.S. in human ecology) at Cornell University; the Graduate Program in Health Administration (M.H.A.) at Duke University; and the Program in Hospital and Health Services Management (M.M.) at the J. L. Kellogg Graduate School of Medicine/Northwestern University. The University of Pennsylvania is now offering an innovative program leading to dual M.D.–M.B.A. degrees, and a similar program is in the planning stages at the State University of New York at Syracuse.[29]

Successful participants in the increasingly popular professional-certificate programs receive graduate credits that frequently can be applied to master's degrees. Examples of such instruction include Executive Administration of Mental Health Programs offered by Graduate Program in Health Services Administration at the School of Public Administration at the University of Southern California, and the Advanced Professional Certificate in Health Policy and Management (for clinicians), sponsored by the Robert Wagner Graduate School of Public Health at New York University. The American Management Association, which is not university affiliated, offers a certificate program in strategic management. Of the many certificate programs listed in *Bricker's International Directory,*[30] most are limited to administrative and clinical aspects of substance-abuse programs.

The Bay Area Foundation for Human Resources, a tax-exempt organization founded in 1969 for research, training, and program development in mental health, health, and other human services, oversees an Institute of Mental Health Policy and Administration, established in 1987 as a result of funding from the National Institute of Mental Health. The Institute of Mental Health Policy and Administration, which serves as the regional training center for administrators of mental health service programs, sponsors a teaching program related to the needs and priorities of mental health administrators in the West.

Resources and references for self-study and course work in mental health administration frequently recommended to clinicians include three major textbooks,[31,32,33] two of which[34,35] (the books by Barton and Barton, and Talbott and Kaplan) include management principles and theory derived from generic and classic literature that are applied to clinical systems. Journal resources include *Administration and Policy in Mental Health;* the *Journal of the American Association of Psychiatric Administrators;* the *Journal of Mental Health Administration;* the *Physician Executive;* the *Journal of Management; Hospital and Health Services Administration;* the *American Journal of Psychiatry;* and *Hospital and Community Psychiatry.* Journals that appeal primarily to administrators who are graduates of degree programs in administration include *Hospital and Health Services Administration, Hospitals,* and *Modern Health Care.*

Residency Education and Administrative Psychiatry: A Survey

A decade ago, a survey of the American Association of Directors of Psychiatric Residency Training indicated that only 30% of psychiatric residency programs had assigned readings or required core training in administration, while 46% offered didactic instruction or seminars.[36] Most programs focused their attention on administrative issues involved in psychiatric practice.[37,38]

In 1989, directors of psychiatry residency education programs were surveyed to determine the current emphasis on administration in mental health.[39] A six-question survey item yielded a response rate of 74.5%. The findings may be summarized as follows:

A majority of residency directors (69.5%) indicated that their programs presently offer some formal education in administration. Of these, 72% plan to continue with their present curriculum, while the remaining 28% plan to expand their curriculum. Of the 47 programs not currently offering formal administrative teaching, 31 plan to add this in the future.

Of the residency programs currently offering administrative teaching, almost all (89%) provide at least part of it during the fourth postgraduate year (PGY-IV); 28% offer experience during the PGY-III year; and only 20% begin their teaching in the initial two postgraduate years. A majority (63%) of the programs offer both didactic and experiential components. The survey indicated that 72% of administrative teaching time was focused on management of systems and organizations, and that an additional 19% of time was focused on administration of the private practice of psychiatry. Residency training directors rated the usefulness of their teaching programs highly, and their residents' receptivity above average.

There appears to be some consistency in the methods used to teach administration across programs. For example, almost all teaching is offered during the final two postgraduate years. Most programs provide both didactic and experiential components, and both residents and training directors generally view the experiences positively.

Among the most popular and successful special programs for residents has been the Annual Chief Resident Conference at Tarrytown, New York, sponsored for 18 years by the Albert Einstein College of Medicine's department of psychiatry, organized and directed by professor Jack Wilder. It is an intensive four-day experience in which all aspects of the chief resident's role are explored and discussed. Reports from chief residents who have attended are enthusiastic. The University of Utah department of family practice also offers an annual conference for chief residents of all specialties, as does the American College of Physician Executives (in collaboration with the University of Southern California School of Medicine and the George Washington Medical Center in 1989). Conferences for chief residents identify and analyze problems of this highly sensitive and specialized middle management role—problems that cause considerable anticipatory anxiety.

Summary and Comments

In the education of the administrator, important questions concern who is to be trained; the nature of the job; and the nature of the training program. Didactic and experiential training are both desired. Backgrounds of trainees, their talents and traits, and their early and recent leadership experiences are relevant. Technical, human, and conceptual skills, as well as skill in listening, are important areas of development. The several roles an administrator must play in the execution of his job can also be used as a framework for the training program. The program must also pay attention to the importance of maintaining health in the face of the chronic strains of office, as well as to possible mechanisms to reduce stress and strain.

EDUCATION OF STAFF: THE ADMINISTRATOR'S ROLE

In this section, let us turn 180 degrees—shifting from education/training of the executive to the role of the executive in fostering and supporting the education/training of his staff.

The Challenge

An ideal view of this challenge would be to think of all the people in the organization as forming a pool of human resources in which the individual members (be they professionals or nonprofessionals) have a desire to learn and grow as intelligent citizens, as therapeutic agents, and as human beings. Then we may ask how the organization constrains or enhances this potential, and what administrators can do to release and gratify the drive for growth. It is assumed here that intellectual and personality growth impact importantly on the treatment of patients, on institutional morale, and on the satisfaction of workers with their jobs.

The challenge that then stretches before us is a large one, indeed. It can be broken down into three main components:

1. Mastery of the technical skills related to direct treatment of patients
2. Personal growth (i.e., movement toward greater maturity, particularly by broadening the span of positive identification with patients and others, increasing empathic understanding of people, and reducing neurotic baggage persisting from the past)
3. General intellectual broadening (i.e., increasing the staff's range of interests and knowledge of the surrounding world)

Technical mastery of the fields directly related to the care and treatment of patients through continuous in-service education is now very much the idiom. Starting in medical school, and including the days when the psychiatric resident enjoys individual patient supervision by four or five clinicians, the young practitioner has inculcated into him the necessity for continuing in-service education and growth. Indeed, in the last decade, continuing education credits have become a sine qua non for continued recognition by professional parent bodies. In most hospitals and clinics, robust teaching programs are now ongoing year-round. On the wards, in endless rounds and patient presentations, the professional sharpens his clinical wits and keeps abreast of the times. Much the same type of education goes on in other professional fields—nursing, psychology, social work, rehabilitation, and so forth. The regular influx of students and trainees from professional schools keeps this educational-training machinery in motion.

It is worth stressing that administrators should be deeply interested in this process. I refer here not merely to administrators from clinical fields, but also to administrators who are not primarily trained in the mental health professions—the professional administrators, per se. They live side by side with highly developed educational systems, and could easily enrich their knowledge and understanding of what their colleagues in the front lines are experiencing. In like manner, caregiving professionals should understand the more strictly administrative aspects of the institution. This two-way exchange will reduce misconceptions about roles, increase respect, improve communication, and help define role boundaries more clearly. Interest in learning about the other person's domain will reduce errors of intrusion that often lead to irritation and animosity.

Administrators should realize that an educational component costs money. One county program of my knowledge was seriously handicapped by lack of stipends and honoraria to build its lecture program. The costs were actually minimal compared to the value to the institution; without such funds, it was well nigh impossible to compete in the lecture marketplace for outstanding teachers.

Sometimes administrators can help a young professional obtain an education by collaborating with outside institutions, as illustrated below.

Case Illustration

Hospital and University Collaborate to Advance the Education of a Social Worker

A brilliant young social worker, age 38, came to her departmental administrator seeking a way to go on to higher education—specifically, to earn a Ph.D. in social welfare—without sacrificing income sorely needed for her basic personal support. She was restless in her present job, not sufficiently challenged intellectually, although her work with mentally ill adolescents was in many ways rewarding. She had explored with the dean of a nearby college the possibility of part-time course study and of scholarship support. He was encouraging. Now, she asked, was it possible for the hospital to help? Her specific suggestion was to allow her one day off per week, but without reduction in pay, provided she worked 10 hours a day for four days (thus fulfilling her 40-hours-per-week obligation).

The first concern of the administrator was that the social worker might overload herself, risking exhaustion and impairment of health. However, the young lady was not dissuaded, pleading that she could handle the challenge and at any rate wanted to try, anticipating that financial help would eventually come from her family after they realized the importance of her ambitions. Thus, upon further reflection, the administrator referred her to the chief social worker and to the psychiatrist head of her clinical service; they were to explore possible ways to provide the opportunity she so fervently desired.

The psychiatrist chief of the adolescent service said she would be happy to further the educational interests of this valued social worker, provided the chief social worker could persuade her staff to fill the needs of patient care and treatment during that day away in school. Finally, after long discussion, the chief social worker reported that her staff agreed to cover the assignment of their colleague one day per week, assuming that similar opportunities to advance education would be forthcoming for all staff members with like ambitions.

Since ward staffing was at best very thin, cooperation in this plan was a true act of generosity. It was made possible by the esteem in which the petitioner was held, the high morale on the ward, and the general attitude of mutual support of those in search of professional improvement. The administrator's willingness to support the plan gave a signal to staff that pursuit of professional and intellectual advancement was an important value in the system.

Education at Lower Levels

Many professionals cherish the personal and intellectual broadening that they enjoyed in their early liberal college education. Many lower-level personnel may not have had the advantages of a liberal education, but yearn for intellectual stimulation nevertheless. These employees may be closer to patients than other workers and play a great role in their lives. About 40 years ago, the development of the attendant became a matter of great importance when it was appreciated how neglected they were and how their fear of patients could make them distant and controlling, inclined to become watchdogs rather than friendly helpers.

Many of the techniques for staff development tried in those days could well be considered for their application today. Whatever the intellectual level of attendants, they are highly intuitive and understanding of patients' behavior, once shared life problems are made part of the educational program.

Space does not permit a detailed analysis of all the modalities that can be used successfully in staff development. A few are outlined below.

Group Therapy by Nurses and Attendants[40]

During World War II, manpower requirements of that great struggle decimated personnel, including professional personnel of many hospitals. Medfield State Hospital in Massachusetts was one of those that so suffered. Undaunted, a courageous, innovative clinical director, Dr. Kaldeck, organized therapeutic groups led mainly by attendants and nurses. The groups met three times a week under appointed leaders, who in turn met once a week with the medical director. With this arrangement, 250 chronic patients were involved in group therapy who otherwise would have been idle on the wards. Gradually, patients learned to talk more freely and to verbalize anxieties instead of acting them out. Attendants learned about the purpose and processes of group therapy, gained insight into their own reactions to patients, and developed insight into patient psychodynamics. Several of the chronic patients showed enough improvement to be permitted to go out with their families; others were transferred to better wards, and some could be discharged on indefinite visits. As morale and interest of attendants improved, new attendants were more easily recruited from the many who had heard of the program.

A similar program, inaugurated by Robert W. Hyde[41] at the Massachusetts Mental Health Center, for the edification of attendants (both day and night shifts) consisted of regular meetings devoted to didactic instruction on technical matters involved in patient care, as well as open discussion of current ward problems, the meaning of patient symptoms, the attendant's role, and problems posed by staff friction. Appreciable learning and emotional growth came from these sessions. The down-to-earth nature of the discussions, and the emphasis on feeling rather than intellectual abstractions, made it possible for all participants to speak a common language, despite widely divergent backgrounds.

Problems-of-Living Seminar

The problems of living seminar arose from a felt need for better interdepartmental communication and morale.[42] It was agreed that the meeting should be social in nature, include employees from all departments at whatever levels, that the proceedings should be in nontechnical language, and that the subjects for discussion would be of common interest. The meetings were held weekly at the end of the day, often stretching over to the evening hours. It soon became very popular, attracting a large audience. A list of common topics follows:

> The Need for Recognition
> The Need for Other People
> Extramural Relationships
> How to Know the Right Man to Marry
> Responsibility to Our Parents
> Problems Confronting the First Child
> Mixed Marriages and a Career
> Can Psychiatrists Get Along with Other People?

Some sessions did, indeed, strike deep chords of feelings. Self-expression gave participants a sense of greater acceptance and belonging. Personal prejudices were often aired. Respect and appreciation of other persons' individuality and work contributions were heightened, and insight into one's own problems was sometimes an unexpected reward.

Psychodrama

The purpose of psychodrama was to enact scenes that were meaningful in hospital life and the lives of patients. Dramatizations were spontaneous and unstructured. Participants could act out something from their own lives, or the lives of important others; then they might see others play the same parts. Many were shocked into sudden realization of their personal contributions to the troubles they were in.

Psychodrama has had many modifications since originally introduced by Dr. Jacob L. Moreno. An interesting related method, originated by the successful television actress Margaret Ladd and her playwright husband, Lyle Kessler, is "imagination workshop." Like psychodrama, it involves both patients and staff in various roles under the supervision of experts.

Patient Government and Therapeutic Community

Two other modalities, also involving patients and staff together, are patient government and therapeutic community. In the former, patients are to a large extent entrusted with governance of their ward affairs. This proved invaluable in teaching patients elements of democratic procedures, and providing an experience in self-management. Therapeutic community was developed during World War II by Maxwell Jones as a way of handling psychopathic and neurotic patients who were otherwise very difficult to manage. Later it became popular in U.S. peacetime hospitals. It is adapted to help patients and staff work together to establish a functioning community that is directed to the greatest good of all. In group sessions, moderated and conducted by nonphysician members of the staff, a very open and candid exchange of feelings, opinions, and ideas is encouraged. Meetings of *all* the members of the ward community are held daily; in addition, subgroups meet often with the objective of working out interpersonal problems.

Summary and Comments

Three main concerns in staff development are:

1. Technical mastery of the areas in which they work
2. Personal growth
3. General intellectual broadening

The first relates directly to the care and treatment of the patient, and is usually assumed under in-service training. The second refers to personal development, for example, moving toward greater maturity, broader empathic identifications, and fewer neurotic hang-ups. The third refers to increasing the range of interest and knowledge of the world in general.

All the above are served by educational programs that include lectures, demonstrations, group meetings, and special seminars on problems of living. Psychodrama and imagination workshops expose personal problems and conflicts. Patient government and therapeutic community (as originated by Maxwell Jones) programs are powerful educational tools for the development of both patients and staff.

RESEARCH: THE ADMINISTRATOR'S ROLE

Dynamic educational and research programs are the sine qua non of medical schools and university hospitals. But a great many other health and mental health organizations aspire to have these elements represented in their clinical facilities. VA hospitals, particularly after World War II, made great strides in linking with medical schools through the instrumentality of dean's committees and various formal and informal agreements and understandings. Many state and county hospitals have vigorous training and research programs, usually in connection with medical schools. Private institutions seek to educate staff and attract quality attending staff via educational programs, and are proud if they can be counted as medical school affiliates.

Establishing a research identity in an affiliating institution is usually a much harder task than developing educational programs, but many VA, state, and county institutions have succeeded in making progress in this direction.

Research is least developed in private for-profit institutions, but some of these institutions have managed to set aside significant resources in order to gain a reputation in this area. Institutional self-worth and self-esteem seem to be dependent, at least partially, on closeness to academe. Dedication of its staff to intellectual development is considered a mark of distinction. Needless to say, the effect on the bottom line of improved self-esteem as well as improved public image does not escape the notice of sophisticated management.

Collaboration with Academe

In developing an institutional research identity, ties with a medical school, health science center, or college should proceed *pari passu* with the development of scientific resources at the affiliating institution. Cultivation of the support and cooperation of departmental chairs and research personnel in the university is a necessary early step. Identification of personnel *inside* the institution who are interested in developing their potentialities as researchers, or actually developing a research career, should be undertaken. Space, laboratories, a vivarium, and assistance in design and methodology in preparation of research proposals will be necessary.

Universities play host to many investigators, some of renown. Their records of original contributions to knowledge and theory brighten the university's name. Many have a secure financial base augmented by grants from federal and private foundations. Their success is often based on two quite different attributes: excellent research, and mastery of the art of grantsmanship. Seasoned investigators can be very valuable in promoting careers of younger colleagues. Not infrequently, they are interested in collaborating with an affiliating institution because they need space for expansion, and access to another, different population. The affiliating institution may offer laboratories and assistants. Also, currently operating clinical laboratories may provide routine chemical and biological tests valuable in clinical research.

Trained clinical laboratory assistants already employed by the affiliating institution can help a project get started, often without additional expenditures.

For its part, in the longer run, the affiliating institution—in order to reap the benefits of research and closer ties with academe—must make a substantial investment. Social research or mental health services research, not requiring wet laboratories, need relatively small outlays of funds, but a fully functioning wet laboratory with a full-time scientist and appropriate technical support may require hundreds of thousands of dollars. One can start with far less by encouraging staff to devote a few hours of their "clinical time" to scholarship and research, adding their own private hours to those allotted by the institution. If the staff person "catches fire" in the excitement of research, it is amazing how both his clinical and research work can get done, particularly if his research is cleverly designed to obtain data evolving naturally from his day-to-day work with patients.

The VA Model

The Department of Veterans Affairs has done a great job in making many of its institutions desirable places for investigators to settle and work. The VA not only has set aside millions annually in research funds for principal investigators with approved proposals and for career support, but also has established research offices with space and salaries for a director and assistants and the paraphernalia needed for computer and statistical analysis. A wise arrangement was made with the National Institutes of Health so that VA investigators may apply there also for funds, without prejudice. A policy that allows professional staff members with research inclinations to devote a significant proportion of their time to scholarship or research has been a boon to creative individuals. For basic research, the VA has also invested in equipment, vivaria, and animals. The device that provides appointments of promising individuals jointly in VA and medical school departments, as well as joint contribution to salaries, completes a system that has been successful in recruiting staff and upgrading the caliber of clinical care.

Functions of Administration and the Research Director

A word about the function of administration in the creation of a research environment is in order. Research and development efforts are more successful when upper management sees value in these pursuits and supports them consistently. It helps if top administration is also creative, intellectually inclined, and carries on its own research programs. A research director can be a great help, provided that the director does not "direct" too much. *Facilitator* would perhaps be a better term than *director*, for no researcher worth his salt wants to be subordinate for long; he strives for independence, the opportunity to follow his own line of thought and to choose his own collaborators. The research director's main functions are to discover talented individuals, to help them obtain the means to prosecute their programs, and then to leave them essentially on their own. The good research director is likened to a benign father, or a painstaking teacher, not an orchestra conductor who rules with an iron baton.

Yet, a research organization does not grow by chance. Someone has to assign space, help raise funds, look after morale, cultivate interdisciplinary communication, and facilitate collaborations with other sources of inspiration.

Leadership is required to develop an environment in which researchers can meet together in healthy exchange and enjoy opportunities to stretch their minds in directions above and beyond their own, often narrow, perspectives. Research workers should not be isolated; opportunities should be provided to mingle with others. Collaboration between clinical and basic science should be encouraged. A critical attitude toward prevailing concepts may encourage more critical thought by clinicians. In return, contact with the clinician reminds the researcher why he is doing research: not only to satisfy innate curiosity but, it is hoped, to contribute to the health and welfare of people.

Are Researchers Different?

Obviously, no sharp line can be demarcated between researchers and other personnel; nevertheless, many individuals drawn to a research career do have characteristics that, to an extent, set them apart. Like artists obsessed with their own thoughts and ideas, they need to create something useful, thus to fulfill themselves. They are often more analytical and critical in their approach to problems than others, and have a nagging desire to move from general concepts to precise measurement and quantification. In the methodological sense, they reduce hunches to hypotheses, which they then test by the orderly accumulation of relevant data, analyzed and reanalyzed to cast maximum light on basic questions. The true scientist hopes to build an intellectual edifice of enduring value; he knows this will require great persistence, patience, and perseverance. To do his very special thing—again like the true artist—he may make sacrifices, and he sometimes travels on a lonely road. Many scientists earn less than their clinical counterparts, and often their salaries or supports are based on soft money; they must win grants in order to survive.

In clinically oriented institutions, basic scientific personnel often tend to become clannish. Clinical personnel may resent the research person's freedom from routine duties of patient care, the massive paperwork, and the rules and regulations of standard-setting organizations. Particularly when work is burdensome, they find it difficult to understand why research personnel are not helping them on the front lines. To administration, however, research is justified because it represents investment in the future. One can point this out to the querulous clinician and also indicate how clinical personnel may profit in the enrichment of the environment, and in advances in treatment developed by research personnel. Clinicians, too, it should be emphasized, are in a position to make important original contributions, as the histories of the Oslers, Corrigans, Heberdens, and a host of other bedside observers attest. The ambitious clinician can receive advice and assistance from his research colleagues in shaping hunches into researchable questions, as well as in the design and selection of methodology appropriate to his problem.

Who Can Do Research?

In a multidiscipline hospital, the question may be asked, "Who can do research?" The answer, I believe, is simple: All disciplines can do research, and ought to be encouraged to do so. The curiosity of the various disciplines is particularly valuable when directed to their own fields, for each specialty has unique questions to ask and a unique contribution to make. It would be foolhardy for a clinical specialty to wait for highly trained experts in research to focus their attention on areas in which they have little familiarity or interest. Sometimes untrained people are in awe of research, which they view with a capital R, as involving mastery of highly technical concepts and methodologies. However, there is methodology appropriate to every question and to every level of sophistication.

Obstacles and Resistances

About 30 years ago, during a period of national expansion of research and clinical innovations, a number of studies on psychiatric residents were generated at Massachusetts Mental Health Center (of which I was chief of laboratories and research from 1943 to 1963) by Levinson and Sharaf.[43,44,45] During that time the Massachusetts Mental Health Center (MMHC), with a total complement of about 70 residents, attracted some of the best and brightest men and women. Interviews were conducted with these residents as to their backgrounds, experiences, and interests in the field of research. During their training period, research was accorded a high value in the curriculum. The field in general was undergoing a massive research development, with increasing amounts of money available from the National Institute of Mental Health (NIMH) and the foundations. Many residents were considering the possibility of making research a serious part of their career. At this time also, NIMH was beginning to award career research grants to promising young investigators.

Briefly, studies revealed that about one-third of the residents became sufficiently immersed in research to produce publishable papers. These residents had research in their blood, and were hell-bent to accomplish something important. And many of them, in fact, are among the most prominent names in psychiatry today.

Another third of the residents came to psychiatric research by adoption, so to speak. Research was in the ambience, a vigorous department of research was growing, and research seemed to be the thing to do to gain "brownie points"—but a full-time research career was not in their stars, and they knew it. The final third of residents either had little interest in research, were intent on becoming first-rank clinicians, or were primarily concerned with becoming proficient psychodynamic psychiatrists or psychoanalysts. Often, their role models were the psychoanalytic teachers in the department of psychiatry, and their chief desire was to be accepted at an early stage into the psychoanalytic institute.

From these residents, we at MMHC learned a great deal not only about their primary inclinations and career dreams, but also about their resistances to research. Sometimes the natural curiosity they possessed was blocked by some attitude or experience that turned them cold. Some were soured by a traumatic event, as was the case with one promising youngster apprenticed to a highly productive scientist who worked him almost to death. Another had an uncle who was the family paragon of success as a scientist, but he hated this uncle. Another could not stand the discipline required to amass data by the repetition of boring tests. Another saw in the research obsessions of his colleagues not a natural expression of their curiosities, but an opportunistic zeal for academic advancement—it was "publishing for publication's sake," the journals were "full of trash," and only a few articles had merit; most were "think pieces" of little value or were methodologically seriously faulted.

F. Lyman Wells[46] used to say that a good researcher had three qualities: he was a "thinker upper," a "worker through-er," and a "getter done-er." Some of the psychiatric residents avoided research because they knew their own limitations: They simply did not possess the qualities necessary to succeed in the demanding field of research. Others realized that their talents did not lie in research, and indeed feared that concentration on the narrow mechanics of research would squelch their other aptitudes. In this latter group were some who displayed exceptionally empathic understanding of the dynamics of mentally ill patients, particularly those who were severely regressed. With the added insight afforded by psychoanalytic training, they hoped to enjoy a career of work with such patients.

Vicissitudes

"The young researcher may think he is all set when he gets his own laboratory, his university affiliation, his equipment, his salary, his secretary, and his assistant."[47] Unfortunately, the realities of the current scene present him with the task of maintaining status in the face of budgetary curtailments, diminished support from funding agencies, and perhaps the practical necessity of shifting his focus to fit the funding policies of foundations. Today, institutions stricken with debts and deficiencies may phase out nonrevenue-producing programs—research being one. Federal and private foundations have had to cut back. Competition for their dollars is fierce; the possibility of a turndown of an application is greater than ever, even after the applicant has expended his best efforts. Almost every researcher of long experience has suffered the deflating experience of rejection by a jury of his peers. After one or two of these, should he then abandon the field? This is where the administrator has to give hard thought to raising tide-over funds until another proposal, incorporating the grant-giving foundation's critique, can be fashioned. Should he also assist the researcher in raising funds from new resources, and perhaps establish a local foundation for this purpose? The dilemma facing the career-oriented investigator is whether and how far to go in assuming a new role as a fund-raiser to support his personal projects. In any event, failure of a proposal does not mean the end of the world, although it does provide a role for someone to help sustain the researcher's courage in the face of a major narcissistic injury.

As if this were not enough, the researcher has to search his soul for justification for a change in direction in order to stay alive in a changing world of finance. The principle here is seen by some as an eminently ethical one: for example, is it morally defensible to abandon the track of one's prime interest, and possibly years of hard work in that direction, simply to pursue the research dollar?

The answer is not an easy one. Before making a final decision, however, the following should be considered:

1. Foundations change their direction in response to community needs. A great deal of research and consultation goes into their decisions as to how they can best serve humanity, given the guidelines provided by donors or by consultants.
2. Imaginative reformulation of research design can frequently allow inclusion of additional concepts and aims more suitable to foundation policies without seriously straining one's principles.
3. Research techniques and skills honed in the service of one set of hypotheses can often be translated to another.

The Clinical Research Center

Let us assume, however, that the researcher continues more or less happily with his career. Along its course, he may come to a point where he tries to develop a clinical research center, or develop a protocol that subordinates much of the work of a ward to his research design. Here he should be aware of how much the clinical functions of the ward may come into conflict with his research aims. Surely, at this point, he needs steadfast support from administration in order to make *any* headway, and he also needs to do a great deal of work with clinical personnel lest his research design be seen as contrary to good clinical care and the patients' best interests. Where the research design involves obtaining data that delays or complicates treatment, or where some patients receive medication that is denied others, the clinical staff may withhold cooperation overtly or covertly. Under such circumstances, either present personnel must be won over or new personnel hired. Do not underestimate personnel's problems in accepting a new equilibrium that puts researchers virtually in charge or imposes a new way of working with patients that has not been fully rationalized to them.

Much experience has been gained since clinical research centers became popular in the 1950s. The following guidelines have emerged: (a) Considerable time for orientation and planning is needed before a research is undertaken; (b) both ward personnel and administration should be involved in the planning stages; (c) repeated ward community meetings will be necessary to resolve resistance to the new pattern of activities; (d) feedback and interpretation of results to ward personnel at intervals will be appreciated; and (e) credit should be given to other than strictly research personnel who have made the program possible.[48]

Multihospital Research

Some research projects, particularly those that require a large number of research subjects who are relatively scarce in any one hospital, may require the collaboration of several hospitals. This increases the number of research personnel involved, as well as the importance of shared participation in design and execution. It also increases the number of administrators whose agreement and continued support become absolutely vital.

Probably the earliest multihospital project was that involving four hospitals on the treatment of depression, steered by the research group at Massachusetts Mental Health Center.[49,50] Approximately 300 hospitalized depressed patients from several different diagnostic groups were treated by a variety of methods. Monoamine oxidase inhibitors, tricyclics, and electroconvulsive therapy were compared, using uniform behavior and symptom scales. This project succeeded only because research leaders accepted a strong managerial role in order to guarantee cooperation, compliance with the details of the design, and careful harvesting of data in a timely fashion. Since then, the VA system has carried out a number of large-scale treatment evaluation projects, and NIMH has funded many more.

Both the clinical research center and the multihospital research program have become standard modern research instrumentalities. They have contributed much to improved patient care and to the institutions that have participated in those large efforts.

Research as an Instrument for Social Change[51]

The mere presence of research workers in an institution can change the ambience significantly. More critical thinking, more attention to observations that are new or instructive, identification of intriguing ideas or hypotheses, greater interest in scholarship, intellectual stimulation—all these and more can occur. Research personnel enrich the teaching program by periodic feedback of progress and results to staff. Seminars and conferences with outside invited experts advance knowledge and practice in the field. Investigators who are experts in given areas are encyclopedias of useful information that can be tapped simply by a telephone call.

Among the more useful aspects of research is its application to social and organizational change. Here social psychologists, sociologists, and social anthropologists have a special role, and through their efforts, valuable bridges can be established to corresponding social science departments beyond the medical school. I have collaborated with social scientists for many years, and in one particular phase of the developing research program, a number of social scientists working at MMHC produced a memorable harvest of insights into the inner workings of mental institutions.[52,53]

Examples of their valuable contributions are numerous: studies of interaction rates of patients on the ward and their fluctuations in relation to interaction rates of patient leaders and their cliques;[54] preferential treatment of patients by staff as related to prognosis;[55] custodialism and humanism as polar ideological belief systems of hospital personnel;[56] ideological polarities in the treatment philosophies of psychiatric residents;[57] how the attendant sees his role and functions;[58] prevention of hospitalization;[59] drugs and social therapy in schizophrenia;[60] the role of college students in the mental hospital;[61] and custodial to therapeutic patient care in mental hospitals.[62]

Also directly applicable to patient care were studies of the day-care program, halfway house, apartment cooperatives, admission procedures, executive succession, rehabilitation, administration, and psychopolitics. These and other studies were often critical in determining policy and in developing priorities in the allocation of resources. It is virtually impossible today to make sophisticated policy decisions without social dynamic studies linked to resource availability and patient flow.

In summary, cultivation of a research atmosphere is a sine qua non in a mental hospital. It is a link to the academic community, a way of looking at ourselves, and a tool for social change. It attracts talented people and outside funds. The task of building a research organization can be immeasurably lightened by a hospital administrator who has had research training and experience and is a constant support of its growth and development.

Summary and Comments

To collaborate with academe and establish a research identity is considered important in upgrading the intellectual climate as well as the care and treatment of patients. Medical school affiliation and the cultivation of research and training programs are widely valued for their contribution to professional development and institutional respect. Often a substantial outlay in space, laboratories, and vivarium support is required. Joint appointments of talented personnel to both university and hospital and joint contributions to their salaries are familiar arrangements that function to bring the two institutions together.

Administrators play a vital role in such aspirations, for research organizations do not grow by chance. In addition to space and equipment, a supportive intellectual environment must be created with time for scholarship and scientific investigation by clinical staff members who possess interest and show promise. The program is significantly enhanced if top administrators, whether clinical or management personnel, are themselves involved in creative activities.

Far from being an esoteric pursuit for a selected group of inspired investigators, individuals from any discipline can be involved, each assisted to advance upward from current levels of interest and abilities. A research director with skill in eliciting and abetting creative potentialities can be a great help.

Studies have enlightened us as to the psychological obstacles and resistances that impede the indulgence of native curiosity, and practical experience informs us as to the vicissitudes of the investigator and the institution in developing vigorous, exciting, and high-quality research programs.

Clinical research centers and multi-institutional collaborations are hallmarks of advanced research programs. They challenge the administrator to achieve cooperation and collaboration with a network of hospitals and policymakers. In addition to its uses for the researcher, research can serve an institution well as an instrument for social and organizational change.

REFERENCES

1. Duval AM, Klein RH, Feldman PE: Must a mental hospital superintendent be a physician-psychiatrist? Hospitals 31:34–38, 1957
2. Barton WE: Vanishing American—mental hospital administrators and commissioners. Mental Hospitals 13:55–61, 1962
3. Barton WE: The hospital administrator. Mental Hospitals 13:259–264, 1962
4. Kolb LC: Who should administer psychiatric facilities? Hospital & Community Psychiatry 20:170–173, 1969
5. Barton WE: Training in administration for psychiatrists. Psychiatr Ann 3:8–26, 1973
6. Gaver KD, Norman ML, Greenblatt M: Life at the state summit: Views and experiences of 18 psychiatric leaders. Hospital & Community Psychiatry 35:233–238, 1984
7. Arnold WN, Rodenhauser P, Greenblatt M: Residency Education in Administrative Psychiatry: A National Survey. Academic Psychiatry 15:188–194, 1991
8. Sherwood E, Greenblatt M, Pasnau RO: Psychiatric residency, role models, and leadership. Amer J Psychiatry 143:764–767, 1986
9. Greenblatt M, Gaver KD, Norman M: Psychiatric leadership. The paths to the summit: The risks and the rewards. Presented at American College of Mental Health Administration annual meeting, October 30–November 1, 1983, St. Petersburg Beach, Florida (unpublished)
10. Greenblatt M, Gaver KD, Sherwood E: After commissioner, what? Amer J Psychiatry 142:752–754, 1985
11. Gaver KD, Norman ML, Greenblatt M: Life at the state summit: Views and experiences of 18 psychiatric leaders. Hospital & Community Psychiatry 35:233–238, 1984
12. Greenblatt M, Rose SO: Illustrious psychiatric administrators. Amer J Psychiatry 134:626–630, 1977

13. Greenblatt M, Rose SO: Illustrious psychiatric administrators. Amer J Psychiatry 134:626–630, 1977
14. Sherwood E, Greenblatt M, Pasnau RO: Psychiatric residency, role models, and leadership. Amer J Psychiatry 143:764–767, 1986
15. Perkins DS: From interviews conducted by Collins EGC, Scott P, with Lunding FJ, Clements GL, Perkins DS, in Everyone who makes it has a mentor. Reprinted from Harvard Business Review, July–August 1978, Number 78403, in Harvard Business Review, Paths Toward Personal Progress: Leaders Are Made, Not Born. Cambridge, Mass., President and Fellows of Harvard College, 1983
16. Livingston JS: Myth of the well-educated manager. Reprinted from Harvard Business Review, January–February 1971, May–June 1971, Number 1108, in Harvard Business Review, Paths Toward Personal Progress: Leaders Are Made, Not Born. Cambridge, Mass., President and Fellows of Harvard College, 1983
17. Grusky O, Thompson WA, Tillipman H: Clinical versus administrative backgrounds for mental health administrators. Administration and Policy in Mental Health 18:271–278, 1991
18. Katz RL: Skills of an effective administrator. Reprinted from Harvard Business Review, September–October 1974, Number 74509, in Harvard Business Review, Paths Toward Personal Progress: Leaders Are Made, Not Born. Cambridge, Mass., President and Fellows of Harvard College, 1983
19. Nichols RG, Stevens LA: Listening to people. Reprinted from Harvard Business Review, September–October 1957, Number 57507, in Harvard Business Review, Paths Toward Personal Progress: Leaders Are Made, Not Born. Cambridge, Mass., President and Fellows of Harvard College, 1983
20. Greenblatt, M: Some ingredients for mental health. Western Journal of Medicine, special issue, Personal Health Maintenance, 141:861–863, 1984
21. Kets de Vries MFR (ed): The Irrational Executive: Psychoanalytic Studies in Management. New York, International University Press, 1984
22. Kernberg OF: Leadership and organizational functioning: Organizational regression. International J Group Psychotherapy 20:3–25, 1978
23. Kernberg OF: Regression in organizational leadership. Psychiatry 42:24–39, 1979
24. Harrison JC: How to stay on top of a job. Reprinted from Harvard Business Review, November–December 1961, Number 61605, in Harvard Business Review, Paths Toward Personal Progress: Leaders Are Made, Not Born. Cambridge, Mass., President and Fellows of Harvard College, 1983
25. Bennis W, Nanus B: Leaders: The Strategies for Taking Charge. New York, Harper & Row, 1985
26. Foley AR: Certification and training in administrative psychiatry. Hosp & Comm Psychiatry 22:69–73, 1971
27. American Psychiatric Association, Committee on Administrative Psychiatry: Information Bulletin for Applicants. Eleventh Edition. Washington, DC, American Psychiatric Association, 1989
28. University of Wisconsin-Madison: Master's Degree Program in Administrative Medicine. Program announcement by American College of Physician Executives, July 5, 1989
29. Henry JF: M.D.–M.B.A.: A dual degree whose time has come. J Amer Med Assoc 257:1727–1728, 1987
30. Bricker's International Directory of University Executive Programs. Princeton, New Jersey, Peterson's Guides, 1988
31. Feldman S: The Administration of Mental Health Services. Springfield, Illinois, Charles C Thomas, 1980
32. Barton WE, Barton GM: Mental Health Administration: Principles and Practices. New York, Human Sciences Press, 1982
33. Talbott JA, Kaplan SR: Psychiatric Administration: A Comprehensive Text for the Clinician-Executive. New York, Grune & Stratton, 1983
34. Barton WE, Barton GM: Mental Health Administration: Principles and Practices. New York, Human Sciences Press, 1982
35. Talbott JA, Kaplan SR: Psychiatric Administration: A Comprehensive Text for the Clinician-Executive. New York, Grune & Stratton, 1983
36. Borus JF: Teaching residents the administrative aspects of psychiatric practice. Amer J Psychiatry 140:444–448, 1983

37. Borus JF: Teaching residents the administrative aspects of psychiatric practice. Amer J Psychiatry 140:444–448, 1983
38. Talbott JA, Sacks M: Teaching psychiatric administration to senior residents. Admin in Mental Health 9:281–288, 1982
39. Arnold WN, Rodenhauser P, Greenblatt M: Residency education in administrative psychiatry: A national survey. Academic Psychiatry 15:188–194, 1991
40. Kaldeck R: Group therapy by nurses and attendants. Diseases of the Nervous System 12:138–142, 1951
41. Hyde RW, in collaboration with the Attendants of Boston Psychopathic Hospital: Experiencing the Patient's Day: A Manual for Psychiatric Hospital Personnel. New York, Putnam's Sons, 1955, pp 208–211
42. Greenblatt M, York RH, Brown EL: From Custodial to Therapeutic Patient Care in Mental Hospitals: Explorations in Social Treatment. New York, Russell Sage Publications, 1955
43. Sharaf MR, Levinson DJ: Patterns of ideology and role definition among psychiatric residents, in Greenblatt M, Levinson DJ, Williams RH (eds): The Patients and the Mental Hospital. Glencoe, Illinois, Free Press, 1957, pp 263–285
44. Sharaf MR, Greenblatt M: Attitudes of psychiatric residents towards milieu therapy. Social Psychiatry 9:142–156, 1968
45. Sharaf MR, Levinson DJ, Greenblatt M: The Psychiatric Alumni of Psycho: Initial Findings. Presented at Semicentenary Anniversary, Massachusetts Mental Health Center, Boston, October 1962 (unpublished manuscript)
46. Wells FL: Personal communication, ca. 1953
47. Greenblatt M, Sharaf MR, Stone EM: Research, Chapter 9 in Greenblatt M, Sharaf MR, Stone EM: Dynamics of Institutional Change. Pittsburgh, University of Pittsburgh Press, 1971, p 224
48. Madakasira S: Integrating research projects into clinical service settings. Hosp & Comm Psychiatry 39:888–889, 1988
49. Greenblatt M, Grosser GH, Wechsler H: A comparative study of selected antidepressant medications and EST. Am J Psychiatry 119:144–153, 1962
50. Greenblatt M, Grosser GH, Wechsler H: Differential response of hospitalized depressed patients to somatic therapy. Am J Psychiatry 120:935–943, 1964
51. Greenblatt M, York RH, Brown EL: From Custodial to Therapeutic Patient Care in Mental Hospitals: Explorations in Social Treatment. New York, Russell Sage Publications, 1955, pp 210–211
52. Kotin J, Sharaf MR: Management succession and administrative style. Psychiatry 30:237–248, 1967
53. Schulberg HC, Baker F: Mental Hospital and Human Services. New York, Behavioral Publications, 1975
54. Boyd RW, Baker T, Greenblatt M: Ward social behavior: An analysis of patient interaction at highest and lowest extremes. Nursing Research 3:77–80, 1954
55. Morimoto FR, Baker TS, Greenblatt M: Similarity of socializing interests as a factor in selection and rejection of psychiatric patients. J Nerv & Ment Dis 120:56–61, 1954
56. Gilbert DC, Levinson DJ: "Custodialism" and "humanism" in mental hospital structure and in staff ideology, in Greenblatt M, Levinson DJ, Williams RH (eds): The Patient and the Mental Hospital. Glencoe, Illinois, Free Press, 1957, pp 20–35
57. Sharaf MR, Levinson DJ: Patterns of ideology and role definition among psychiatric residents, in Greenblatt M, Levinson DJ, Williams RH (eds): The Patient and the Mental Hospital. Glencoe, Illinois, Free Press, 1957, pp 263–285
58. Wells FL, Greenblatt M, Hyde RW: As the Psychiatric Aide Sees His Work and Problems. Genetic Psychology Monographs 53:3–73, 1956
59. Greenblatt M, Moore RF, Albert RS, Solomon MH, et al: The Prevention of Hospitalization. New York, Grune & Stratton, 1963
60. Greenblatt M, Solomon MH, Evans AS, Brooks, GW: Drug and Social Therapy in Chronic Schizophrenia. Springfield, Illinois, Charles C Thomas, 1965
61. Umbarger CC, Dalsimer JS, Morrison AP, Breggin PR, with assistance and supervision of Kantor D, Greenblatt M: College Students in a Mental Hospital. New York, Grune & Stratton, 1962
62. Greenblatt M, York RH, Brown EL: From Custodial to Therapeutic Patient Care in Mental Hospitals. New York, Russell Sage Foundation, 1955

10

Relation of the Organization to the Outside World

Ever since the "bold new approach" (1963) launched by President Kennedy with the support of the American Psychiatric Association, the National Institute of Mental Health, and numerous other organizations, we have become increasingly conscious of the larger community in which mental health service organizations are imbedded and on which they depend for their viability and success.

If we think of a mental institution as the hub of a wheel (see Figure 10-1), its spokes extend outward to the body politic; labor unions; the media; regulatory agencies; licensing and accreditation bodies; citizen groups; professional organizations and boards; educational institutions; foundations and grant-giving agencies; surrounding clinics and facilities; and private mental hospitals. Communication between the hub and these outer agencies and facilities is a two-way phenomenon. The scene is constantly changing. The network of outside agencies is of great interest to the administration of any mental health institution, for a poor relationship with any of them can cripple or even destroy the healthy functioning of the hub institution. Good relationships with all of them, highly desired, come only at the expense of careful planning and hard work. As the administrator is drawn into interaction with these outside agencies, he tries to delegate his inside functions to trusted deputies. Sometimes this dilemma is solved by apportioning functions to two top administrators—one dedicated mainly to harmonizing the institution with outside agencies, the other attending primarily to inside demands. The two functional areas, however, must be integrated smoothly by executives who are compatible and work together harmoniously.

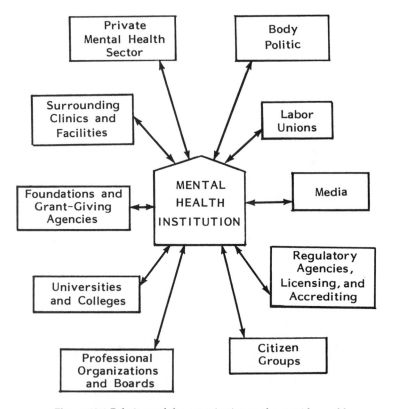

Figure 10-1 Relations of the organization to the outside world.

THE BODY POLITIC[1]

Deserving of our first attention is the body politic. The network of mental health facilities—state, county, VA, or university—is highly dependent on the body politic. A given institution may be robust if adequate resources are supplied, anemic if financial support is thin, or phased out altogether if its support system collapses. We have seen how in the deinstitutionalization period, many governmental hospitals were reduced in size, and some closed entirely.[2,3]

The Political System[4]

How may one best characterize the political system? Many books and treatises have been written on the subject. My observations here are based on the experiences of directors of institutions related to, and at least partially dependent on, the body politic.

An administrator who moves into a political system may be surprised to learn how different that system is from the academic and clinical systems in which he has previously worked. The pursuit of politics is an intensely adversarial game; opposite parties are in perpetual war for power and control. Each politician belongs to a party that is seeking to diminish, embarrass, or unseat members of the opposite party. In this game, truth and justice may be sacrificed to personal ambitions. Often, *ad hominem* charges and accusations take the place of the search for truth, and service to one's constituents may take a back seat to gratification of narcissistic needs for power and acclaim. The administrator thrust into this world must understand how this system works, and realize how difficult it is to change it to a more professionally oriented system. Under no circumstances can he discard the values of his own profession and descend to political gutter tactics. How can he be most effective in his task of promoting interest and attracting resources on behalf of the mentally ill, retarded, chemically dependent, and all those crippled by neurotic defenses or character disorders? That is his challenge.

Characteristics of the Political System

The administrator will note that the political system is characterized by three elements: (a) the search for power, (b) an ambience of suspiciousness, and (c) an ambience of materialism.

Power is often the dominant motif in the political system. Power resides in voter strength and in the politician's reputation as able fighter. Power is accrued by membership on important committees, particularly those that allocate resources (ways and means), decide crucial questions (judicial), or investigate wrongdoing. Power is enhanced by increasing one's name recognition and developing a positive image through appearances before the public; therefore, newspaper, radio, and TV coverage are much coveted. Fortunately, the need for power competes to a greater or lesser degree with the desire to serve one's constituents and to hew to the ideals of true statesmanship. These in turn must be achieved while mastering the complicated structural/functional aspects of the political system, the many new laws and initiatives coming up for votes in the immediate future, and the forces active in one's own local electoral district.

In the political system, suspiciousness concerning the motives of the various other office seekers is rampant. Each person is assumed to be interested primarily in serving himself or his immediate band of supporters, and higher motives are regarded with skepticism. The climate of suspiciousness is linked with an ambience of materialism. In political/governmental systems, people work primarily for material gain—money, security, higher position, vacations, and the accoutrements of status—whereas altruism, love of scholarship and learning, the search for truth, or dedication to the health and welfare of one's fellow man are more highly valued in hospitals and academic settings.

Psychiatric administrators are challenged to accept this state of affairs and to maintain their own value systems intact while they do business with political types who march to another drummer. They cannot show disrespect or play holier-than-thou to politicians, for most politicians believe that they, too, are professionals who wish to serve their public well. However, in order to do so, they feel they must first earn a secure place for themselves in the rough-and-tumble world of politics.

Founded on competition and rivalry, the political system is full of tensions and unrest. Actually, the winner in an election is never fully secure, for public attitudes shift rapidly, and at any moment a more attractive candidate may threaten the politician's hard-won place in the system. The incumbent's desires are to be reelected and eventually to win higher office; therefore, to all intents and purposes, he is always running for office. It is perilous to go against the public's priorities. Quite the opposite, it is imperative to please the people here and now in order to amass the votes necessary for survival and ascendancy.

The Politicians[5]

Politicians are of many breeds; there are at least five major types. The most common brand includes those who rise through party ranks by working on behalf of others seeking office, and thus gain experience in getting out the vote. They may work for years before they get the chance to run on their own. They are practical, down-to-earth, and opportunistic.

A second brand of politician gains recognition by rising in the hierarchy of a public service agency, such as those handling roads, parks, law enforcement, education, or business administration. The position he has achieved is often an appointive one, probably protected by civil service, but he may decide to try his hand at an elective office, skipping all the lower rungs of the political machine. Such individuals, during their years of running a professional agency, may therefore become partial to the mental health agency, which is parallel to their own. This shift of an agency head from a professional branch of government to an elective office, however, rarely occurs in the careers of heads of mental health or public health agencies.

A third group of politicians—a small group—seeks office because of a family tradition of public service. They usually have independent means of support, are well educated, and possess high ideals. They can resist being coopted by power seekers, and in the long run, exert an uplifting influence on other colleagues. They are open to the importance of mental health and are often quite interested in trying to raise its priority in the public mind.

A fourth group of individuals has become so well-known and liked in another field that the public is willing to endorse them for political office. The first one that comes to mind is Lee Iacocca of Chrysler Corporation, who sparked the public's imagination by the dramatic rescue of his company from debt and the speed with which he paid back a humongous federal loan; for a time, he was regarded as possible presidential timber. Of this same genre are Ronald Reagan, who became governor of California without ever having held public office; and Ted Kennedy, youngest son of a famous Massachusetts family and brother of a president and a senator, who was elected senator from his state without previous elective credentials. It is possible for these folks to pursue a more independent course than the average politician, who may be bound by his party backers to the rigid tenets of the party machine.

Finally, there are the defenders of the republic who have heroic records of performance on the field of battle and are, therefore, warmly regarded by a grateful people. In modern times, it has been Eisenhower; in previous times, Washington, Jackson, and Grant. One might argue that the ability to lead hordes of men in battle is not necessarily the best training for the responsibilities of government; nevertheless, some of our great soldiers appear to have been equal to the task.

How Politicians Relate to Mental Health

Whatever the type of politician an administrator of a psychiatric facility may meet, such contacts will surely be important. Local political officeholders are almost always interested in institutions serving their own district, and often seek active contact with directors of such institutions. They may visit and/or inspect the facility; they are interested in developing positive communication in case constituents come to them for help with health problems. Indeed, a compassionate politician functions at times as a pseudo–social worker, referring many needy people for treatment, especially those who are down and out.

On the other hand, politicians may make unwarranted demands on hospital administrators for special attention to constituents who helped get them elected. As commissioner of mental health in Massachusetts, I was on one occasion asked (perhaps *ordered* would be a more accurate term) by a senator to move a mental patient belonging to a distinguished supporter's family from one ward of the hospital to another. In another instance, an official at the very top echelon of government wanted me to appoint a friend as steward of a state hospital over candidates who I believed were better qualified. In still another case, much political pressure came to bear to admit developmentally disabled patients to schools for the retarded when all such schools in the state were hopelessly overcrowded. A final example: The chairman of the powerful state senate ways and means committee made it clear that he expected the department of mental health to change the mental hospital serving a variety of patients in his district to one dedicated exclusively to geriatric patients.

Such demands were a signal for very careful discussion and reasoning with these politicians, to explain how the hospitals were run, how difficult it was to recruit and retain good hospital superintendents unless their authority over their institutions was properly respected, and how unwelcome were political "orders" from outside. Two techniques I learned from wise counselors were (a) to appeal for support to the leadership of the Mental Health Association, a highly respected and important nongovernmental body dedicated to the welfare of the mentally ill, and (b) to mobilize support from more enlightened members of the party, or the governor's office, to prevent meddling in a professional state service organization. The overriding consideration in such cases was to resist as much as possible political control of the operations of the department of mental health. The commonsense principle was that if the commissioner got a reputation for yielding to politicians' demands, soon the department as a whole would be corrupted.

The utmost in tact and patience was required when the so-called "State Office" (actually a patronage office answerable to the governor) requested a change in the way the department was to do business in the future in hiring new people. Specifically, when the party in power was girding for reelection in a tight race, the state office sought to screen all applicants for non–civil service positions in the department of mental health. The situation was delicate, indeed, because the commissioner owed his appointment to the governor and served at the latter's pleasure. The difficult task was to convince the governor's advisers that their effort to capture and fill all vacant positions could be read by the people as interference with the integrity of a professional department, and could lose more votes than it would gain. Here, too, the upright citizens of the Mental Health Association, hinting at a bad press for the governor if he pursued this course, brought about a slow phaseout of this hiring program. It was a welcome return of control of the mental health department to its professional managers.

At this point, it should be noted that allocations of resources to mental health in almost all states come directly from the legislature to the department of mental health, based on a budget drawn up and submitted to the legislature by the executive branch. Thus, in most states, the state system of mental health is under direct control of the legislature and the governor. How different this is from the state department of education, which receives its funds and policy directives from a board of education, a regency, or some such body interposed between the governor and legislature, on the one hand, and the educational agencies (the universities and colleges) on the other. This buffer keeps the educational system one step away from direct manipulation by the political branch—a blessing that may someday come true for the state departments of mental health.

Disjunction between State and County

Another source of difficulty has recently been identified and analyzed by J. R. Elpers,[6] himself a former mental health commissioner for Los Angeles County. Unlike Massachusetts, where the state government deals directly with the cities and towns, in California, 58 county governments operate between the state and the mental health agencies that serve the people. The state allocates funds to the counties and then holds them responsible for providing services. What can happen then, especially distressing in times of austerity or financial crisis, is that the county supervisors face the heavy responsibility of providing services without adequate resources necessary to do the job. Such a crisis came to pass when, despite an increase of 19% in the population of Los Angeles in 17 years (from 7.0 million in 1970 to 8.4 million in 1987) and a concomitant increased demand for hospital services, a draconian reduction in hospital beds was effected, leading inevitably to great distress in the many emergency and crisis-intervention facilities of the counties. As a result, thousands of patients in need were turned away—many onto the streets. Many were handled under the penal code. A large number of those fortunate enough to gain admission to emergency facilities, for lack of beds, were forced to sleep on the floors of these units.

Elpers points out that developmentally disabled patients of California—whose funds, in contrast to those for the mentally ill, are allocated on a per capita basis directly from the legislature (probably as the result of a more powerful and persistent lobby)—have fared much better than the mentally ill in competition for state dollars.

Legislative Investigations

At all times, mental health facilities are vulnerable to legislative investigations because (a) they serve sick patients, many of whom are angry, bewildered, emotionally unstable, and out of touch with reality; (b) their family members, too, suffer from emotional stresses and strains, to a considerable extent related to the fear, disappointments, frustrations, and guilt attending the unwanted role of caring for sick relatives; and (c) the mental health facilities, particularly those in the public sector, are chronically underfunded. Treatment, therefore, is far from satisfactory, and the needs of the patient and family at best only partially met. Under these conditions, complaints and litigations increase, and the institutions in question are called to task by the media, the courts, citizen groups, or legislative investigators. Legislative investigations are more likely to occur during an election year, when politicians strive to be viewed as knights in white armor, tracking down evil. They may be precipitated by death or suicide of patients; complaints of assault and battery; complaints of discrimination; or accusations of malpractice, misfeasance, or malfeasance.

An administrator must react by welcoming the investigation, since as a conscientious executive and a person of moral rectitude he has nothing to hide. However, the threat to stability and even the tenure of the administrator is a very real one, for few organizations that are chronically underfunded—no matter how well run—can withstand detailed, intensive scrutiny, let alone ruthless searching for faults, errors, and oversights. The legislative investigating committee is apt to interview disgruntled employees, among other personnel, as well as patients and families who have complaints—often reaping a veritable harvest of discontents. When the results are finally in, the upshot may be negative press releases that demoralize dedicated employees working under hardship conditions; the scapegoating of an executive, including his removal from office or transfer to another position; or a change in institutional policy or procedures. But rarely is the financial support forthcoming to produce a fine hospital with quality service and high morale. There are notable modifications of this bleak scenario, as when a federal inspection reports so many deficiencies that millions of dollars in federal funds may be withdrawn unless immediate corrective actions are instituted. Then the state or county government will find a way to meet the federal criteria, although rarely rising above the minimal standards necessary to restore the flow of federal funds. A parallel event is when an inspection by JCAHO reveals so many faults that withdrawal of accreditation is threatened.

The new administrator soon realizes that he is under constant surveillance by patients, family, staff, standard-setting bodies, the superior officers of his department, the media, the legislators, and interested citizen groups. Of these, no agency has a combination of power, aggressiveness, and control of purse strings equal to the body politic.

One final element in the political constellation of bureaus must be mentioned, and that is the office of the auditor. State and county auditors are usually elected by the people, not appointed by the governor; therefore they are answerable only to the electorate and not likely to be held in check from powers above. There is much wisdom to this arrangement, but one point of vulnerability remains—namely, that the auditor, too, looks for publicity at election time. That publicity is his for the asking, for his army of auditors examines public facilities throughout the year, with a yield of negative findings ready to be released to the media whenever it is timely in terms of a bid for reelection.

THE MEDIA

Relations with radio, television, and the press should be supervised directly by the chief executive; however, it may be assigned operationally to others who can report quickly to top administration. Top administration must be involved actively in shaping public relations policy, for the simple reason that the life of the institution may depend on what the public thinks of it. Further, the top administrator is regarded by the public as the chief spokesman and representative of the institution to the people. It should be carefully noted that there is little he can say in a public forum that the media respect as off-the-cuff, even if he specifically asks the media not to quote him. Not only are his remarks assumed to carry official significance, but also an ardent young journalist intent on delivering a juicy morsel to his editor may forget to respect a request for silence—or if he represents a yellow journal, he may distort remarks or embellish them to suit his own purposes.

> The power of the press is formidable and frightening. It can make or break. It can elevate a politician or other public figure to the skies or crash him to the earth. It can be a vital force in the passage of laws or in their

defeat. It can concentrate attention on any issue of its choosing and ignore others. It can stimulate and enhance, or it can harass and irritate. It can be a great respecter of the truth, or it can be sloppy with the facts. It can probe and uncover, or it can gloss things over.[7]

Journalists often say "We do not make the news, we only print it." This, unfortunately, is only a partial truth, for among the events of the day, some are selected, others rejected, and the method of handling the event and expressing the so-called facts varies with the integrity and intelligence of the medium representative, the policy of the medium, and its economic needs. Journalists vary greatly in talent and integrity. I have known a journalist of a poor newspaper who rarely got the story straight, even when it was written down for him. And I have known a journalist of a great newspaper who appeared to be taking sketchy notes, but could produce a better, more eloquent statement than was originally provided.

When news is thin, a small story may be spread large. When news is abundant, a big story may emerge as a short précis on the last page. If the newspaper is threatened by diminishing circulation, it may exaggerate and sensationalize. Finally, the owner may have a set of values, concepts, and goals that the staff from the editor down must respect or lose their jobs.

In a hospital, a set of policies and procedures must be made clear. Remember that in dialogue with the media, two goals are simultaneously served: first, to tell the truth, and second, to respect the institution's basic mission—that is, to give the best possible service to the patients and their families within the sources provided. Since the truth is many-sided, it pays to think through carefully what is to be presented so that both aims are successfully served. Be brief; do not expand remarks inappropriately or elaborate beyond that which has been asked. Remember also that questions asked by media representatives may be strategically loaded so as to catch the unwary. Try to anticipate questions, and think carefully about the best phraseology to reflect your point of view.

The media are always avidly searching for stories of human interest, and what goes on in mental hospitals and clinics fascinates their readers. Not infrequently, complaints by relatives or by disgruntled staff are investigated, resulting in a negative report. Then that negative story is repeated in follow-up articles, for the readers' orientation, each time the original event is referred to. It may take many positive references to the institutions' good work to counter a single negative release; moreover, positive material released to the press is less likely to be printed than negative.

A steady stream of information of potential interest to the public should emanate from the front office: important appointments on the staff, awards and honors, new programs, research findings of interest, activities of volunteers, developmental campaigns, new buildings, and banquets and testimonials honoring hospital staff or community citizens. Many of these will be picked up by media people, who at times of low news input may be glad for a few "fillers." To facilitate two-way communication, personal relationships with media personnel ought to be assiduously cultivated. What ought to be just as assiduously avoided, on the other hand, is any direct feuding with the press—for the press, as is well-known, always has the last word.

A final comment applies to the phenomenon wherein hospital personnel are asked to give their slants on human interest topics of the day. Sometimes it concerns a scientific discovery just reported in the *New England Journal of Medicine* or the *Journal of the American Medical Association,* where the opinions of leading scientists are indeed newsworthy. Sometimes it concerns a debate of public interest, such as "Why are celebrity children so often drug addicts?" or "Why are some Nobel laureates and Oscar winners disdainful of receiving prizes?"

Since many of these opinion-type questions do not bear directly on hospital policy or practice, they may be answered without referring to the hospital public relations department for guidance. However, the wary respondent often wonders whether anything is truly served by speculating on questions where few data are available.

PROFESSIONAL ORGANIZATIONS AND BOARDS

Mental health organizations are unique in terms of the involvement of professional associations and boards in their structure and function. The members of the multidisciplinary team—the psychiatrists, psychologists, nurses, social workers, rehabilitation specialists, nurse counselors, and clergy—all owe their training to university programs that bestow upon them degrees they value highly. The conferring of degrees is accompanied also by special rites of passage that have great emotional value and bind them to the tenets and beliefs of the specialty. Ideals and standards inculcated during the training years are then brought into the treatment institution. Thus, professionals who make up the treatment team have double loyalties: one to the values of their profession, and the other to the needs and values of the therapeutic institution. When professional ideals are compromised (as by progressive erosion of the quality of services through budgetary reductions), professionals become dissatisfied. They attempt to right matters by reporting to important people in academe who trained them, by advising new trainees to steer clear of the questionable hospital, by reporting to influential political persons or the press, or by activating the union representing their professional association. Finally, they may resign from the institution in question when their tolerance is exhausted.

The most acute distress the treatment organization can suffer is through the strike, an example of which is given in this chapter. But the gradual erosion of confidence in an institution by spreading the word that its level of moral commitment to patient care is unacceptable also can cripple programs.

Mental health systems recognize professional attainment through their pay scales. Years of study and success in passing the board exams of their specialty pay off in larger salaries and higher appointments. Thus, the director of a psychiatric training program must be board certified, and the vast majority of psychiatric residents desire to pass their boards as soon as possible. A psychologist who leads a training program must have proper credentials before his students can receive academic credit for time spent in his program, or before they can accumulate approved supervised hours permitting an application for a license to practice. A psychiatrist giving testimony in court may find that his board certification is given additional weight. The percentage of board-certified people in a given specialty in a hospital is often regarded as a rough measure of the quality of its staff.

Most hospitals are not only desirous of technical affiliation with academic institutions, but also willing to provide training opportunities for students in the several specialties. If the students have had a satisfying experience, they often opt to stay with the mother institution; high quality of staff can thus be assured by choosing the best from those trained. Worthy of emphasis are the boost to prestige afforded by university affiliation, the positive effect on staff from the interaction with bright young minds, and the recognition by the public that affiliated institutions may offer better medicine than the nonaffiliated.

However, special obligations come along with the virtues of training programs. The specialty boards do have rigorous rules and standards, which they enforce by periodic inspections. The American Board of Psychiatry and Neurology, together with the American Medical Association, establishes a residency review committee that promulgates rules relating to the size of training programs, curricula, the diversity of areas to be taught, periodic internal review, and testing of trainees before graduation. Over the years, board examinations have grown greatly in importance, so that now the vast majority of psychiatrists in training plan on sitting for the board exam early in their careers.

EDUCATIONAL INSTITUTIONS

Hospitals and clinics have found that it can be good business to hitch up to institutions of higher learning.[8] The advantages are many. Teaching hospitals find that training physicians, nurses, and other health care professionals expands their patient pools. As it becomes known that their staffs and equipment are superior, capable of dealing with every level of clinical complexity, patients come from far and wide. Teaching hospitals also develop medical research centers that are early aware of new advances in diagnosis and treatment, or may even be pioneers in developing new advances. Teaching hospitals become specialists in areas of medicine that help mold the hospital's reputation in the community. Teaching hospitals win supporting funds from foundations that help pay administrative costs and add clinicians and scientists to the roster of those caring for the sick. Scientific advances pioneered by development of teaching/research programs form the basis for fund-raising that may intrigue a philanthropist. Research funds can pay for costly drugs and equipment, bed costs, space renovations, and information systems that improve statistical control over treatment systems.

However, training programs in hospitals and clinics are not without their drawbacks. Stipends for psychiatric residents, for example, were once generously supplied by the National Institutes, then withdrawn over a period of a few years, thus forcing hospitals to assume the costs. The same applies to instructors of trainees—their support has been freezing up. Overhead on training grants is not as generous as for research grants and may not fully cover hospital indirect expenses. Then there is the time necessary to write up excruciatingly detailed applications, or requests for renewal; in some demonstration proposals, particularly, there is the necessity for the applicant institution to raise a matching contribution.

For research and training grants, space and animal care in approved vivaria managed by certified veterinaries are a necessity. A research-and-education administrative entity ought to be set up from the very beginning to keep track of funding sources, to administer funds, and to monitor use of equipment. Also, it is necessary that patients' rights be suitably protected and the hospital suitably insured against damage suits if anything goes wrong. The expenditure of time and money just to administer a research department may be considerable.

As funds for research and training fluctuate over time, or even dry up, there is the unhappy consequence of phasing out a research team to which the institution feels committed. Finding funds to bridge to the next project or program is not easy. Nor is it easy to find regular hospital employment for researchers who for some time have been funded by outside sources. This is, in fact, a serious reality of our times—for not only have there been deep slashes in research and education funds, but also the shift of training costs to other patient care items has been resisted by third-party payers.

Nevertheless, the participation of hospitals in research and education is absolutely vital to the health and welfare of our citizens, and the struggle to find resources is critical in such a great cause. At this time, roughly one in every four hospitals trains health professionals. Not only doctors are represented in this group but also nurses, social workers, psychologists, rehabilitators, occupational therapists, and pastoral counselors. Field training of public health administrators has also become a familiar activity.

A special problem arises with respect to regularly employed members of staff who wish to devote part of their time to scholarly or research goals, but who themselves are not recipients of outside research or educational funds. How much encouragement should they receive, and how much time may they be allowed—time obviously drawn from providing units of service that form the basis of hospital revenues? Practices vary greatly. In universities dedicated by charter to scientific and scholarly attainment, a great deal of time is granted for teaching, pursuit of knowledge, and development of theory. In many medical schools approximately one-half time of the faculty member is supported in this manner; the other half time devoted to practice, consultation, and so forth, sufficient to make up a competitive total income. In many VA hospitals, up to 25% of a physician's time may be devoted to creative activities approved by the individual's supervisor. County and state hospitals are finding it necessary to allow time for creative activity in order to attract competent staff, despite the fact that they are so heavily revenue dependent. Private hospitals generally do little research and development, although they like to have trainees around to promote an academic climate and to honor academic values.

It should be noted that when a university medical school commits itself to collaboration with a hospital (be it state, county, VA, or private), it has specific practical interests above and beyond altruistic public service. The university needs space for expanding research facilities, which are expensive to build; it can use hospital salary funds to supplement its own funds in recruiting renowned scientists and teachers; or it may require broader and richer clinical populations to improve both teaching and research. Clinical pathology may be found in county and state hospitals that is not matched by the university population (usually selected from a higher socioeconomic level). As an example, in one great university teaching hospital of my knowledge, there is a gross shortage of obstetrical cases to support the teaching program; in another, emergency cases and adolescent mentally ill are lacking. It is a great help not to have to pay for real estate, bed costs, or administrative overhead, or to have to do battle directly with political bodies related to the affiliated institutions.

From the hospital's side, the gains are very important, although less tangible. University collaboration raises the intellectual and scholarly level, makes it possible to recruit better staff, and focuses greater interest on the patients, particularly those with complicated secondary and tertiary illnesses. The availability of the library facilities of the university, its special expertise in important clinical areas, and a general aura of dedication to high standards of care and treatment are important values to be gained by affiliation with a university.

REGULATION: LICENSURE AND ACCREDITATION

Licensure and Accreditation[9]

The costs and quality of health care are the two variables in clearest focus nowadays. Annual health care costs consumed 11% of the gross national product (GNP) in 1986 ($458 billion), as compared to 6% ($255 billion) in 1966. Despite drastic steps taken by government agencies, insurance companies, and corporations, costs of health care continue to spiral. The inevitable result of strategic efforts at cost containment is increasing concern for quality of care.

At what point, one asks, do progressive funding restrictions impact so seriously on quality of care as to prick the conscience of professionals, cause errors in diagnosis and treatment, prolong illness of patients, and place hospital staffs and hospitals in legal jeopardy?

Professional Licensure and Credentialing

State licensing of medical practitioners has for generations been one form of protection of the public. Because of public concerns about unqualified professionals engaging in practice and occasional lurid press stories about fraudulent doctors,[10] state licensing procedures have become much stricter in recent years. The concern is about physicians who falsify their credentials; practice under the influence of alcohol or drugs; or, through the prescriptive process, in effect act as drug pushers. The states' licenses are generic; the state depends on professional specialty board examinations to identify qualified specialists. In recent years, most specialty boards have been moving toward reexamination and recertification for maintenance of specialty status. Psychiatry, however, does not currently require recertification, although this has been an active topic of discussion in the circles of the American Board of Psychiatry and Neurology and the American Psychiatric Association for years. Psychiatry, instead, depends on evidence of continuing education—the merits of which need much further research.

The Joint Commission on Accreditation of Healthcare Organizations (JCAHO) requires health care facilities to present their procedures for credentialing and privileging of health care professionals at each survey. This applies not only to doctors but also to nurses, social workers, and psychologists. The information must be approved by the chief of the service and by quality assurance committees, usually after initial approval by the applicant's professional peers. This form of self-policing should be seriously undertaken by professionals, for the alternative—namely, greater government control—is highly undesirable. All physicians are expected to report evidence of unprofessional or unethical practices of their colleagues as part of this self-policing policy.

Allied professionals also are subject to the credentialing and privileging process. Clinical psychologists, for example, may obtain state license to practice their specialty after appropriate academic attainment and supervised clinical experience with patients. They, too, in working with hospital patients must undergo credential and privilege screening before independent work with patients is allowed. Hospitals differ in their views regarding to what extent clinical psychology practice must be subordinated to medical supervision. Medical clearance of patients is, however, usually required; consultation with physicians and treatment of medical complications by M.D.s during the patient's hospital stay make sense. In recent years, hospitals have accepted qualified allied professionals into their professional staff organizations to help in both policy development and governance of their treatment programs.

Many hospitals now accept direct referrals of patients for admission from allied professionals without the intermediation of M.D.s.

Joint Commission on Accreditation of Healthcare Organizations[11]

To correct poor conditions in health care hospitals, the American College of Surgeons (ACS) made valiant efforts during the period from 1918 to 1951 to develop standards and to review general hospitals. In 1951, they were joined by the American College of Physicians, the American Hospital Association, the American Medical Association, and the Canadian Medical Association to form the Joint Commission on the Accreditation of Hospitals (JCAH). (The Canadian Medical Association withdrew in 1959.) Standards developed by JCAH were applied mainly to medical and surgical hospitals. They included also psychiatric hospitals, but the reviews (conducted usually by non-psychiatrists) were often less than satisfactory; the reviewers were not in touch with psychiatric thinking and developments of the times.

In the 1950s, the American Psychiatric Association published standards for psychiatric facilities—both hospitals and clinics. In the 1960s, JCAH accreditation became a requirement for Medicare and Medicaid reimbursement and, in various states, a requirement for facility licensure. In the late 1960s, an Accreditation Council on Psychiatric Facilities was formed that formulated standards for psychiatric hospitals and clinics, as well as programs for alcoholism, drug abuse, children, and adolescents. Later (in 1977), standards for community mental health centers were established. In 1979, the JCAH Consolidated Standards for Child, Adolescents, Adult, Alcoholism and Drugs were adopted; further efforts in 1981 improved standards of professional and medical staff responsibilities. This latter revision broadened the concept of the organized medical staff—the important element in hospital governance—to include non-M.D. professionals. It should be noted that JCAHO (renamed in 1987 as the Joint Commission on Accreditation of Healthcare Organizations) has become increasingly powerful over the years. JCAHO approval is now required for academic affiliation, recognition by professional organizations, approval of training programs, and reimbursement by third-party payers.

JCAHO's financial support is obtained on a voluntary basis from the very institutions it surveys. Today, JCAHO hospital surveys are conducted by trained teams of inspectors on a triennial basis; their inspections are events of major importance. Literally thousands of standards have been enunciated, covering every facet of institutional functioning from administration to departmental organization and governance, patient rights, professional privileges, treatment plans, food services, and fire safety. A new departmental entity has developed in most hospitals, dedicated to utilization review and quality assurance (two major components of JCAHO inspection). It is also fair to say that this whole accreditation development has led to the founding of a new specialty in medicine—that of *quality assurance*, which has its own base of literature and requires specialized study and field experience. Altogether, counting the cost of these new departments plus the work of all other services in the institution, many thousands of hours are spent in preparing for inspection by JCAHO. Costs of such preparations are widely estimated as upward of one-half million dollars a year, and this is probably a conservative estimate.

How have hospital personnel taken to these periodic evaluations? Basically, there is a lot of grumbling, although with management's help much of this is suppressed by the hard necessity of meeting the standards (or else). Staff persons often see the preparations as a resented addition to their normal work load and as carrying an unwarranted emphasis on exacting paper documentation, without which inspectors tend to believe "it didn't happen." A regrettable withdrawal of attention from patients while knuckling to the demands of an outside body that "doesn't really understand what is going on" is often the complaint.

In fairness to JCAHO, however, it must be said that, generally, inspectors are out to help the hospital make the grade—and without JCAHO, quality care in many hospitals would certainly slip dangerously. The potential situation is comparable to what happened in 1910 with the Flexner Report; as a result of that report, medical schools were forced to meet stringent requirements in the training of doctors, and some "doctor mills" were phased out altogether. That program did a great service to the profession of medicine throughout the county and, as a consequence, protected the lives and safety of countless patients. It also raised greatly the public's confidence in its medical institutions.

But the worries of administrators of mental health facilities do not end with JCAHO inspections alone. There are also periodic inspections in regard to patient rights, building safety, and food services. Hospital records, treatment planning, patient records, and reports of staff conferences may come in for a battering, as patients' safety and rights are subject to local checkups at intervals before the triennial inspections are instituted. Not infrequently, the management of an institution may be racked by a JCAHO survey that may conclude that a given building does not meet safety standards and must be replaced, although it requires an expenditure of millions of dollars. Recently, in Southern California, the Martin Luther King, Jr., Medical Center was found so deficient by a JCAHO committee that federal inspectors (who arrived hard on their heels) declared that $60 million in federal money was in jeopardy unless radical changes were made. A shakeup of hospital administration was instituted immediately by the county board of supervisors, and millions were sought to try to remedy a chronically underfunded situation.

These are some of the problems that relate to the regulation, licensing, and accreditation of health and mental health facilities. They are a constant headache to the conscientious manager. A quality assurance system must be set up that *functions throughout the year*—for, after an accreditation survey, there is too often a letdown in interest and attention. Much work must be done, particularly with department chiefs, to help them and their staffs accept exacting standards, and much paperwork that they may regard as unnecessary and boring. It should be recognized, however, that JCAHO standards are not necessarily set in concrete and may be modified if proper representations are made.

What happens if accreditation is denied? Each hospital or facility is given ample opportunity to study and correct recommendations made by JCAHO in its last survey. It is important that attention be given as soon as possible to these recommendations before the next survey. Only if recommendations are ignored, or inadequate progress made after repeated warnings, is total denial of accreditation likely. This event is truly a disaster and should be avoided like the plague.

One can do no better than to quote Ethel Bonn, a surveyor of great experience, on the consequences of denial:

1. The governing body loses confidence in and seriously "wonders" about the capability of the psychiatric administrator and staff.
2. The funding source withholds funding for new programs and/or pay increases for management and/or clinical staff; third-party payors withhold reimbursement.
3. The press has a field day, with headlines, about the loss of accreditation and hints at the need for an investigation.
4. The news media give the facility long-overdue visibility but at a time of embarrassment and crisis.
5. The public—including prospective patients, staff and citizen volunteers—loses confidence in the facility, which, in turn, may lose income and have trouble recruiting staff and volunteers.
6. The morale of staff sags; many raise questions about the competence of administration.
7. The patients lose confidence in the quality of care.[12]

Professional Standards Review Organizations (PSROs)

Established in 1973 and supported by the federal government, these cost containment–oriented organizations are regional mechanisms for monitoring providers to Medicare and Medicaid recipients through review of medical necessity, length of stay, and utilization of ancillary services. Generic screening is first provided by nursing personnel; problem charts are referred to physician reviewers. Problems uncovered may be handled by education, intensified review of individual physicians or hospitals, or withholding of payments. As with JCAHO surveys, PSROs are often resented as another intrusion upon professional autonomy because of burdensome paperwork, lack of confidence in surveyors' judgment, and disagreement with standards per se.

VOLUNTEERISM AND CITIZEN INVOLVEMENT[13,14]

Citizen participation in mental health has burgeoned in recent decades, although volunteerism itself goes back to the early years of our country's history. It is part of the American heritage. The administrator of today should know and appreciate what volunteerism has done in the past, how much it can contribute today, and how essential a part of the mental health scene it has become. To my knowledge, no community has yet exploited the *full* potential of citizen support of mental health efforts; the more we try, the more people come forth to help.[15]

In 1974, it was estimated by the Agency for Voluntary Action[16] that one in every four Americans over the age of 13 engaged in some volunteer work, totaling at that time 37 million people. Thirty percent of Americans between 25 and 44 were volunteers; 12% of those with a household income below $4,000 were part of the volunteer force; and volunteer services yielded the equivalent of 3.5 million full-time workers for one year. Of these volunteers, 15% were in the health services. Nationally, the work of the Peace Corps and of VISTA volunteers gave great impetus, dignity, and legitimacy to the whole volunteer movement.[17,18]

The enormous versatility and capability of volunteers are shown by the tasks they have undertaken: identifying therapeutic and rehabilitative potential of patients; contributing to policy development; providing direct services; raising funds; interpreting programs to the public; reporting on community reactions; serving as advocates for the poor; and promoting public action.

Volunteers in mental health were sparse in state hospitals before 1945, but VA hospitals had enjoyed vigorous programs for at least two decades before. In Massachusetts, state volunteer efforts were pioneered by a "Grey Ladies" group during World War II, when contributions to the war effort were fashionable. (The state hospital had been steadily losing staff to the general mobilization.) After the war, the Grey Ladies were absorbed into a hospital auxiliary, which made itself felt in many ways: improvement in ward decor, establishment of a gift shop, founding of a hospital canteen manned by patients, and sponsoring of an annual dance. Funds were raised and donated for coffee and tea for patients and families at admission, as well as for research on adolescents, movies for children, and community education. The experienced hospital administrator knows how valuable these flexible funds are, particularly in public hospitals where funds are not only limited but also tied to specific functions. Often the niceties of patient care can only be provided through the efforts of private citizens.

The success of such programs in hospitals throughout Massachusetts led to the establishment of a director of volunteer programs in the state department of mental health, with similar positions in each mental hospital and school for the retarded. A landmark in citizen contributions to mental health and in citizen–professional collaboration, this proved a boon not only to patients, but also to the volunteers themselves, who profited and grew through the enjoyable giving of themselves to others.[19]

By 1973, in Massachusetts, there were more individual volunteers working in the far-flung system than employees. Patients welcomed them warmly as persons whose interest was not based on a paid job, but came "from the heart," so to speak. Although employees were sometimes wary of these "strangers," they soon learned to respect the work that volunteers did to fill in the voids in patient service of which the employees had long been aware.

The Span of Volunteer Projects

The imagination and ingenuity of volunteers are impressive. Unfortunately, only a few selected projects can be mentioned here, but the enterprising administrator today—increasingly constrained by limited budgets—can exercise his own ingenuity in utilizing this almost limitless supply of openhearted citizens.[20]

In Switzerland, the postman checks on health and welfare of older people on his route.[21] In England, Samaritans provide support, comfort, and preventive services for depressed persons who may be at risk for suicide.[22] In America, the widow-to-widow program has prospered.[23,24] This offers assistance to acutely grieving widows through the services of other widows who have been through the experience and recovered. In Los Angeles, there is a group called the Older Women's League[25] that comes together for social, recreational, and occupational diversion. In Los Angeles again, there is also Stepping Stone, a small residential facility for runaway adolescents—and for the senior group, the Senior Health and Peer Counseling Center, where hundreds of older volunteers give of themselves to help other elderly persons in distress. These organizations try to raise funds through both public and private sources. A new entity that recently moved into Los Angeles is the Covenant House, a charity ministering to runaway homeless or destitute youths. Efforts of this sort are literally legion, a most impressive contemporary example being the many thousands of charitable efforts that have sprung up in the last dozen years on behalf of homeless adults, adolescents, and homeless women with young children. It is difficult to leave this subject without mentioning self-help groups: Recovery Incorporated, Alcoholics Anonymous, Parents Without Partners, Schizophrenics Anonymous, Gamblers Anonymous, Project Return, and Parents of Abused Children. Katz's[26] comprehensive report shows the remarkable spread of self-help groups in America and throughout the world.

Student Volunteers[27,28,29,30,31]

Never to be overlooked are student volunteers. About one-half of the 400 volunteers at the Neuropsychiatric Institute in UCLA are students. Highly adaptable, student volunteers work on wards and in laboratories, take patients out to ballgames, teach languages, and work and play with patients individually and in groups. Historically, the most impressive milestone in the history of student volunteering involved the students at Harvard and Radcliffe who, in 1954, began to work with the mentally ill on the back wards of the Metropolitan State Hospital in Waltham, Massachusetts, a few miles from Harvard Square. These students—in the hundreds each year—were fascinated by patients, excited about the opportunity to bring them "back to life," enthralled by the discovery of therapeutic powers that existed within themselves, and anxious to transform the patients' barren environment into a more meaningful, homelike place.[32]

Their activities at Metropolitan State Hospital were soon copied by nine other colleges in the Boston area. Halfway houses, home treatment service, and community clinics benefited from their students' enthusiasm, goodwill, and optimism. One of the noteworthy accomplishments was the development of a halfway house for chronic patients wherein patients and students lived together under the same roof;[33] the superintendent of the hospital and the dean of Harvard encouraged the project at a time when some prominent members of the psychiatric profession were concerned that the patients would be damaged by contact with untrained persons, or that students would suffer from traumatic relationships with psychotic patients. This particular venture successfully rehabilitated a number of chronic patients who, without the students' attention, would surely have languished for many months or years on the wards.

Another exciting student venture was the project aimed to give hospitalized chronically ill patients a break from the tedium of hospital life by taking them on a vacation to Cape Cod during the summer of 1968.[34] The accomplishments in connection with this enterprise were extraordinary. Encouraged by the superintendent of Boston State Hospital and the commissioner of mental health, the students obtained a $30,000 grant from the Boston Permanent Charities, convinced the town fathers of Barnstable to let them rehabilitate an old abandoned poor house, and transported 30 patients from a chronic ward of the hospital to the new location. Patients and students lived together in this setting for seven eventful weeks during that summer, carrying out chores in the morning, going to the beaches in the afternoons, and carrying on numerous rap sessions that explored in depth the backgrounds and lives of both patients and students. To make a long story short, the patients began to move forward rapidly in their rehabilitation, and at the end of the summer not one wanted to return to the hospital. Quickly, other arrangements were made for them, including halfway houses, independent living in the community, or return to relatives or friends. The majority of patients succeeded in adapting to such new situations; a small group, unfortunately, had to return to the hospital.

This was an extraordinary accomplishment by determined, enthusiastic students at a fortunate time in history that encouraged experimentation with new modalities of treatment. This experience taught many seasoned psychiatrists a lesson, namely, what could be accomplished by highly motivated, intelligent youths—novices, without formal training. (They were, to be sure, supervised by an unusually wise and dynamic social worker, David Kantor, whose permissive and highly participatory style attracted hundreds of student volunteers.)

These were days when the field of mental health was looking for recruits, and the federal government was awarding grants for training of social workers, nurses, psychologists, and psychiatrists. More than a few of the students caught up in volunteer adventures soon turned to professional training in one or another area of mental health.[35]

Volunteers from the Business Community

Public hospitals had long used patients as unpaid employees to assist in various functions of the institution: in the kitchen and dining room, laundry, the farm, garage and grounds, and occupational shops to learn shoe and clothing repair, sewing, and so forth. With shortages of paid staff, these patients became valuable assets to the departments in which they worked, and not infrequently this fact alone slowed their progress toward discharge. When this type of institutional peonage was banned, Boston State Hospital managed to attract a group of businessmen from the community who organized a program of *paid* work for hospital patients based on contracts they negotiated with various industries.[36] It was an enormous success, and demonstrated the great power of work rehabilitation when the patient's productive effort was immediately remunerated. The dignity of a steady job, the possibility of escape from institutional poverty, and the freedom to spend their own money as they wished were for many patients the most powerful treatments the hospital had to offer.

Voluntary Citizen Organizations

These are of two types: (a) independent citizen groups formed for the purpose of advancing the cause of the mentally ill and developmentally disadvantaged, and (b) citizen groups with similar goals appointed by governmental authority.

In the first category would fit the business group mentioned above, which had voluntarily and independently organized to help chronic patients at Boston State Hospital. More conventional groups include the various mental health associations, mental retardation associations, and alliances for children. Recently, the national and state alliances for the mentally ill, (NAMI, and in California CAMI), made up primarily of relatives and friends of the chronically mentally ill, have been growing rapidly, and they have succeeded in influencing public policy. It behooves administrators to cooperate with these community forces—desperately needed where the consumers (because of illness) are not able to organize in their own behalf—as they are a leading hope for a higher priority for the mentally ill in the future.

The second category includes formally appointed members of hospital boards of trustees, advisory boards to the state office of the commissioner, and regional and area boards. Altogether, the number of citizens appointed to these positions, usually by governors or commissioners, is quite large. They generally serve staggered terms, with part of the board replaced each year by new appointees. If these boards are properly oriented and given opportunities to learn by active participation, mental health and retardation programs profit greatly from their support and strength.

Implications for Mental Health Leaders

In summary, there exists in the community a great reservoir of individuals who—if properly cultivated, oriented, and supervised—can be of great help to the vast number of programs for the mentally disabled that need (a) community support, (b) fiscal support, and (c) willing hands to assist overburdened staff. The motivations for volunteering are varied, ranging from lofty, altruistic idealism to curiosity about one's own mental health and/or a search for help for mental illness, alcoholism, or drug abuse in friends or loved ones. Volunteers possess energy, talent, and a high potential for accomplishing things when properly motivated; to the patients, they represent a hopeful link to the community. The administrator who wishes to take advantage of this potential army of voluntary employees must invest much time and energy in planning and implementation. Projects for volunteers (interesting rather than boring, and fostering growth and change rather than stagnant repetition of meaningless tasks) must be fitted to the volunteers' interests and abilities. Volunteers must be carefully integrated into the family of workers on a given unit, with clear expectations and appropriate rewards. At the same time, they like to belong to their own identifiable volunteer service that has its own director and staff. Planned and implemented along these lines, volunteer programs become invaluable assets in a vast array of mental health programs.

SURROUNDING CLINICS AND FACILITIES

The proliferation of clinics and facilities surrounding mental hospitals has been one of the most gratifying developments in recent times. Their numbers and diversity defy the imagination; they are a great credit to the many inspired citizens and public-minded groups that have been unwilling to leave the care and treatment of our mentally ill entirely to government. In many instances, they fill in voids in services of state and county institutions, and in others they are manifestations of citizens' desire to gratify personal needs for better programs for loved ones who are afflicted.

During the period of deinstitutionalization, many of these facilities spread outward from the hospital into the community as means of providing aftercare for discharged patients, whose numbers were growing exponentially. They were primarily transitional programs—to a large extent hospital inspired, hospital administered, and serving formerly hospitalized patients. Day-care programs were initially housed in the hospital, or established on hospital grounds; later they were sited in the community. Many halfway houses started as "community preparation wards," then were located near the hospital and later deeper into the community, away from the hospital. As they moved away and multiplied in numbers, the patients became less and less dependent administratively and financially on the hospital.

In early years, these facilities served mainly discharged patients who were sufficiently integrated to adapt to community living. Later, patients served were community mentally ill cases whose expected clinical course might have taken them to the hospital if not for their placement in a community facility. The two-way function of these community facilities was utilized more and more as their therapeutic programs evolved.

The early community entities fell generally into the following categories: outpatient programs, day-care facilities, halfway houses, cooperative apartments, sheltered workshops, supervised jobs in the community, supervised "independent" living, group homes, board and care homes, ex-patient clubs and programs (such as Alcoholics Anonymous, Recovery Incorporated, and Project Return), and storefronts with usually both referred and walk-in admissions.

Administrative authority was often centered in nonmedical individuals who had originally provided the enthusiasm, initiative, and fund-raising talents to make the facility go. Funding sources varied from primarily government support to mainly or exclusively community support. As a rule, however, necessity dictated multiple sources of financing to ensure relative stability.

Community programs and facilities have been discussed here as though they were limited to patients moving out of the hospital toward the community or moving toward the hospital from the community. However, most seriously mentally ill patients today are not in hospitals or in hospital-sponsored programs but in the community, essentially homeless and unsheltered. Yet, for this group, largely abandoned by the governmental sector, it was reported in 1984 that approximately 111,000 community services had been established in the last few years—ranging from soup kitchens, temporary shelters, and single-room occupancies to jerry-built camps and tent cities. (See "Homelessness: The New Epidemic" later in this chapter.)

Finally, one of the most striking phenomena of recent decades has been the proliferation of private facilities. The significance to the administrator is that the facilities and clinics surrounding him have three types of decisions to make relevant to his institution: whether to refer patients to his organization; whether to receive patients from his organization; and how to characterize his organization to their publics.

Referral of patients to hospitals is vital to all hospitals that depend on revenue for viability. With competition as rough as it is—and increasing with the reduction of benefits—the lifeblood of many hospitals is threatened. This applies more or less to private facilities, university hospitals, and VA, county, and state facilities. Increasingly, public facilities (in this respect, not unlike private facilities) depend on third-party payers. As public support has diminished, today many public facilities need paying patients almost as much as private facilities. The development of multiple funding streams is the imperative rule today.

Within limits, surrounding facilities have discretion in deciding whether or not to receive discharged patients from a given public hospital. On the other hand, the private patient who has exhausted his funds must be referred elsewhere—usually to a public clinic, board and care home, or county hospital. In such cases, social workers must often plead for a "place" or bed with the gatekeepers of still another service. Often, in such negotiations, the goodwill of personnel in the other programs is tested; policy barriers and unconscious resistances operate if interfacility personnel relationships are not satisfactory. Hours of professional time may be wasted searching for a place for a patient who with every passing hour is eating up local resources.

The image of a given hospital in the community arises from the seeds planted in the minds and hearts of community citizens. The average citizen listens with special attention to those who actually are at work in systems of psychiatric care and whose opinions are not easily swayed by the media. The conscientious administrator strives to cultivate the goodwill of surrounding agencies through personal visits and regular interagency conferences, thus to promote the smooth flow of patients and information among interdependent institutions.

LABOR UNREST AND THE STRIKE*

"Labor law as it is known is essentially the child of successive industrial revolutions from the 18th century onward." Limitations on the hours of work, sickness and workmen's compensation emerged first in Germany in 1883 and 1884. Compulsory arbitration was first adopted in New Zealand in 1890. Protection of the young was adopted in Zurich in 1915. The bulk of legislation in the United States was adopted after the 1929 Great Depression; a major right—that of freedom of association—was restrained by political and legal injunctions until the 1930s. In 1913, the Department of Labor was established in the United States, responsible for the effective administration of labor legislation.[37]

In recent decades, labor has won many benefits, such as guaranteed vacations and sick leave, improved conditions of work, grievance rights, higher wages, and retirement allowances. Collective bargaining laws have been adopted widely as labor has grown in strength and in the recognition and use of its power.

*I am indebted to Douglas D. Bagley, hospital director, and Marianne Kainz, director of nursing, at Los Angeles County–Olive View Medical Center for sharing their knowledge of labor relations and their personal experience with actual strikes.

It is unwise for the administrator to neglect worker complaints, or to fail to meet with labor representatives; indeed, the executive must participate in planning meetings with labor representatives in order to feel the pulse of his workers and to avoid job actions and strikes. Binding contracts may be negotiated for many months before a new agreement can replace the old; then it is necessary that the administrator look after the rights of labor as a necessary element in the maintenance of morale and productivity. In bargaining sessions, the top administrator may accede to many of the requests of labor, but he must steadfastly hold to those management rights and prerogatives that make it possible to fulfill his obligations to patients, staff, and the general missions of the facility. When labor and administration are not in good relationship with each other, it is an invitation to costly work slowdowns and stoppages.[38]

In 1987, the National Labor Relations Board (NLRB), because of constant litigation, abandoned its traditional practice of case-by-case determination of appropriate bargaining units in acute care hospitals and substituted instead a rigid set of rules calling for eight different appropriate bargaining units: physicians, registered nurses, all other professionals, all technical employees, all skilled maintenance employees, all business office clerical employees, all guards, and all nonprofessional employees (service workers). Hospital administrators opposed these rules, which they believed would make unionization of their institutions easier, lead to higher costs, and increase the probability of strikes.[39]

In fact, work stoppages and union militancy have increased in the 1980s. Since the introduction of diagnostic related groups (DRGs) in 1983 as a basis for reimbursement, the average hospital's profit from Medicare reimbursements declined by 31%; hospital administrators have been forced, therefore, to reduce lengths of stay. Private insurers, too, have moved aggressively to control costs through health maintenance organizations (HMOs) and preferred provider organizations (PPOs). Nevertheless, health care costs have escalated, defying all attempts at containment.[40] In this particular climate, work slowdowns, job actions, and strikes are particularly unwelcome.

Varieties of Job Actions

Blue Days and Work Slowdowns

Blue days refers to days in which the individual calls in sick but in fact may be able to work. Oftentimes, as has been mentioned, these absences occur on Friday and/or Monday, when the employee gives in to a strong desire to have a long weekend. Only if such excuses are flagrant does administration do anything about it; usually, this takes the form of a request to produce a doctor's certification for the workdays missed.

Beyond such individual "blue days" are *work slowdowns* that affect a whole ward, or department of the facility. Two examples are as follows.

Case Illustrations

Work Slowdowns

ILLUSTRATION A: In a well-staffed university hospital with four residents per ward of 25 patients, the faculty assigns all patients in rotation to the residents while they function as teachers or ward managers and pay attention as much as possible to their research—the principal road to academic promotion. When a resident is absent for sickness or whatever, ward admissions are automatically reduced. Since revenue depends on turnover, the hospital director puts a stop to it, asking the faculty members to fill in at the front lines.

ILLUSTRATION B: This heavily burdened county hospital imposes a constant work load on its staff physicians (most of whom work at the front lines, admitting and treating patients in rotation), although psychiatric residents help to a degree. Control of inflow can be effected to a great extent by keeping patients longer before discharge. Average turnover time varies by as much as 70% from one doctor to another; each defends his style as most appropriate for the welfare of his particular patients. Turnover time also varies as a function of the number of patients admitted, patient needs for clinical attention, chronicity of illness, and the ability of social workers to arrange proper outflow referrals. Slowdowns therefore can occur by manipulating a number of factors that are under the control of ward physicians.

Rolling Sickouts

The *rolling sickout* is usually engineered by a union as part of a job action. The union keeps management off guard, not knowing what area will be hit next, but guessing that in all probability the most vulnerable area will be the next target.

Informational Picketing

Informational picketing is that form of job action in which employees carry signs and distribute handouts to patients, visitors and staff, usually at lunch time. No official picket line is established, and no official union strike is declared. No loss of work time is involved; therefore, no sanctions are applied.

Strikes

Most feared of the job actions, most costly, and most distressing to all parties is the open strike that pits management against labor and one worker against another, and tears at the most important functions of the institution—the care and treatment of patients. Strikes, although infrequent, are increasing in number in recent times. They necessitate planning by administration at many levels, in the same manner that management plans for fires and earthquakes. The anatomy of a recent nursing strike in a 300-bed county general hospital is illustrative.

Case Illustration

Saga of the Nurses' Strike

Nurse shortages in this facility had been a major problem for years. Wages were far below compensation in the private sector. Additionally, nurses often worked extra shifts, and tasks inimical to their sense of professionalism had been forced upon them. Their benefits package was not satisfactory; they had less choice in health coverage, and high premiums had caused hardships, especially for those with dependents. Respect from physicians was often lacking. Too often, nurses were not asked for their opinion. They felt it was often impossible to provide that quality care to patients expected by their profession. After many months of negotiations, the union declared a strike.

On the morning of the strike, picket lines of placard-carrying nurses formed outside the hospital. A high percentage of nurses joined in the strike. Patient load was reduced 50% overall, and in some areas by as much as 100%. Sympathetic technicians, students, and some residents joined the action.

How the Strike Was Handled. Everything was immediately put on an emergency basis, subject to the decisions of a command post that monitored the actions on a moment-to-moment basis, receiving all information necessary for reasonable decisions. Vital information included: Who could you count on? What resources in manpower and supplies could be mobilized? What advice and counsel was there from the department of health and hospitals, the county supervisors, the county's chief administrative officer, county counsel, and other county hospitals involved in the strike? What word was there from the wards as to nursing and other staff coverage in relation to patient needs, and what success in discharging or transferring patients to other facilities?

All "nonrepresented" employees were mobilized, including nurse supervisors, physicians (including interns and residents), psychologists, social workers, and pharmacists; they were deployed for maximum coverage of patient care and treatment. Personnel were put on two daily shifts of 12 hours (or even longer), rather than the regular three daily 8-hour shifts. Registry nurses were called upon for help.

Patients who could possibly get along without hospitalization were discharged. Many were transferred to VA hospitals, private hospitals, board and care homes, or other facilities.

Personnel who gave extra time were paid overtime. Personnel on strike were denied pay for time on strike; sick time *was* allowed for striking personnel, but only on strong and specific documentation by a physician. Sickouts were carefully reviewed in the hope of forestalling long and often acrimonious grievances that might later be forthcoming—grievances that in turn might compromise future work relationships or impair ability to recruit.

Of the many contingencies, food service was a most important consideration, both for patients and for working employees. Fast food companies, airline food services, and outside contractors were contacted to keep the food chain moving.

An open dormitory for women who were staying on the job was made available, with meals, showers, and sleeping accommodations to make them comfortable.

End of the Strike and Aftermath. After four days, county lawyers obtained an injunction based on "detrimental impact." Picketing ended, but intense negotiations continued, leading to improvement in both wages and conditions of work. Afterwards, a countywide nursing advisory board was established to study support services and environmental issues, and to formulate a compensation plan for the future. Probably the major accomplishment was that the union riveted the attention of county and state officials onto the serious nursing problems that had not been fully addressed before.

The financial cost of the strike was in the millions; human costs were more difficult to estimate. In an effort to restore equilibrium, groups were formed and moderated by a psychiatrist. The anger and bitterness of those nurses who refused to strike and stayed behind to cover wards of very sick patients under extreme hardship conditions were ventilated against the striking nurses who left the bedsides, the administration for not supplying help, and the radiological and laboratory technicians who had joined the dissenters. The ethical dilemma was intense and at times seemed unsolvable—between the ideals of the nursing profession (the Florence Nightingale tradition) and the hardships and deprivations of contemporary work life that motivated the strike in the first place. These "therapeutic" sessions helped greatly to defuse anger and to promote respect for the courage of those who joined the picket line, as well as for those who rose to the overwhelming challenge intramurally.

Prevention of Strikes

Imberman[41] compared 31 health care institutions throughout the nation that experienced multiple instances of labor walkouts with 31 institutions that had a history of living peacefully and profitably with their unions. Differences are discussed in four areas:

1. *Grievance Handling.* In the strike-free institutions, employees seldom pursued grievances beyond the level of the department head. In the strike-prone hospitals, grievances were delayed or stonewalled by administration; people were treated with less respect, like "things."
2. *Overtime and Weekend Duty.* The troubled hospitals preferred overtime to hiring more employees.
3. *Degree of Employee Participation/Involvement.* In the strike-free hospitals, new ideas and upward communication were encouraged. In strike-prone hospitals, good efforts were often sabotaged by department heads and by union officials who feared threats to their authority.
4. *Perception of Management.* Strike-free hospitals extended the professional environment to include every nonprofessional area. Employee recognition programs, one-to-one relationships between administrators and workers, and tours by senior officials were encouraged. Joint labor—management problem-solving and safety meetings were also required by labor agreements.

The formula for prevention seems to be: Keep tuned to labor unrest; handle employees with respect and understanding; encourage two-way communication; and take early remedial action. Since strikes are infrequent, and professionals are generally unsophisticated in strike-response technology, it further behooves management to develop plans in detail for all foreseeable job-action contingencies.

HOMELESSNESS: THE NEW EPIDEMIC

Christ made the prescient prediction: "The poor will always be with us." It is said that in America some 34 million people live below the poverty line; what is more, the gap between the rich and the poor seems to be growing. Certainly the War on Poverty did not succeed in dissipating the ranks of the poor. Can it be that a wealthy nation—by virtue of its having a capitalistic economy—will not phase out the poor, simply because a significant number of unemployed are necessary to keep a pool of workers available to industry and thus to hold down the level of wages?

In ancient times, people with little means, or unemployed, were designated as vagabonds, loiterers, rogues, beggars, or inebriates—and were subjected to the harshest punishments. In America, after the Civil War, many young men released from military duty who roamed the country on the way to their homes were called "hobos," "bums," and "drifters." During the Great Depression of the 1930s, the ranks of the poor and homeless in America swelled enormously; unemployment was at an all-time high, and the country was in its worst slump in history. Until World War II was launched, it seemed that the Depression would drag on endlessly. (Strangely, the war appeared to be the cure.) In those days, it was poverty or hard times for people in all walks of society; today, it is quite different—it is poverty and homelessness in a climate of relative prosperity.

How did this homelessness in the midst of plenty come to be? Who are the homeless, and what can be done for them? What role can psychiatry and psychiatric administrators play?

Parallels between the homeless of today and the epidemics of yesteryear are not hard to find. The homeless condition affects masses of people, particularly in the inner cities. If we define homeless people as those who spend one or more nights per month out of their homes (or other usual and natural habitats), the estimates are as many as 2 million adults; another million adolescents, it has been estimated, are today "on the streets." Whatever their numbers, the "epidemic" includes men, women, adolescents, and children. The majority of homeless suffer from physical and/or mental illness. Increasing in numbers, the homeless spread from the inner city—the skid-row areas and the barrios—to suburban communities. They are shunned by a large segment of society. And as of this moment, a cure for this epidemic has not been found.

Why is the general population revolted by the sight of the homeless? Fear of poverty and homelessness threaten many; few feel totally invulnerable. Many are on the edge, and many people know that with a few bad breaks they, too, could fall into the state of poverty and homelessness. Further, the homeless are disheveled, decrepit, often unclean, and in many cases infested. A significant proportion have active tuberculosis. Sexually transmitted diseases (including AIDS) are a serious threat, and chronic infections are indigenous.

The homeless beg, panhandle, sleep in doorways, interfere with the normal flow of business, overrun parks, and sometimes urinate and defecate in public places. Thus, the public reacts to these unfortunate people as if they were victims of a plague.

As compared to yesteryear, the homeless of today are better educated. Blacks, Hispanics and women are overrepresented compared to the general population. The homeless population also includes many veterans of recent wars—Vietnam and Korea—and a relatively high proportion of addicted individuals. Many mentally ill are found in samples of homeless individuals, a significant proportion of whom may be considered casualties of the deinstitutionalization period. It is also reported that women with small children are the most rapidly growing subgroup of the homeless.

Farr and Koegel's[42] epidemiological survey of homeless adults in the Skid Row area of Los Angeles is one of the best in the literature. According to their figures, approximately 28.3% suffer from severe chronic mental illness (of whom a diagnosis of schizophrenia is made in 11.5%; depression, 15.5%), and another 46.2% are addicted to alcohol and/or drugs. Altogether, 74.5% are persons with chronic mental disabilities. As to the remainder, what can be said of them is that most of them are certainly not well. They suffer from anxieties, depression, loss of self-esteem, poor nutrition, character disorders, and a host of medical illnesses ranging from cardiovascular and respiratory disorders to skin diseases.

More recently, attention has been directed to homeless adolescents. Their numbers are large, their mental and emotional disorders numerous, and their alienation from mainstream values almost total. They have been referred to as "aliens in their own land,"[43] for they do not vote, have no fixed address, are often hungry, find shelter in abandoned buildings (squats), and encounter great difficulties finding legitimate jobs because of their age. They avoid established social and medical agencies unless forced by necessity; they also avoid the police and other legally constituted representatives of the establishment. If apprehended—and many are guilty of breaking and entering, pushing drugs, stealing, engaging in fights, or possession of dangerous weapons—they fear incarceration or remand to detention facilities. The large majority left their homes of their own choice and do not wish to return to them.

Just as the population of the homeless is diverse, so are the causes of homelessness. The homeless of today are caught in a complex economic, political, and social maze. Among the major causes of homelessness are the following:

1. The elimination in the last dozen years of approximately $34 billion of federal support from welfare, education, and nutrition.
2. The trickle-down economic theory, which holds that to encourage prosperity, increase employment, and foster innovation, the shackles must be removed from industry. The theory has been that economic growth would then be sufficient to foster both prosperity and employment and to make the nation militarily secure. Unfortunately, the large appetite of the war machine has thrown the nation into overwhelming debt, trade imbalance, and increasing poverty and homelessness.
3. Lack of affordable housing is a proximal cause. Far too many low-cost rooms or apartments have been bulldozed, making way for units far beyond the means of the poor.
4. The deinstitutionalization movement, which in depopulating the mental hospitals discharged many mentally ill into the community without appropriate facilities to take care of them. In studies throughout the nation, it has been shown that approximately 25% of the homeless have had previous histories of hospitalization for mental disorder.
5. Although the overall unemployment rate is not what it was during the Great Depression, there appears to be a general unrest in industry as restraints have been removed and competition has become more intense. Employee turnover has been rapid, with many workers eventually drifting downward to homelessness.
6. The breakup of family relationships yields a relatively high rate of divorce, abandonment, and single-parent families. Interpersonal stresses, alcoholism and drug abuse, and physical and sexual abuse have caused many thousands to sever ties with their families. These persons seek solace with friends or relatives; failing this, they enter life on the streets.
7. Public apathy. In a democracy, the will of the people must be mobilized in order for the legislature and the executive branch to move aggressively on a great problem. Either the public clamor must be very great, or a sufficient number of politicians must be in jeopardy before a task of great magnitude can be successfully confronted. However, some encouragement is afforded by the fact that public and political interest have been excited in the last few years by the sizable media attention to the homeless. The fear of spread of tuberculosis and AIDS from the ranks of the homeless has also played a role.

In considering the challenge of homelessness, the psychiatric administrator should know that there are more seriously mentally ill persons on the streets, so to speak, than in all the state and county hospitals in the nation. But whereas there are few professionals engaged in looking after the homeless mentally ill on the streets, by comparison a veritable army of professional and nonprofessional caretakers are congregated in the mental hospitals. The private sector, intent on the bottom line, wants no part of the homeless problem, but public hospitals and clinics have increasingly felt the pressure of the homeless. The Department of Veterans Affairs has developed a program to alleviate the stress. New public beds have opened up in many communities to accommodate the mentally ill homeless. In some states, legislation has been adopted to mandate treatment of mentally ill homeless individuals in clinics, and if treatment is refused, involuntary admission to mental hospitals can be effected.

Very important in any program to treat the mentally ill homeless is the need to reach out to them where they are. Many are reluctant to give up the freedom of their life-style for the confines of a hospital. If and when mental hospitals and clinics take up the task more boldly, they will move even deeper into the community than was the idiom during deinstitutionalization. Personnel will have to be carefully selected, trained, and/or retrained to withstand the frustrations of making therapeutic relationships with chronically ill patients.

Above all, it should be emphasized that many thousands of homeless— particularly the newly homeless—can be reclaimed by a job, an affordable residence, attention to medical problems, pharmacotherapy, and the psychosocial and rehabilitation techniques available today in the armamentarium of psychiatry. I believe that there are many dedicated people who await the nation's mandate for action, and who hope for an organized effort they can join.

In summary with regard to homelessness, the following must be considered by hospital/clinic directors:

I. Hospitals and clinics are feeling the pressure for service to this population. Admissions of mentally ill homeless individuals are increasing in many facilities.
II. Funds for treatment of the mentally ill in the form of demonstrations, research projects, and block grants to the states are increasingly available. Federal, state, and county governments are allocating monies for this purpose.
III. In some jurisdictions, obligatory treatment in community clinics and hospitals has been initiated.
IV. Increasingly, administrators of mental health programs are being involved in planning services for the homeless mentally ill. Outreach will be an important element in such plans, as will recruitment and training of personnel for the arduous tasks of working with very hard-to-reach patients.

V. Many forms of emotional stress arise from the sheer humiliation and debilitation of the homeless life-style.

VI. Since mentally ill homeless patients are a very diverse population, treatment strategies must be tailored to different clinical groups:

A. The adult chronic psychotic mentally ill, including patients with schizophrenia, depression, and/or brain damage.

B. Adolescents with a variety of disorders: depression, anxiety, conduct disorder, and dissociative reactions.

C. Mothers with children—the latter requiring attention for varying development disorders, the former for depression and chronic stress reactions.

D. Patients with mild to moderate emotional maladjustments (with promise of response to pharmacotherapy and/or occupational and social rehabilitation) are prevalent in the homeless population. Many of the "new" homeless fit into this category; affiliation with some healthy group and professional follow-up is a basic treatment requirement.

E. Programs for the chemically dependent and those with multiple diagnoses will be needed for one third or more of the population.

SUMMARY AND COMMENTS

Mental health organizations exist within a larger community and are related to many surrounding institutions and agencies. Laws governing the operation of institutions emanate from the *body politic,* which provides the institutions with their mandates and the resources to accomplish their missions. The characteristics of the political system and the nature of the relationship between lawmakers and the institutions in their districts are often critical to the health and welfare of the institution. Legislative investigations when something goes wrong can be very distressing to administrators and damaging to institutional morale. Meanwhile, the *media* are alive to stories about what goes on in mental institutions. Thus, it behooves administrators to cultivate good relations with the media.

Professional organizations claim the loyalty of professionals who turn to them for standards, legitimacy, and support in times of crisis. *Educational institutions* may maintain field training stations within hospitals, supply manpower, and confer academic prestige. Affiliations with professional schools are highly desired; the long payoff is that the affiliating institutions can usually provide a higher quality of care and treatment to their patients and enjoy a better reputation in the community through their collaboration with academic centers.

Regulatory bodies confer licensure upon individuals and institutions through laws, regulations, periodic surveys, and the application of sanctions when their standards are not met. Powerful among these are the Joint Commission on the Accreditation of Healthcare Organizations (JCAHO) and patient-rights organizations, but many other groups regulate other subjects such as food, safety, and patient involvement in research.

Voluntary groups include citizens who serve the institution or its hospital board, or who contribute personal time to the hospital's volunteer organization. Community voluntary groups such as mental health associations and alliances for the mentally ill have gained prominence and effectiveness in recent years. They monitor the work of the institution and develop liaisons with local political bodies, federal health agencies, and private foundations. The range of volunteer projects is very great, and the good that they do is almost incalculable.

The hospital does business constantly with *surrounding hospitals and clinics.* Many patients may be referred by members of this community network, and many patients discharged from the hospital are placed through the efforts of these facilities. Good relations with these facilities and satisfactory two-way communication are necessary at all times.

Labor organizations look after the working conditions of employees, and are deeply concerned with salaries and rights of workers. Work slowdowns and stoppages can be the price paid for poor worker morale or the mishandling of complaints and grievances. When workers are seriously aggrieved, labor can wield the mighty weapon of the strike, with crippling force.

Finally, in relating to the outside world, a group that arrests our attention is an unorganized mass of *homeless* people, many of whom are mentally ill, chemically dependent, alienated from society, and an embarrassment to the public. It is fair to predict that the administrator of tomorrow will be much more involved in planning and serving this population.

REFERENCES

1. Greenblatt M: The nature of the psychopolitical system. Chapter 2 in Greenblatt M: Psychopolitics. New York, Grune & Stratton, 1978, pp 9–29
2. Greenblatt M: Historical forces affecting the closing of state mental hospitals, in Plog Research, Inc., and Stanford Research Institute (Preparers): Proceedings of a Conference on the Closing of State Mental Hospitals: "Where Is My Home?" Menlo Park, CA, Plog Research, Inc. and Stanford Research Institute, April 1974, pp 3–17
3. Greenblatt M, Glazier E: Some major issues in the closing of the hospitals, in Ahmed PI, Plog SC (eds): State Mental Hospitals: What Happens When They Close. New York, Plenum, 1976, pp 127–139
4. This section adapted almost verbatim from Greenblatt M: The nature of the political system, Chapter 2 in Greenblatt M: Psychopolitics. New York, Grune & Stratton, 1978, pp 9–17
5. Greenblatt M: The nature of the political system, Chapter 2 in Greenblatt M: Psychopolitics. New York, Grune & Stratton, 1978, pp 17–18
6. Elpers JR: Public mental health funding in California, 1959 to 1989. Hosp & Comm Psychiatry 40:799–804, 1989
7. Greenblatt M: The nature of the political system, Chapter 2 in Greenblatt M: Psychopolitics. New York, Grune & Stratton, 1978, p 27
8. McCarthy CM: Viewpoints: Teaching hospitals' varied missions make funding vital. AHA News 25:4, Issue No. 1, October 9, 1989

9. Simon N: Regulation and review of psychiatric services in the United States. Psychiatr Annals 19:415–420, 1989
10. Smith D: Rise and Fall of Dr. Boggs. Los Angeles Times Magazine, 6–16, 38, October 20, 1989
11. Bonn EM: Accreditation and regulation of psychiatric facilities, Chapter 21 in Talbott JA, Kaplan SR (eds), Psychiatric Administration. New York, Grune & Stratton, 1983, pp 299–310
12. List quoted from Bonn EM: Accreditation and regulation of psychiatric facilities, Chapter 21 in Talbott JA, Kaplan SR (eds), Psychiatric Administration. New York, Grune & Stratton, 1983, p 303
13. Fulton JR, Greenblatt M: Volunteerism in American psychiatry, Section 45.6 in Kaplan AM, Freedman HJ, Sadock BJ (eds), Comprehensive Textbook of Psychiatry/III. Baltimore, Williams & Wilkins, 1980, pp 2885–2887
14. Greenblatt M: Volunteerism and the community mental health worker, Chapter 43.4 in Kaplan HI, Sadock, BJ (eds), Comprehensive Textbook of Psychiatry/IV. Baltimore, Williams & Wilkins, 1985, pp 1893–1897
15. Greenblatt M, Schulberg HC: The mental hospital and its links to community systems. Canadian Psychiatr Assoc J 15:615–623, 1970
16. Agency for Voluntary Action: Americans Volunteer 1974. Washington, DC, Agency for Voluntary Action, 1975
17. The Peace Corps. House of Representatives 7500, Public Law 87-293, September 22, 1961
18. National Volunteer Antipoverty Programs. Part A—Volunteers in Service to America. Senate 1148, Public Law 93-113, Sections 101 through 107, October 1, 1973
19. Greenblatt M, Hinman FJ: Citizen participation in community mental health and retardation programs, Chapter 34 in Grunebaum H (ed), The Practice of Community Mental Health. Boston, Little, Brown, 1970, pp 769–785
20. Greenblatt M, Chien C-p: Depression in the elderly: Use of external support systems, Chapter 13 in Breslau LB, Haug MR (eds), Depression and Aging: Causes, Care and Consequences. New York, Springer, 1983, pp 193–207
21. [No byline]: Outreach: Sweden. Ageing International 5:8, 1978
22. Fox R: The recent decline of suicide in Britain: The role of the Samaritan Suicide Prevention Movement, in Shneidman ES (ed), Suicidology: Contemporary Developments. New York, Grune & Stratton, 1976, pp 499–524
23. Silverman PR: The widow-to-widow program: An experiment in preventive intervention. Ment Hyg 53:333–337, 1969
24. Silverman PR: Widow to Widow. New York, Springer, 1986
25. [No byline]: Older Women Unite to Cope with Aging. Older Women's League. Los Angeles Times, Section 5:32, September 4, 1980
26. Katz AH: Self-help and mutual aid. Ann Rev Sociol 7:129–155, 1981
27. Greenblatt M, Kantor D: The College Student and the Mental Patient. Presented at Third World Congress of Psychiatry, Montreal, June 4–10, 1961, and published in Proceedings, 1964, 1219–1225
28. Umbarger CC, Morrison AP, Dalsimer JS, Breggin PR (Prepared with the assistance and supervision of Kantor D, Greenblatt M): College Students in a Mental Hospital. New York, Grune & Stratton, 1962
29. Greenblatt M, Kantor D: Student volunteers in mental health. Pennsylvania Psychiatr Q, No. 1, 43–48, Winter 1961
30. Dohan JL: Development of a student volunteer program in a state mental hospital, Chapter 35, Part II in Greenblatt M, Levinson DJ, Williams RH (eds), The Patient and the Mental Hospital: Contributions of Research in the Science of Social Behavior. Glencoe, Illinois, Free Press, 1957
31. Kantor D: Use of college students as "case aides" in a social service department of a state hospital: An experiment in undergraduate social work education, Chapter 35, Part III, in Greenblatt M, Levinson DJ, Williams RH (eds), The Patient and the Mental Hospital: Contributions of Research in the Science of Social Behavior. Glencoe, Illinois, Free Press, 1957
32. Dohan JL: Development of a student volunteer program in a state mental hospital, Chapter 35, Part II in Greenblatt M, Levinson DJ, Williams RH (eds), The Patient and the Mental Hospital: Contributions of Research in the Science of Social Behavior. Glencoe, Illinois, Free Press, 1957
33. Kantor D, Greenblatt M: Wellmet: Halfway to community rehabilitation (A cooperative student–patient halfway house for chronic mentally ill). Ment Hosp 13:146–152, 1962

34. Greenblatt M: Lombard Farm: The summer of '68. Hosp & Community Psychiatry 28:589, 1977
35. Greenblatt M, Kantor D: Student volunteer movement and the manpower shortage. Amer J Psychiatry 118:809–814, 1962
36. Greenblatt M, Sharaf MR, Stone EM: Rehabilitation service, Chapter 6 in Greenblatt M, Sharaf MR, Stone EM, Dynamics of Institutional Change: The Hospital in Transition. Pittsburgh, Pennsylvania, University of Pittsburgh Press, 1971, pp 106–129
37. Labour Law—Historical Development, in Encyclopaedia Britannica, 15th Edition, 10:570–571, 1979. Chicago, Encyclopaedia Britannica
38. Greenblatt M: Administrative psychiatry, Chapter 51 in Freedman AM, Kaplan HJ, Sadock BJ (eds), Comprehensive Textbook of Psychiatry/II. Baltimore, Williams & Wilkins, 1975, p 2448
39. Imberman W: R_X: Strike prevention in hospitals. Hosp & Health Service Admin 34:196, 1989
40. Imberman W: R_x: Strike prevention in hospitals. Hosp. & Health Service Admin 34: 197–198, 1989
41. Imberman W: R_X: Strike prevention in hospitals. Hosp & Health Service Admin 34:195–211, 1989
42. Farr RK, Koegel P: A Study of Homelessness and Mental Illness in the Skid Row Area of Los Angeles. Los Angeles County Department of Mental Health, Los Angeles, California, March 1986
43. Miller D, Miller D, Hoffman F, Duggan R: Runaways—Illegal Aliens in Their Own Land: Implications for Service. New York, JF Bergin Publishers/Praeger Press, 1981

11

Power and Decision Making in Organizational Context*

The uses and abuses of power have fascinated men and women for generations. In 1532, Machiavelli[1] outlined the use of guile, deceit, and opportunism
in the pursuit and maintenance of power. His cynical view of man justified his
efforts at their domination and subjugation:

> Men in general . . . are ungrateful, voluble, dissemblers, anxious to avoid
> danger, and covetous of gain; as long as you benefit them, they are en-
> tirely yours; they offer you their blood, their goods, their life, and their
> children . . . when the necessity is remote; but when it approaches, they
> revolt.
>
> Abstain from taking the property of others, for men forget more easily the
> death of their father than the loss of their patrimony.[2]

Power is a fascinating, complicated, and troublesome area. It enters into
all social behavior and is a vital element in the behavior of leaders. With the
growing emphasis in modern management on the quirks and aberrations of
leaders (see Chapter 5), their power drives, conflicts, and hangups have become fashionable areas for analysis. Assuming that power is a subject whose
time has come, its study will increasingly absorb attention in the future. If so,
the reader may welcome a discussion of power and its accoutrements, including its developmental and theoretical aspects, in a book dedicated to practical
and theoretical problems in administering therapeutic systems.

*This chapter is adapted in part from Psychopolitics and the Search for Power: The
Meaning of Power, Chapter 13 in *Psychopolitics*, by Milton Greenblatt. New York,
Grune & Stratton, 1978, pp 210–226. Reprinted with permission of The Psychological
Corporation.

POWER, AUTHORITY, AND INFLUENCE

Machiavelli was concerned with power in the political sphere, at a time when Italy was composed of a number of small states at war with each other. He was advising the Prince on the maintenance and aggrandizement of his power. To this end, he said, the people could be manipulated and even sacrificed, if necessary, while the Prince negotiated and conspired with rival factions to increase his power.

Power is a concept used across a variety of social and natural sciences. It has application in law, political science, military science, and religion, as well as in mechanics, mathematics, and physics. Bertrand Russell's[3] definition of power is short and succinct: *Power is the capacity to produce intended effects.* As such it applies to functions of the administrator in a very cogent way.

Power may be differentiated from *authority* and *influence*, with which it is closely related. *Authority* is permission granted by statute, court, ruling, or title implying the right to determine, adjudicate, and settle issues. It is a responsibility granted by rank or office to control projects, issue commands, or punish violations.[4] It has an eminently legal connotation. *Influence* is a personal, unofficial power dependent on deference of others to one's character, ability, or station. It may be exerted unconsciously, invisibly, or insensibly, or it may operate through persuasion.

Administrators are given considerable implied power in the authority granted them to get their jobs done. In addition, power may be enlarged by virtue of strength of personality or charisma. Expert knowledge, high intelligence, and roles as social leaders, avuncular or paternal objects of identification, and norm setters for social, moral, and ethical standards of behavior further enhance their power and influence. However, to exercise wisely the power, authority, and influence they do possess, it is important that administrators work through and resolve their own psychological conflicts or hang-ups in relation to power/authority figures in their past. Ideally, they should reach a point in self-understanding such that they can be comfortable as either *superordinate* or *subordinate*. The administrator is the authority in his own system, but he is also inevitably a subordinate in a larger system. His authoritative role should not be complicated by ambivalence, tentativeness, guilt, or fear, nor his subordinate role by anxiety, anger, or excessive competitiveness.

Once freed to the extent possible of emotional/neurotic baggage, the person in authority perceives more clearly that employees in the organization orient themselves in many different ways toward him as an authority figure. The blinders are off. Some workers assume an unnecessarily subservient or fawning attitude; others show open hostility and seek to challenge his authority, while some see him as a potential aggressor and want to join him for their own protection. Fortunately, there are many people in the system who are not overly threatened by authority, and for whom the subordinate role, too, may be no major problem. If they are given sway over others, they do not suffer from crippling tensions, and as subordinates they cooperate happily.

Nevertheless, although many emerge relatively healthy in this respect in adult years, conflicts about the possession and use of power are ubiquitous, for all of us have the experience of being subordinate to others—whether to our parents, teachers, or the body politic. Many who eventually attain positions of power in their adult years are still constrained by these conflicts, which are largely unconscious. Thus, problems regarding power may be denied or downplayed. Indeed, it has been said that although the concept of power has long been central in the social and political spheres, in the field of clinical psychodynamics, power is too often denied or downplayed. In relationships with patients, the therapist is clearly the power figure; as the process of therapy unfolds, his power generally increases, while the client becomes more dependent.[5]

In an amusing book, *Power: How to Get It, How to Use It,* Korda[6] predicts that the drive for power will be the last of the psychological mysteries to be unraveled.

DEVELOPMENTAL VIEW OF POWER

In analyzing our earliest struggles, psychodynamic theory ascribes to the infant strong drives for omnipotence and control of his environment, eventually tempered by the realization that he is not the master of the universe. At an early age, battles take place between mother and child in the areas of feeding, toilet training, and cleanliness. During the oedipal phase, a critical struggle occurs for possession of the parent of the opposite sex. From all these experiences, pitting innate narcissism against hard realities, deep emotional attitudes are established in relation to power, authority, and influence. They may be further molded and tempered in school, sports, jobs, and social relationships, but basic structures from childhood may persist. Developmentally, with mastery of these challenges, feelings of competence (power) emerge.[7] Then the individual is free to use his energies for personal creativity and social good.

Viewed from a social perspective, power needs are unevenly distributed in a population. There are those who possess strong innate drives to be leaders and to possess power, and those who are more or less content to follow. Presumably, executives belong to the former group, many of whom clearly manifest leadership potentialities in their earliest years. Leaders seek to create organizations or to become heads of organizations where power can be grasped and used. But power tends to corrupt, as Lord Acton[8] has stated; and "lust to rule,"[9] if unchecked, can ruin an organization.

The modern hospital administrator, then, has authority given to him as one of the tools of leadership. It is his responsibility to understand it, appreciate its limitation, and use it to gain power, not for personal gain but for public good. He is entitled to use his power in the search for resources needed to make the organization more efficient and effective, within the scope of humanitarian purposes and objectives.

AUTHORITY

Although authority is that which is *granted* to the individual by virtue of statute, court ruling, rank, or office, one discovers that power presumably possessed by the authority figure is inherent in the individual who determines which laws or rules he will obey.[10] Only when a command is accepted is power bestowed upon the designated authority. Thus, as has been so often said, power derives from the "consent of the governed."[11] We owe to Barnard,[12] in his famous chapter 12, the insight that there exists a "zone of indifference within each individual where orders are accepted without conscious questioning of authority." This zone of indifference is established over time by conditioning and practice so that the good soldier unquestioningly accepts commands from his superior officers, even those that may lead to his death. As for the executive, Barnard cautions never to issue orders that are unlikely to be obeyed, for that will weaken authority; therefore, in making organizational changes that evoke resistance, it is prudent to test the waters first. Make sure that the lines of communication are clear, and that the competence of individuals issuing the orders is unquestioned.

ADMINISTRATIVE THERAPY

Since the administrator has multiple roles in relation to his employees, it is only natural that they turn to him at times of stress. Many of the problems presented call for him to exercise his decision-making functions, but it is not only decisions that people desire from contacts with their chief. It is also an opportunity to *be* with him, to "feel" his presence, to affirm once again in their minds his image as a benign, thoughtful, and caring father figure. Should he be a less appreciated leader, the image may not be so complimentary. The "decision asker" is then wondering, "Has he changed?" or "Where do *I* fit in his esteem and in his affections?"

In small organizations, strong affectional ties may build up between a boss and workers; in large organizations, impersonal relationships between boss and worker are more the rule. But under such conditions, close ties are often established between workers and their immediate unit chiefs. In either case, an image of the top executive is introjected, and it usually is very meaningful to the worker.

The question before the administrator in relation to persons who seek his counsel in personal matters may be formulated as follows: In a therapeutic system serving sick patients, how "therapeutic" should the system be toward its workers? Since the administrator's primary responsibility is to the goals and purposes of the organization, and since his time is limited, he ordinarily must refer workers with clinical problems to others. However, for workers facing problems of living, or manifesting minor (less than clinical) character difficulties, is there something he can do? For example, can the overly subservient one be taught to be unafraid? Can the hostile one be taught to control his anger? Can the one who identifies strongly with power figures be given an opportunity to exert command (under appropriate supervision)? By recognizing these types of behavior, or the nature of workers' transferences, the administrator can influence the channeling of energies and drives in favorable directions.

The unit or team in which the individual inevitably acts out his personal problems also has a decision to make as to how far it should go in attempting to assist the individual. In this, the unit takes its clue from the leader—whether to persist in trying to help the person change, or to throw up its hands and close ranks. The latter will greatly increase the probabilities that, in the long run, that worker will either leave or be terminated.

There are no hard-and-fast guidelines in this subtle area. However, apart from humanitarian considerations, the administrator will find himself wondering: How important is this individual to the mission of the institution? How difficult would it be to replace him? What will be the effect on morale and efficiency of the organization of my level of concern for the individual worker's welfare? Perhaps even more important, what are my reasons for being involved in this person's personal problems?

TAXONOMY OF POWER

The *taxonomy of power* has long held great fascination for many thinkers. It is important that the administrator appreciate the variety of choices open to him in relation to the appropriate and effective use of whatever power he possesses. Here I refer briefly to three classifications of power: one that derives primarily from studies of influence on educational and medical organizations; one that views power from the perspective of the administrator responsible for a huge agency; and one that views power from the perspective of the political scientist. (I will also point out where these views overlap.)

Bertram Raven's[13,14,15] taxonomy recognized six basic sources of power:

1. *Coercive power* stems from the belief that the leader can exact punishment for nonconformity. Coercion may lead to public change in behavior but exert a negative influence on private feelings and attitudes.
2. *Reward influence* results when the leader can benefit or reward the individual for conformity. The resulting influence is also public. In coercive influence, the person may leave the group rather than continue to conform; in reward influence, the group member will be encouraged to remain in the group and accept its leadership.
3. *Expert influence* of a leader stems from the group members' feeling that the leader has superior knowledge or skill of direct bearing on the members' welfare. An example is so-called Aesculapian authority—the authority of the physician whose special knowledge can help pre-

serve or enhance the health and welfare of the individual. Thus, a president can be ordered to bed by a physician without anyone feeling that the president's authority has been undermined.

4. *Referent influence* of the leader arises when the group member identifies with him and wishes to be closer to him. This may also relate to the psychological mechanism often referred to as "identification with the aggressor." It also operates where the leader is much admired for exceptional gifts or personality traits, or exudes a charismatic, uplifting effect on group members' morale or self-esteem. Many teachers have exerted great influence on their students because of their unique ability to inspire intellectual excitement and joy in learning.

5. *Legitimate influence* results from acceptance of the right to prescribe behavior or opinions. A minister, for example, is seen as having the right to suggest standards of ethical behavior in relation to one's neighbors, as well as rituals in conformity with systems of worship.

6. *Informational influence* results when the leader presents information effectively in a factual and organized fashion that then results in a change in behavior or opinion.

Employees tend to believe that all forms of influence reside to a great degree in the administrator. It is generally agreed that he can exert more influence than anyone else in the organization. The administrator, in turn, must understand exactly how much power he possesses, both formal and informal—on the one hand so as not to exceed his limits, and on the other hand not to be restrained from using judiciously what powers he does possess. Since his power is often viewed by subordinates and the public as inseparable from himself as a person, the administrator's every utterance, however casual, may be interpreted as a statement of policy. The administrator may precede his remarks by saying, "I speak not in my role as authority but in my role as an average citizen," but his listeners too often will construe his remarks as coming *ex cathedra*. This is a caveat particularly pertinent when the administrator confronts audiences or cooperates with the media.

The second classification of power arises from my experience as commissioner of mental health in the commonwealth of Massachusetts, where there were 17,000 employees and hundreds of programs, large and small. Here the purpose was to gain influence and support for a large organization dedicated to treating more patients more adequately. Power in this context was often a function of competition with other major programs of government—public health, welfare, correction, roads, commerce, veterans' affairs, and so on. Often, the benchmark of success was how much influence one carried with the governor, the legislators, major committees, and the citizens at large. Success was also measured by one's ability to acquire resources for the department's mission.

In relation to this type of experience, the following classification of power seemed pertinent:

1. *Structural (statutory or legitimate) power* is the power conferred upon the head of the agency by law. It is the basis of all activities and outlines both responsibility and authority and the limits thereof, as well as the penalties for breaching those limits. Its closest relatives in Raven's schema are coercive and reward power. Insofar as the statutes allow final decision in hiring and firing, and on policy formation, the powers of such a post are very large.

2. *Sapiential power* is power conferred by special knowledge and expertise. It is identical with Raven's expert power. In the context of the role as commissioner of mental health of a state, it was assumed that problems related to the care and treatment of patients who are mentally ill would be decided by the commissioner or his appointees, and that no other agency or arm of government would ordinarily do a better job. The possession of the M.D. degree, together with specialty training and experience in the field of psychiatry, was not infrequently the ticket to respect.

3. The *power of excellence* arises from the recognition that a department or agency has achieved a very high quality of service, has recruited an excellent group of individuals who work together smoothly, and enjoys high morale. As a result, that department gains an extra measure of support—enhanced also, it should be noted, by credit reflected upon the legislature, the governor, and the state.

4. The *power of broad-based support of programs* develops when a program advanced by an agency excites the imagination of and achieves broad support from citizens, legislature, and the governor. As a result, that department gains increased clout in competition for scarce resources. The administrator of an agency of government is therefore constantly searching for the fortunate formula that will unite a wide variety of constituencies in favor of his programs. In the mid-1960s, the "bold new approach" to an overhaul of the mental health systems of the states, inspired by the federal government and backed up by their funds, gave the programs of the state great prominence in the public eye and led to many reforms. This was a brilliant example of how an inspired concept that promised to do away with the "shame of the states"[16] stimulated massive coalition building and much effective action for mental health.

Finally, from the standpoint of an economist and political scientist, Galbraith,[17] in his *The Anatomy of Power*, defines three instruments of power and three sources of power. "*Condign power* wins submission by inflicting or threatening appropriately adverse consequences"; it is similar to Raven's coercive power. "*Compensatory power* . . . wins submission by the offer of affirmative reward"; it is similar to Raven's reward influence. "*Conditioned power* is exercised by changing belief. Persuasion, education, or the social commitment to what seems natural, proper or right causes the individual to submit to the will of another or of others." This is much like Raven's legitimate influence. (Emphasis added in all quotations.)

According to Galbraith's schema, behind these instruments of power lie three sources of power: personality, property, and organization. *Personality* is the quality of leadership that gives access to one or more of the instruments of power; in some ways, this resembles the charismatic aspects of leadership as defined by Weber.[18] *Property* or wealth accords an aspect of authority insofar as it provides the wherewithal to purchase submission. *Organization* is the foremost source of power in modern societies and is related to conditioned power, to condign power, and to compensatory power.

Galbraith's reflections on the *use* of power in modern society are worth noting. Power is pursued for many reasons, but also for its own sake, for there are emotional as well as material rewards in its possession and exercise. However, the purposes for which power is sought are often artfully hidden. Command is a mountaintop; the air breathed there is different from that of the valley of obedience. "Yet, power, per se, is not a proper subject for indignation. . . . Power can be socially malign; it also can be socially essential."[19]

MODIFICATION AND CONSTRAINT OF POWER

As indicated above, psychodynamicists declare that deprivations suffered in childhood determine one's drive for power and how such power, once gained, will be used. Lasswell[20] affirms this in his formula for political man: "Private motives displaced onto public objects and rationalized as in the public interest equals political man." Many powerful figures in history suffered from low self-esteem. Power holders may feel superior to others and develop social distance from their fellows. The power holder may surround himself with a coterie of admirers who serve the purpose of isolating him from his constituents. Some may begin to assume they are exempt from common morality. The overemphasis on the importance of power may preclude an intimate and loving relationship. Deference and servility on the part of those selected to surround him feed into the narcissistic self-image. For the administrator, this kind of self-deception will ultimately be destructive and lead to his downfall. Close touch with all that is going on may be impossible, but the constant and necessary striving of the administrator is to keep a sensitive finger on the pulse of his living system as far as is possible.

Some persons in a system may have their powers augmented by delegation from high formal sources; others may acquire informal power by addition of knowledge, experience, or seniority. Some persons in positions of *formal* power may suddenly be downgraded because they have lost the confidence of a higher-up, perhaps through bad judgment, misbehavior, misfeasance, or malfeasance. Persons in positions of very high authority in a hierarchy may employ outside consultants, or confer on volunteers a great deal of delegated authority, thus downplaying reliance on formal sources. An outstanding example of the latter was the conferring of extraordinary power onto Colonel House by President Wilson.[21] House became Wilson's close friend and, on occasion, informal ambassador in strategic international relations, although he was never formally employed. Another fascinating example was the shift of presidential power to Mrs. Wilson during the time of her husband's cerebral vascular accident. Mrs. Wilson probably assumed more presidential authority during that worrisome period than any woman in history before or since. Michael Medved[22] has published a fascinating book, called *The Shadow Presidents*, that describes the heavy reliance of almost all presidents on persons in whom they had great confidence, whether these persons were elected officials or not.

Not all power, by any means, resides in the individual at the top, although that individual may possess the greatest share of power in formal terms; often, that power is shared within an executive constellation (see "Executive Constellation in Organizational Leadership" in Chapter 2). But still other modifiers of power must be mentioned. For example, the top administrator in a given organization is himself a cog in a larger system. He is beholden to the appointing official(s) in that larger organization and to other checks and balances provided in the larger system. Then there may be an advisory or trustee group with whom he must share power, if only to solidify his hold on his job (see Chapter 5). Other individuals or agencies—such as comptrollers, auditors, fire and safety inspectors, food and sanitation standard setters, and policymakers of many descriptions—modify, control, and limit power possessed.

Beyond the larger organization of which the administrator may be a part are still other agencies to which he must pay heed. I refer to such influences as the Joint Commission on Accreditation of Healthcare Organizations; patient-rights advocates; labor unions; professional societies and associations that set standards for their members; various research and training departments of universities with which an organization may be affiliated; federal and private foundations that support research, training, and clinical programs; various citizen groups; the legislators, courts, and attorneys general's offices; the grand jury, with its investigatory powers; and finally, whatever community groups claim a stake in the programs and policies of the institution—the administrator must take notice of all of these (see Chapter 10).

Even more, there are major trends in society that impinge upon the administrator's actions. As examples of these, I cite the rising tide of color—the rapidly growing minorities clamoring for improvement in their socioeconomic status, their health services, and their share of the nation's wealth. In the selection of a new employee, for example, the administrator must consider carefully current minority rights and the pressure to bring more minority individuals into the organization, particularly at higher levels.

ABUSE OF POWER

Administrators are entrusted with power; they are expected to wield that power with honesty, integrity, intelligence, and wisdom. Any deviation from these standards constitutes a breach of trust and a less than optimal use of power. Indeed, the (often unwritten) contract that gives the administrator his power includes expectation of good performance "in sickness and in health." The able administrator senses when to accept power, when to delegate it to others, and when to give it up. As Bennis and Nanus[23] have put it, the leader rarely openly asserts that power. He lets it remain implicit, for "leadership is like the Abominable Snowman, whose footprints are everywhere but who is nowhere to be seen."

Galbraith[24] wisely observed, "We may lay it down as a rule that almost any manifestation of power will induce an opposite . . . manifestation of power." Not only does resistance to power develop almost automatically, there are also often highly organized efforts to achieve its total dissolution on the basis that its exercise may be improper, illegitimate, unconstitutional, oppressive, or evil. Moreover, Galbraith again reminds us, there is a tendency to symmetry between the magnitude of power developed and the force of resistance mounted against it. The greater the power, the greater the checks and balances, including penalties against its malignant use. "This symmetry is affirmed in a dozen aphorisms: one fights fire by fire; force begets force; those who live by the sword, die by the sword."

"Power tends to corrupt, and absolute power corrupts absolutely" (Lord Acton[25]). But power does not *necessarily* corrupt, for there are many checks and balances. There are many mature, responsible people who—after a taste of power—realize that its rewards are not as great as anticipated and that its potential for misuse must always be controlled. Executive/administrative positions may carry with them so many constraints that continuing in office becomes a real headache. It is also true that responsibility over people's health and welfare *can* produce more compassionate and understanding leaders. Some agencies, such as the Supreme Court, function by law largely to discourage an imbalance of power between other great agencies.

In a democratic society, the common sense of the group influences the nomination and election of political leaders. Unfortunately, with the use of large-scale image-making techniques, speeches drafted by professional writers, and public presentations tailored to the latest opinion poll, the true personality of a candidate may not emerge; but with the exposure provided by the media, this danger may be mitigated to a large extent.

Checks and balances are numerous, but perhaps the greatest deterrent to the abuse of power is still the maturity and emotional balance of the individual, based upon self-understanding, a respect for others, and a desire to be of service to the public. When asked, as is often the case, "How many people work for you?" I have heard an excellent executive reply, "I really don't know, but I do know how many *I* work for."

What is the significance of all this for the administrator? The bottom line is that hostility against authority—whether from unresolved conflicts with parents, unresolved sibling rivalries, or omnipotent dreams of freedom from all restraints—is part of the human condition. Some of the force of these unresolved conflicts will be directed against the person in charge; it is then his job to keep these forces within bounds. Understanding oneself, as well as the dynamics behind the behavior of the other person, is an invaluable asset in the maintenance of organizational equilibrium. Finally, limits placed on abrasive behaviors depend not only on the administrator's personal tolerance but also on the organization's ability to absorb disruption and chaos.

DECISION MAKING

In the flow of documents that come across the administrator's desk are items requiring little attention—where, for example, merely a quick reading and a signature are all that is required. Then there are many items that are simply informational, with no action expected. And then there are items that require thought and the assembling of additional data; they alert the administrator to a problem that requires concentration, conceptualizing, and a plan of action. Many problems surface via direct communications from colleagues inside or outside the organization. Which ones should the executive attend to first? Should he or an assistant or a subordinate handle the problem? In what time frame should it be solved? Indeed, can it be solved at all?

In order for organizations to function, decisions have to be made in a wide variety of areas. Here are a few:

1. The purposes and goals of the organization
2. Program and budgetary priorities and resource allocations
3. Space allocations
4. Organization of work, supplies, and equipment
5. Establishment and maintenance of organizational structures
6. Planning, development; maintenance and alteration of programs and of the physical plant
7. Human resource management: hiring, assignment, training, evaluation, promotion, leaves, and discipline
8. Relations to outside agencies and organizations

No single individual can have the knowledge and experience to make wise decisions in all these areas. Thus, decisions have to be "composite"[26]— that is, made up of components traceable through formal and informal chains. A multitude of small and large decisions may be made before some final authority signs his name authenticating a policy.

Where does the impetus for decisions come from? Some arise from higher authority, as when a manager enunciates a policy affecting a number of divisions. Some decisions arise from the interests and needs of the workers in the organization, where a judicious choice between alternatives or between subordinates must be made—so-called appellate cases. Finally, cases originate from the executive of the organization himself in relation to his role as a leader, planner, organizer, and implementer.[27]

Since decision making depends on the organizational context in which the problem arises, on the definition and dimensions of the problem, and on the available resources for its solution, it is very difficult to spell out precise guidelines for arriving at a solution. The administrator, however, can certainly consider the problem with the following questions in mind:

- Why did this problem come to me? Why at this time? Has lower authority been bypassed? If so, why? Look for both immediate, remote, or hidden causes. (A companion question might be: Why did this problem, which may have been kicking around for some time, *not* come to me *before?*)
- Do I, personally, *have* to render a decision? Perhaps a decision should be made *not* to make a decision, or at least not to indulge in any action. This could be indicated because the timing is wrong, the data are inadequate, the base of participation has not been sufficiently inclusive, the people involved have not been properly prepared for their part in its implementation, or the remote consequences of the action need to be better envisioned. Avoiding premature decision making avoids future prejudice and resistance. Decisions that turn out to be resisted or neglected by subordinates tend to undermine both power and authority. The art of leadership is, therefore, often the fine art of rejection of decisions and/or actions that in the short or long run may be injurious to the purposes of the organization.[28]
- If I do render a decision, will it encourage other problems of this kind to come to me? How much of my time and energy am I, therefore, committing to this category of issues?
- To whom or to what group can I refer this problem for help in decision making? If I, as the administrator, refrain from making decisions that others should make, will this help to preserve morale and authority, develop competence, and fix responsibility? Decisions made by higher authority that could well be made at a lower level may suggest that the lower level cannot be trusted—and that level may believe it is more competent to make such decisions than any other level.
- What time frame is appropriate for a solution to this particular problem?
- What level of participation of my staff should I encourage (along Tannenbaum's[29] guidelines—see below)?

- Do I want feedback on staff's progress in arriving at a decision? If so, in what form and at what intervals?
- Following the decision, how do I reward those who contributed to the solution?

Since intelligent decisions cannot be made except in the context of the goals and purposes of the institution, all decisions, small or large, relate ultimately to the achievement of final goals. Decisions are basically of two types, as Simon[30] reminds us: value judgments, and factual judgments. Factual judgments are validated by agreement on the facts of a case. Value judgments, which lack the kind of objectivity enjoyed in the natural sciences, concern choices among alternatives that have ethical, normative, social, or political valence. They eventually are promulgated by consensus, edict, or fiat.

A matter of considerable importance in decision making is the base of participation of staff persons and consultants, and the degree of decisional power that is delegated to them. Here Tannenbaum[31] helps us with his description of the range of behaviors available to the manager, along an authoritarian–democratic continuum:

1. The manager makes the decision and announces it.
2. The manager "sells" his decision; he takes the additional step of persuading his subordinates to accept it.
3. The manager presents his ideas, and invites questions. Here he provides his subordinates with an opportunity to get a fuller explanation of his thinking and intentions.
4. The manager presents a tentative decision, subject to change. Here subordinates can exert some influence on the decision, but the initiative for identifying it and diagnosing the problem remains with the manager.
5. The manager presents the problem, gets suggestions, and then makes his decision. The subordinates get first chance to bring their ideas to bear on a problem; then a final decision is made by the manager.
6. The manager defines the *limits* and requests the group to recommend a decision. He has, however, defined the problem and the boundaries within which the decision must be made.
7. The manager permits the group to actually *make* final decisions that will be followed. This is an extreme form of delegation not usually encountered in formal organizations.

Tannenbaum further comments on a group of important questions related to the choice of one or another of the above techniques. First, the manager can never relinquish responsibility for the quality of decisions made, no matter how fully he delegates the process of decision making. Second, he advises that the leader consider carefully whether his presence will inhibit or facilitate the problem-solving process. Next, the leader should carefully explicate the kind of leadership behavior he is using, because the relationship between leader and subordinates to an extent depends on how much his subordinates can trust his word. Confusion and resentment may arise if the boss says he will delegate a certain degree of decision making, but actually makes the decision himself. The subordinate group will usually prize the opportunity to participate, but sorely resent it if their efforts are meaningless. Finally, it is not the number of decisions delegated that reveal the manager's confidence in his group's participation in decision making, but the significance of those decisions.

Apart from the manager's stylistic preference for one or another approach to working with his subordinates, there are characteristics of the subordinate group that help determine the appropriate leadership style. Generally speaking, says Tannenbaum, greater freedom can be allowed if the subordinates:

1. Have relatively high needs for independence
2. Have a readiness to assume responsibility for decision making
3. Have a relatively high tolerance for ambiguity
4. Are interested in the problem and feel it is important
5. Understand and identify with the goals of the organization
6. Possess the necessary knowledge and experience to deal with the problem.
7. Have learned to expect a share in decision making.

Other relevant considerations may be the values and traditions of the organization, the anticipated effectiveness of group members in working together, and the pressures of time.

> Thus the successful manager of men can be primarily characterized neither as a strong leader nor as a persuasive one. Rather, he is one who maintains a high batting average in accurately assessing the forces that determine what his most appropriate behavior [and decisions] at any given time should be, and in actually being able to behave accordingly.[32]

Case Illustration

Unwise Use of Power in a University Department of Psychiatry

The director of a famous psychiatric institute was renowned for his ability to recruit remarkable individuals to his department of psychiatry. His goal was to build the greatest possible research and educational institution; and in the years of his tenure he did, indeed, make outstanding progress toward this goal. In the course of time, however, it became apparent that sufficient *consultation in depth* with faculty members heading important subdivisions of the institute was sometimes lacking. This was a crucial matter, particularly as funds to support new recruits were often drawn at least in part from *their* budgets. When complaints of these professors that they had not been fully consulted did not result in a satisfactory change in the director's operating style, members of the faculty charged loss of confidence, and appealed to the dean for guidance.

Consultation in depth is the key phrase here. The director has authority to bring in new people and to arrange financing for them; however, in this case, he asserts his authority beyond the willingness of his associates to comply. Because they have not been convinced of the desirability of diminishing *their* budgets to accomplish *his* aims, the situation quickly and dramatically escalated.

Another psychiatric phrase for consultation in depth might be the "working through of the resistances"—a process prudently adhered to, lest decisions be labeled unilateral. "Working through" in this context means repeated discussion of the views and sentiments of involved colleagues until a reasonable consensus is reached. Expecting associates to agree with one's plans without such due process risks three R's—resentment, resistance, and rebellion.

Two interesting questions arise:

- How much effort and time must the director put in to win over his staff, that is, to work through the resistance? A rule of thumb is "as long as it takes." Usually, the recruiting of a new person is not an emergency; time spent working with staff builds morale and better understanding. In the end, it usually saves time and effort.
- In a persistent difference of opinion, or impasse, should the director yield? But yielding is not the issue if the people believe that the director really wants to utilize the collective wisdom of his staff to arrive at a superior decision. In doing so he does not alienate them, but rather conveys a message of unity, harmony, and respect. Whoever sets up a confrontation, as Galbraith[33] has taught us, encourages the development of an equal and opposite show of power. In this case, consultation with the dean encouraged the director to modify his leadership style to fit the imperatives of his organization.

Case Illustration

Power Squabbles Based on Ignorance and Naïveté*

The following is an interesting example of the kinds of squabbles about power and turf that a naive new superintendent can get into when he neglects rules of procedure and angers other departments within a complicated bureaucracy. It occurred in the year 1964, shortly after I had been appointed superintendent of a state hospital. My background had been essentially in research and development; I was poorly prepared for the bureaucratic complexities I was soon to face.

Breaking with long-standing tradition, my wife and I decided not to move into the superintendent's house on the grounds of the hospital. Instead, based on successful experiences with two halfway houses for chronic patients established in the community,[34,35] we decided to convert the superintendent's house to a halfway house for chronic hospitalized patients. It was an exciting opportunity to

*This case illustration is adapted from The Establishment of Transitional Facilities: The Psychopolitics of a Halfway House, Chapter 9 in *Psychopolitics*, by Milton Greenblatt. New York, Grune & Stratton, 1978, pp 121–128. Reprinted with permission of The Psychological Corporation.

establish the first state-supported halfway house in Massachusetts and to teach the advantages of a "new" therapeutic modality. Halfway houses were then in the early experimental phase, and Massachusetts had pioneered in their development.

Occupants of the house included the following: (a) chronic patients who could be expected to profit by close living together in a surrogate family; (b) students who would lend their youth and enthusiasm to the care of the patients (the use of college students had already been successful in the early experiments); and (c) parent surrogates who would be responsible for "bringing up" the family.

As housefather and mother, I chose the Protestant minister of the hospital (at this point a consultant) and his wife. He agreed to take on responsibilities as housefather in exchange for economical living accommodations for himself and his spouse. His wife was appointed a member of the nursing staff, and thus drew a modest salary for a difficult job. Her previous training and experience in child care fitted her to assist chronic mentally ill patients to develop basic skills: eating properly, bathing, grooming, and carrying out necessary chores. Thus, the first state halfway house was set up in the commonwealth of Massachusetts.

Soon after its opening, criticisms were voiced to the effect that a small group of patients (about one dozen) was enjoying much personal attention amid plush surroundings, while back on the wards, where literally many hundreds of patients were domiciled, the environment was drab and the staffing meager. The superintendent was charged with improper allocation of resources. I remonstrated that we were testing out a new modality for the rehabilitation of chronic patients who, on the custodial wards, had been hospitalized for years without making significant progress.

The events that transpired were a stunning lesson in sociopsychopolitics. We were not prepared for the sudden recalcitrant attitudes of the maintenance crew, which now failed to cut the lawn, trim the hedges, or repair the plumbing. They had been trained to do such chores for the superintendent and his family, but not for chronic schizophrenic patients or students, and not for the minister and his wife. The patients, suddenly thrust from dull and drab surroundings of the back ward to the affluence of the superintendent's house, reacted with a mixture of confusion and paralysis. They were expected to show respect and consideration for others, keep neat and clean, attend to social amenities, participate in conversation, carry out chores, and maintain the environment. It was made clear that one's time in the house was not eternal; each patient was expected to move into the community in the near future, with the support of family, friends, and social workers—or face the grim alternative of a return to the chronic wards. Faced with this choice, the patients began to show improvement, and in a few short months the house demonstrated the results predicted initially.

About five months after the house opened, an official of the Personnel and Standardization Bureau of the State Office of Administration and Finance informed me that I had violated an important regulation: I had failed to obtain approval for a new use of state property. The state investigator also indicated that for a group of chronic mentally ill patients, occupancy of such a superb residence seemed an unnecessary luxury. Further, religious discrimination was charged; it was gossiped that since the minister was Protestant, he would favor Protestant patients over Catholics or Jews. Another rumor was that the superintendent was receiving a "kickback" from the minister for allowing him and his spouse to live in the posh surroundings.

I was further shocked by still another regulation of which I was totally ignorant. Although it was proper to offer living accommodation for his wife, since she was a regular employee in the nursing service, it was improper to offer accommodations to the minister, who was classified as a consultant.

"Do you mean that I am improperly allowing the minister to live with his wife?" I cried. "Yes," was the answer, "and you will have to close up immediately." In the meantime, one newspaper hinted at corruption and criminal misuse of state resources. The following headline appeared in one of the papers:

HOSPITAL MINISTER FREELOADING ON THE COMMONWEALTH

Immediately, a peremptory order from the comptroller demanded we close the house, or state troopers would be sent in to evict all tenants forcibly. It was, indeed, a hard blow. What had seemed a very good idea that promised substantial benefits to patients was about to be wrecked by bureaucratic complications I had obviously failed to foresee.

Such was the state of affairs when the commissioner of mental health (my appointing officer) arranged a meeting with the deputy commissioner of administration and finance, a career government employee of great experience. In short order, these two wise heads converted what had loomed as an unmitigated disaster into a minor annoyance. First, the deputy commissioner of administration and finance satisfied himself that the house was being used for legitimate purposes. He immediately sensed the possibilities for patient rehabilitation through development of a new kind of facility. The commissioner of mental health indicated that he wanted his superintendents to exercise their imagination and initiative, and that whatever supervision appeared necessary should come from his office rather than from other branches of government.

Next it was established that some of the patients who lived in the halfway house were already working outside, actually paying one-fourth of their earnings to the state for room and board. Happily, the sum total of monies paid to the commonwealth by these working patients exceeded what the former superintendent had paid when he occupied the property. Financially, then, the state was coming out ahead.

Third, it made sense to the deputy commissioner of administration and finance that the minister and his wife should live together in the house; since a proper rental deduction was being made from the wife's salary, he saw no particular problem there. He also informed us that although a regulation existed that a consultant could not live on the grounds, the fact that this particular consultant was married to an employee who *was* permitted to live on the grounds—and that he was to function as head of a "family" of patients requiring his presence at all hours—seemed to him sufficient reason to make an exception to the rule (which was a prerogative of the office of administration and finance). He recognized that the minister was performing gratis an indispensable service as housefather, and that the whole success of the enterprise as an experiment in living depended on keeping the "parents" together.

Then we came to the distressing problem: the fact that the comptroller had ordered eviction and was about to send in state police to carry out his command. Here the answer was almost too simple. In the state system, the comptroller reported to the office of administration and finance; he was actually exceeding his authority in assuming that he could order the state police to do anything, for the state police *also* reported to that office. We were advised that the comptroller was bluffing and that the state police would not listen to his command. The comptroller was coming up for reelection and was possibly seeking a way to keep his name in the newspapers.

The deputy commissioner wound up his very helpful consultation by indicating two possible ways to proceed: (a) write a letter to the comptroller, telling him in effect that it was none of his business and that his threats would be ignored; or (b) do nothing and let it all die down. The final advice was to do nothing.

What was the result? No state police showed up, and there were no more letters from the comptroller's office or traumatic visits of officials. The house continued its work, and eventually demonstrated outstanding success in the rehabilitation of chronic state hospital patients.

What did we learn? First, when one is a new superintendent in a state organization, one's actions are carefully watched not only by higher authority, but also by workers at any level. Many governmental employees may view themselves as proper monitors and/or critics of the behavior of public servants.

Second, the media are quick to sensationalize anything that may stir up their readers. Allegations may be reported before facts. Denials by public officials may or may not be printed. And newspapers always have the last word.

Third, politicians, hungry for votes, need exposure and welcome an opportunity to get their names in the newspapers.

Fourth, if one wishes to break through bureaucratic rigidities in the trial of a new treatment modality, it helps immeasurably to have a commissioner of mental health and a deputy commissioner of administration and finance who are highly knowledgeable and sophisticated in the affairs of state, and who are supportive of new enterprises.

Fifth, the combination of a superintendent who is naive in the ways of bureaucracy and bureaucrats who are anxious to arrogate power can cause much friction and damage to worthy programs. Therefore, a new administrator would do well to learn all about the system in which he operates, its rules and regulations, the loci of power (formal, informal, and assumed), and the functions of personnel in vitally related agencies—or it may cost him his job.

SUMMARY AND COMMENTS

Inasmuch as administrators are granted considerable authority in order to get their jobs done, resolution of one's personal conflicts and hangups in relation to the power and authority figures in one's past is most desirable. Thus, one can feel more comfortable with the exercise of power/authority as well as with one's role as subordinate when others are in a power position. This is all-important for administrators who, above all, are expected to make wise decisions affecting people, resources, and the future of enterprises.

Power should be differentiated from authority and influence. A succinct definition of power (by Bertrand Russell) is the capacity to produce intended effects. Authority is permission granted by statute, court, and other formal bodies; influence is unofficial power dependent on deference to one's character, ability, or station.

Several varieties of power are recognized in modern taxonomies. They include coercive power and reward power, as well as expert, referent, legitimate, and informational power (Raven's classification). To this may be added the power of excellence, and the power of broad-based support of programs. Galbraith identifies three sources of power: personality, property, and organization. Power may be modified upward or downward by contingent circumstances. In the case of executives in large organizations, the power of a leader may be shared in an executive constellation, or with advisory or trustee groups; it may be significantly influenced by accreditation and regulatory bodies. The legislature, courts, community groups, universities, and professional bodies may also have a say in modifying power.

Abuse of power is always a risk and a threat. It is counteracted by the modifiers above, existing checks and balances, and by the innate tendency of society to erect opposite and equal power structures to those prevailing. Insight, maturity, and the emotional balance of the individual are inherent safeguards to the excessive use of power.

The administrator's role as decision maker is pervasive. Eight questions that an administrator might ask before rendering a decision have been offered, and seven behaviors suggested in considering how much authority to delegate to others (per Tannenbaum). These guidelines may be of use to decision makers; sometimes, however, the decision to make *no* decision may be the best judgment in an individual case.

REFERENCES

1. Machiavelli N: The Prince. New York, New American Library, 1952
2. Machiavelli N: The Prince. New York, New American Library, 1952, pp 55, 56
3. Russell B: Power: A New Social Analysis. New York, W. W. Norton, 1938
4. Schwartz DA: A précis of administration. Community Mental Health Journal 25:229–244, 1989
5. Gadpaille WJ: The uses of power: A particular impasse in psychoanalysis, in Masserman J (ed): Dynamics of Power. Scientific Proceedings of American Academy of Psychoanalysis. New York, Grune & Stratton, 1972
6. Korda M: The Power Game, Chapter 1 in Korda M: Power: How to Get It, How to Use It. New York, Random House, 1975, pp 3–16, esp. p 8
7. Salzman L: Compulsive drives for power, in Masserman J (ed): Dynamics of Power. Scientific Proceedings of American Academy of Psychoanalysis. New York, Grune & Stratton, 1972
8. Lord Acton (Dalberg-Acton JEE): Letter to Bishop Mandell Creighton, April 5, 1887. Quoted in Bartlett's Familiar Quotations, 14th ed. Boston, Little, Brown, 1968
9. Nietzsche F: The Will to Power. New York, Vintage Books, 1968
10. Barnard CI: The theory of authority, Chapter 12 in Barnard CI: Functions of the Executive. Cambridge, Mass., Harvard University Press, 1938, 1968, pp 161–185
11. Jefferson T: Declaration of Independence, July 4, 1776
12. Barnard CI: The theory of authority, Chapter 12 in Barnard CI: Functions of the Executive. Cambridge, Mass., Harvard University Press, 1938, 1968, pp 161–185

13. Raven BH, Litman-Adizes T: Interpersonal influence and social power in health, in Salisbury Z, Kar S, Zapka J (eds), Advances in Health, Education, and Promotion, Vol. I. Greenwich, Connecticut, JAI Press, 1985
14. Raven BH: Interpersonal influence and social power, in Raven BH, Rubin JZ, Social Psychology, 2nd ed. New York, John Wiley & Sons, 1983, pp 399–443
15. Raven BH: The dynamics of interaction between individual and group, Chapter 19 in Weiner B, Runquist W, Runquist PA, Meyer WJ, Leiman A, Kutscher CL, Kleinmuntz B, Haber RN (eds), Discovering Psychology. Chicago, Science Research Associates, 1977, pp 631–706
16. Deutsch A: The Shame of the States. New York, Harcourt, Brace, 1948
17. Galbraith JK: The Anatomy of Power. Boston, Houghton Mifflin, 1983
18. Weber M (translated and edited by Henderson AM, Parsons T): The Theory of Social and Economic Organisation. New York, Free Press, 1947
19. Galbraith JK: The Anatomy of Power. Boston, Houghton, Mifflin, 1983
20. Lasswell HD: Psychopathology and Politics. New York, Viking, 1960, pp 74–77
21. George AL, George JL: Woodrow Wilson and Colonel House. A Personality Study. New York, Dover Press, 1964
22. Medved M: The Shadow Presidents. The Secret History of the Chief Executives and Their Top Aides. New York, Times Books, 1979
23. Bennis W, Nanus B: Leaders. The Strategies for Taking Charge. New York, Harper & Row, 1985
24. Galbraith JK: The Anatomy of Power. Boston, Houghton Mifflin, 1983
25. Lord Acton (Dalberg-Acton JEE): Letter to Bishop Mandell Creighton, April 5, 1887. Quoted in Bartlett's Familiar Quotations, 14th ed. Boston, Little, Brown, 1968
26. Simon HA: Anatomy of organization, Chapter 11 in Simon HA: Administrative Behavior. New York, Macmillan, 1957, pp 220–247
27. Barnard CI: Decisions, Chapter 13 in Barnard CI: Functions of the Executive. Cambridge, Massachusetts, Harvard University Press, 1938, 1968, pp 185–199
28. Barnard CI: Decisions, Chapter 13 in Barnard CI: Functions of the Executive. Cambridge, Massachusetts, Harvard University Press, 1938, 1968, pp 185–199
29. Tannenbaum R: How to choose a leadership pattern. Harvard Business Review 36:95–101, 1958
30. Simon HA: Decision-making, in Simon HA: Administrative Behavior. New York, Macmillan, 1957, pp 215–217
31. Tannenbaum R: How to choose a leadership pattern. Harvard Business Review 36:95–101, 1958
32. Tannenbaum R: How to choose a leadership pattern. Harvard Business Review 36:95–101, 1958
33. Galbraith JK: The Anatomy of Power. Boston, Houghton Mifflin, 1983
34. Landy D, Greenblatt M: Halfway House: A Sociocultural and Clinical Study of Rutland Corner House, a Transitional Aftercare Residence for Female Psychiatric Patients. Washington, DC, Vocational Rehabilitation Administration, 1965
35. Kantor D, Greenblatt M: Wellmet: Halfway to community rehabilitation (A cooperative student–patient halfway house for chronic mentally ill). Ment Hosp 13:146–152, 1962

12

Executive Careers

PSYCHIATRISTS IN LEADERSHIP POSITIONS

As was stated earlier, in psychiatry the importance of the art and science of administration has been relatively underplayed due largely to the discipline's emphasis on clinical services on a one-to-one basis in a close physician–patient relationship. Recent reports suggest, however, that of the approximately 37,200 psychiatrists who belong to the American Psychiatric Association, thousands spend at least part of their time on administrative duties. A strong case can be made in support of the view that administrative abilities are necessary in any psychiatrist's career. For example, young residents working with patients in a complex clinical milieu must integrate the skills of a number of professionals and paraprofessionals. Those who supervise wards assume executive responsibilities for many patients and personnel; they must become concerned with the relationship between the ward they supervise and other parts of the institution. Soon they become aware of extrainstitutional pressures and forces that impinge on their work. By the time a young psychiatrist takes charge of a teaching program, day-care facility, or outpatient department—or steps up even further to director of education or clinical director of a facility—he necessarily becomes enmeshed in a whole range of administrative functions and activities.

A profound shift in leadership of mental health institutions and systems has taken place within recent decades. Over a 10-year period (1971 to 1981), the number of psychiatrists serving as state commissioners of mental health has fallen by 56%, while the number of nonpsychiatrist commissioners has risen by some 78%. In 1971, there were 41 psychiatrists, 6 nonpsychiatrists, and 7 nonphysicians serving in the various states and territories;[1] in 1981, there were 18 psychiatrists, 4 nonpsychiatrists, and 32 nonphysicians.[2]

This change has arrested the attention of many leaders within the psychiatric community. Whether or not a psychiatrist is likely to be a better head of a major agency than any other professional, this trend heralds a serious loss by psychiatrists of their influence on mental health policy and practice. We know, too, that with respect to the community mental health center movement of the last 20 years, which has produced more than 750 new centers, the majority now are without top-side psychiatric administrative leadership.

Another example: The President's Commission on Mental Health, appointed by President Carter, counted only 3 psychiatrists among its 20 members—a far cry from the first Joint Commission on Mental Illness and Health of 1955 to 1961, which was almost entirely in the hands of psychiatrists (and in general was dominated by psychiatrists belonging to the American Psychiatric Association and by psychiatrist officials of the National Institute of Mental Health).

Former American Psychiatric Association President Donald G. Langsley recognized not only that the psychiatric grip on mental health systems had been weakening, but also that the role of administrator of a mental health organization had in general been given a bad name, and that young psychiatrists were being scared away from a potentially rich, enlightening, and immensely important experience. In 1981, he appointed the APA Ad Hoc Committee on Psychiatrist Leadership in Public Mental Health Programs to study what opportunities exist for psychiatrists for executive training and experience, how negative attitudes toward administration might be changed, and what incentives might attract capable psychiatrists into the field.

Some of the common negative feelings of psychiatrists in administrative roles, especially those in quasi-political jobs, are that salaries are low; ties with teaching and research become attenuated; the work is endless, the jobs thankless, and political pressures overwhelming; tenure is short ("You can't get anything done"); and there is "no future" in administrative work. (See "Stresses and Strains" later in this chapter.)

What Does Administration Offer the Mental Health Professional?

The mental health professional who ventures into the field will find that, assuming he does a creditable job, his colleagues will have considerably more respect for him. They realize he has served and survived in a tough arena. They respect the fact that he has accepted a large challenge, honed a new set of skills, and has been exposed to a range of experiences that have added to his knowledge and wisdom.

The administrator has the opportunity to develop a broader and more sophisticated view of the world. His judgment becomes correspondingly more objective, critical, and balanced. He is likely to have a better understanding of the democratic process, and of the sources, uses, and abuses of power. He develops a better perspective on the place of psychiatry in the professions. He understands the need to change systems and yet how systems resist change; and he has a more realistic view of what is possible.

What Can Psychiatrists Bring to the Executive Role?

Physicians in general are interested in the individual patient's biological, psychological, and social welfare; they are taught that to fully understand his illness, he must be viewed in his total ecological context. Thus, while the early years of medical education focus primarily on the individual, as time goes on one gains increasing respect for the patient's family, background, childhood, education, place in society, aspirations, philosophy, and desire for a meaningful existence. In the course of his career, the physician takes on numerous roles—he may become a ward doctor, a leader of a treatment team, a coordinator of education, an outpatient director, or a top executive in one of myriad different programs and institutions.

Inasmuch as the psychiatrist is a physician, he carries the authority of that role (the so-called Aesculapian authority), which evokes respect and regard in many quarters. Among his credits is his long formal education, which teaches him to take responsibility over matters of life and death. Sensitivity to personal dynamics and competence in handling crises are further assets. When individuals are feuding and factions are battling, he may be effective in helping them work out their differences. Although in recent years, public regard for the authority of many professionals has declined, the doctor of medicine still retains a relatively high place in the public's esteem.

The above is not to suggest that nonpsychiatrist or nonmedical executives lack necessary elements of leadership, or that their educational or career pathways are irrelevant to the administrative role. I suggest only that a further decline in the involvement of psychiatrists in administration may be a disservice to the field.

STUDY OF TOP-LEVEL ADMINISTRATORS

The striking decline in psychiatric leadership prompted a series of studies on "illustrious" administrators, including a number of current and past commissioners of mental health.[3,4,5,6,7] The goal was to gain an understanding of their backgrounds, interest, and experiences relative to the field of administration.

Incumbent psychiatric commissioners[8] had a wide range of prior experience in public mental health, including previous service as deputy commissioners, superintendents, and directors of mental health or mental retardation facilities. Some commissioners had been assistant ·superintendents in public institutions, while others had held high administrative positions in the private sector. One had been chief of service in a VA hospital, and another had been director of a public mental health clinic. Almost without exception, all respondents had held a high-level position in a federal, state, or county mental health program before becoming state mental health commissioners.

What type of formal training did "illustrious" administrators have before assuming their posts? In 1977, findings from a study[9] of 20 prominent psychiatric administrators concluded that

> as a group the individuals did not learn their work from formal sources, either course work or books on administration. . . . Most . . . did not receive formal training to prepare them for their work as chairmen, deans, commissioners, or directors of major mental health programs. . . . All of them recognized that they learned primarily by doing.

The determinants leading to careers in administration for these illustrious psychiatric administrators included "enjoyment in running things," expressed often in their earlier lives in leadership positions in Boy Scouts, high school, or college activities. Some simply offered themselves for work they felt had to be done. A number came from families with strong social consciences and concerns for the problems of the underprivileged. Military service played a significant role; some of the subjects, during their military service, were assigned to administrative jobs and eventually learned to enjoy the experience. Some came to administration because of a sense of dissatisfaction with private practice—they felt they were limited in the help they could provide the few patients they treated.

An important factor in the lives of many were teachers, role models, or mentors whom they met in medical school or in psychiatric training.[10] As one put it, the giants that were admired were often department chairmen whose lives were largely involved with administration. The researchers were also surprised, in questioning a large group of psychiatrists (an average of nine years out of training) who eventually took up careers in administration, at how many (80%) indicated that a prominent if not critical role in their lives was played by senior administrators whom they had adopted as mentors early in their careers. To quote from an article out of the business world, entitled "Everyone Who Makes It Has a Mentor,"[11] in which chief executive officers of large and successful companies were studied, one said:

> I don't know that anyone has ever succeeded in any business without having some unselfish sponsorship or mentorship. . . . We've all been helped. For some the help comes with more warmth than for others, and with some it is done with some forethought, but most people who succeed in a business will remember fondly individuals who helped them in their early days.

What are the requirements of a good administrator? Are the skills innate, or can they be learned? What varieties of administrative styles or techniques can be identified, and what information is available on efficacy of specific leadership styles?

Personality is certainly essential to success, but what kind of personality? The older literature[12] has called attention to imagination, courage, and ability to work with a variety of people—some at peer level, some superior, and some subordinate. High energy and drive, robust health, maturity, intelligence, flexibility, creativity, steadfastness, and tough-mindedness are all extolled. Many other traits could be mentioned. The critical problem here is, however, that we are not enlightened as to exactly when and how to utilize each trait or to what degree. Further, how do these traits work together in proper harmony and effectiveness under challenge situations? A simple listing of traits is therefore not very helpful. Indeed, I suspect that good administrators may come in a wide variety of personality packages.

Katz[13] has directed efforts away from identifying personality traits of the ideal executive toward the more useful question: What observable *skills* does an effective executive need? He identified three basic interrelated skills—technical, human, and conceptual.

Technical skills are concerned primarily with information and with specific knowledge and ability to work with "things." *Human skills* refer to the executive's ability to work effectively as a group member and to build cooperative effort. Such skills imply that the individual is aware of his own attitudes, assets, and limitations, and can create an atmosphere of security and approval. Subordinates feel they can participate without fear or censure, and thus enrich the climate of mutuality and creativity. *Conceptual skills* involve the ability to see the enterprise in its entirety, the interdependence of its parts, and the relationship of the individual business to the community as a whole. At lower levels of the organization, technical skills and human skills are of primary importance; at top levels of management, conceptual skills become essential. Katz's contribution lies in his conviction that these skills *can be learned,* although endowment and aptitudes do make a difference. He recommends case examples with impromptu role-playing as one approach to improving human skills. Coaching of subordinates, trading jobs, and study of specific complex management situations can assist in the development of conceptual skills.

In all this, it is important that the leader learn how others perceive him. He will find a surprising difference between how he views himself and how others view him. Indeed, such revelations may be both critical and threatening, calling upon his tolerance of his own inadequacies, and upon his ability to modify his behavior. This kind of learning is never easy and never to be neglected, for understanding and tolerance of the other's point of view are essential to cooperation and teamwork.

One of the skills that is particularly stressed by some consultants is skill in listening to people. After the average person has listened to some talk, he remembers only about half, and thereafter there is a rapid decline in material recalled. Yet it can be shown that through training and practice, the amount recalled can be greatly increased. "In general, people feel that concentration while listening is a greater problem than concentration during any other form of personal communication."[14] Because we think at high speed and the spoken word proceeds at usually only about 125 words per minute, a severe gap develops that requires forced concentration. If the speaker is not discussing something in a way that rivets our attention, our acrobatic minds tend to wander and lose the sense of what is said.

A good listener thinks ahead of the talker, weighs what is being said as support of an idea or point of view, periodically summarizes the points made, and in particular, "listens between the lines"[15]—that is, he gets cues that add meaning or modify what is being said.

Most difficult is to *hear the person out,* for the normal, almost reflex tendency of a person is to jump in with comments, questions, advice, and counsel. The withholding of interpretations is for most people a difficult task, for the tendency is to "project" onto what the speaker is saying our own interpretations reflecting our own needs. Thus, if the speaker is saying something in opposition to our own ideas, our tendency is to oppose him, however gently we formulate our demurrers. Or if the speaker is saying something that is directly critical—or is even construed as potentially critical—one rises to one's own defense according to traditional habits developed over a lifetime. Thus, communication is dominated by projections of the personality, by transference forces rather than objective listening with concern for how we can help the other person. Clearly, good listening requires a thorough understanding of oneself, something that cannot always be achieved without help from a psychologically sophisticated person. Without good listening, the flow of communications is either shut off, distorted, or shaped to serve irrelevant needs and purposes.

But there is another subtle problem that has to do with the nature of the multiple messages that the speaker brings to the discourse. The messages contain not only what the words per se convey, offered apparently in impartial and objective fashion, but perhaps also a great deal more. In a sense, there are messages behind the messages—several levels of meaning may be communicated at once. For example, a speaker is evaluating the performance of a subordinate working in his area. Does he also then somehow convey hostility against that person, or contrariwise, his affection? Is he inserting a message from some other person in the organization into his supposed independent evaluation of another? Or is he presenting his message in a form designed to win favor with the listener?

Thus, normal interchanges may carry information on several levels—some overt and some covert, some conscious and some unconscious. In this sense, the art and science of administration embraces all the mechanisms and interactions that are normally played out over longer periods of time in the psychotherapist's consulting room.

In their recent provocative book, *Leaders: The Strategies for Taking Charge,* Bennis and Nanus[16] summarize their study of 90 executives from a variety of occupations. They see power as a basic energy needed to initiate and sustain action. Leadership is the wise use of power; it gives an organization its vision, which is then translated into reality. Leadership should be differentiated from management. Management conducts the daily affairs; leaders concern themselves with basic purposes and directions. Leaders are vision oriented, attending to the growing edge of the organization.

Successful leaders have strong views of where the organization should go; they give undeviated attention to their goals, and they "burn" with high intensity. The leaders convey a "compelling image of a desired state of affairs—the kind of image that induces enthusiasm and commitment in others" (Mary Parker Follett[17] referred to this as the power of ideals). Further, the leader not only makes his position known, but also presents a stable set of coordinates over time, which promotes a feeling of his reliability and predictability and evokes trust.

Bennis and Nanus make a great deal of the trait of persistence, apparently prominently mentioned by their subjects as one of the necessary keys to success. In this regard, a cogent quote from Calvin Coolidge[18] is worth noting:

> Nothing in the world can take the place of persistence. Talent will not; nothing is more common than unsuccessful men with great talent. Genius will not; unrewarded genius is almost a proverb. Education will not; the world is full of educated derelicts. Persistence, determination alone are omnipotent.

THE MULTIPLE ROLES OF LEADERS

Just as leaders are endowed with multiple talents, so in the course of their tenure do they fill multiple roles—managerial and executive roles; paternal or avuncular roles; judicial roles; roles as teachers, scholars, and researchers; social roles; and community roles. We have seen that the *managerial and executive roles* pertain to the operations of the organization on a day-to-day basis, and to the planning and implementation of change, growth, and fulfillment of organizational mission.

The *paternal or avuncular role* of the administrator flows naturally from the tendency of employees to project their feelings about authority onto the person with seniority and power. A sensitive administrator feels this and knows that the nature, form, and intensity of the identification varies with the individual. It is the natural result of their early life and upbringing and tells a story about early family relationships.

For some employees, the transference is positive, warm, and loyal. For others, it is complicated by unresolved hostility, anger, and suspiciousness. Experience in hiring employees teaches us that if the prospective employee has had a pleasant and satisfying relationship with his parents, his transference is likely to be of the first type. If his relationship with his parents has been negative and hostile—and particularly if he has projected this onto society—then let the administrator beware.

In turn, the paternal and/or avuncular qualities that the administrator exudes are highly meaningful to his subordinates. They play a primary role in determining the morale and affective climate within the institution. They also become known outside the institution and influence the desirability of a job in his facility and the kinds of people who are attracted.

Judicial functions are exercised when fine judgments have to be made in areas of values, ethics, and morality. What should be done about the formerly excellent worker who comes to work with alcohol on his breath and whose performance is deteriorating? To what extent should the organization bend itself to help him out of his dilemma? To what extent should the organization donate its resources to his medical and psychological diagnosis and treatment? What is the organization's responsibility to promote political action on behalf of workers' welfare? In negotiating with labor, how much should the organization concede to the union's pleas for worker welfare where such may interfere with management prerogatives?

The leader's role as *teacher, scholar, and researcher* arises from the necessity to inform and educate himself and his staff as to the care and treatment of patients and the changing goals and functions of the institution. Intellectual growth is a vital moral value in any human group; certainly, no dullard can be a leader. The many problems that present themselves to the administrator require clear conceptualization, the gathering and analysis of data, and then implementation calling on the skills and abilities of others. Independent critical thinking is a sine qua non, for otherwise the leader becomes overly dependent on other minds.

The *social role* is ubiquitous. Not only is the leader's behavior often a standard for employee deportment, but in the long run, his values system tends also to affect the whole institution. In this sense, Emerson[19] tapped a great truth when he said, "The institution is the lengthened shadow of the man." Crudely put, if the leader has had four wives, his subordinates may be influenced to regard marriage as less than eternal. If the leader shows great interest in the extrainstitutional lives of employees; if he notes with pride those who have won honors or distinctions in extramural or civic activities, sends flowers at funerals, rejoices at marriages, and shows compassionate understanding during times of sickness or bereavement—his humanity will sooner or later influence the whole organization. The leader's more formal social role in parties, celebrations, and other honorific occasions may also influence morale and loyalty significantly.

The leader's *community role* arises from the fact that he is viewed as the organization's figurehead, the boss of its programs. Inevitably, he is asked to explain what the organization is doing, to defend its goals, and to show how services to the people warrant their continued confidence and support. If he employs a large number of individuals and thus adds significantly to the prosperity of the community, he is viewed in a positive light as a supporter of the community's welfare. He must try to mold the community's image of his institution and put himself out to cultivate goodwill and improve that image.

Important communications to the public are often through the media. Here, public relations and communication skills are tested. Openness of communication and the ability to translate intramural activities into simple language, and to achieve and develop a reputation for honesty and integrity, are the essential requirements of good public relations.

ADMINISTRATIVE STYLES

Administrative styles vary with personality; there may be as many styles as there are personalities. Indeed, administrative styles are often characterized by terms usually employed to describe personalities. Thus, one hears of authoritarian styles of administration, for which the opposite would be egalitarian styles. There are dynamic-aggressive leaders, and then those who are mild-mannered, soft, and "non-pushy." Imperial and autocratic may be opposed to democratic, and intimate versus aloof, controlling versus laissez-faire, seductive or "favoritistic" versus even-handed, and anxious versus unflappable.

A dichotomy of administrative style proposed by Kotin and Sharaf[20] (1967) is that of "tight" versus "loose" style, which they applied both to individual psychology and to organizational leadership. In tight organizations, authority and hierarchy are clearly defined, information flows mostly downward through written communications, role boundaries are carefully delineated, and role functions are spelled out through precise job descriptions. In loose style, the opposite is true: Authority and hierarchy are downplayed, communications are personal and verbal, and upward communication is encouraged. Job descriptions are not cast in cement. Most students believe that the loose type of administrative style is conducive to successful patient care and treatment, because it allows freedom of expression, rewards initiative, and encourages creativity.

Still other styles have been characterized as "win over" versus "take over." The former applies to the executive who bides his time (before taking definitive new actions to change a system) until he has won the confidence of a sufficient number of people to be assured that his programs will be accepted. Patiently, he cultivates goodwill, trust, and mutual regard. As confidence and security spread, he then cultivates the group's interest in moving ahead with new ideas, always keeping change within the capacity of the groups' tolerance. The "take over" executive, on the other hand, comes in with a prepared agenda, often shared first with his own lieutenants; together they announce and then implement the agenda, making sweeping changes in the old system—perhaps without sufficient consultation in depth, or satisfactory participation of organizational members.

PERSONAL FACTORS RELATED TO ADMINISTRATIVE PERFORMANCE

Personal factors affecting administrative performance may be considered under three headings: (a) motivation, (b) health and welfare, and (c) psychodynamic.

Motivational factors that play a critical role in administrative performance include the administrator's personal goals that led him to accept the job in the first place. Is it a promotion, a lateral slide, or a downgrading? Is he thinking of a short-term or a long-term commitment? Is it a temporary resting place until something better comes along, merely a stepping stone to other employment? Is this job a dead end, or can it lead to something better? Is his family satisfied? The salary adequate? The task suitable to his skills? Finally, is the administrator totally dependent on this job, or does he have an outside income?

Health and welfare factors, too, are critical. Many administrative jobs require a very high degree of energy output, long hours, and responsibility that can take a toll on personal health and on family life. Some administrators drink too much for their own good, and some may live beyond their means. Administrators are not immune to separations and divorces, nor to illnesses of any types. As age advances, illness tends to be more frequent and severe, recovery more prolonged. How well is the office staff trained to navigate through a period of his disability?

Several significant studies[21,22,23,24,25,26,27] have been made about physical and mental impairment of people in power, the most striking of which recount stories of presidents, prime ministers, or other high officials whose disabilities threatened the stability or even the existence of nations. In our country's history, we can note that Grover Cleveland was secretly operated upon for mouth cancer; Woodrow Wilson suffered a severe paralysis the last 18 months of his tenure that forced the nation's business into the hands of his wife and secretary; Franklin Delano Roosevelt's hypertension and cardiac disease played a historic role during the fateful negotiations in Yalta with Stalin and Churchill; Dwight Eisenhower was hospitalized for regional ileitis, coronary thrombosis, and stroke; and John Fitzgerald Kennedy's Addison's disease and back problems caused much pain and suffering during his brief term in office.

Perhaps even more important are the "lesser" forms of disturbances—the character defects that corrupted the administrations of Warren Gamaliel Harding and Richard Nixon, and the paranoid fixations of Adolf Hitler that brought the world to disaster. When we consider the physical and emotional vulnerability of our leaders today, who hold nuclear power at their fingertips and the fate of the world in their hands, we have cause to shudder.

Perhaps the most baffling problem arises from the operation of subtle character traits that prove inimical to the welfare of both leader and organization. This is the problem of warped character or unresolved neurotic conflicts whose effects become enormously exaggerated when played out in the organizational arena. Men who seek power often have suffered badly from deprivations or abuses of childhood; in their mature years, the organizations they head may pay the price in destructive management.

Thus, the man with bright ideas and ingenious schemes but who never follows through may be the one whose home life was so unsatisfactory that he kept himself busy rushing from one extramural activity to another, his frenetic cleverness a futile attempt to make up for isolation and emotional emptiness.[28] Or again, the boss who is unsure of his authority and anxious to please everyone may be threatened and overauthoritative when differences of opinion arise, yet often overagreeable when discussing problems with an associate. When the next person comes in with an opposite but equally convincing story, he may change his views, throwing his organization into confusion. This unfortunate administrator may have been reared by cold, controlling parents who set him apart from his juvenile confreres and convinced him he was destined to be great. He missed the give-and-take of life with youthful equals that might have taught him to tolerate differences. His double hunger for superiority and for affection undermines the organization's need for a stable, wise, and consistent policy. A final example is the executive reared in a spartan tradition with the model of a father who succeeded against great physical odds. He is full of suppressed rage at a younger brother, who got favors not granted him by throwing tantrums so violent that their sick mother catered to his whims. This executive could not abide anyone whom he considered self-centered or demanding, or who had difficulty with the spartan rules he promulgated.

Such examples, quoted by Cohen and Cohen in their admirable paper,[29] could be multiplied many times. The reader may have had similar experiences with coworkers whose characteristics and styles of working with others have impressed him as odd and made him speculate what conflicts lay behind the odd behavior. After long contact, one may learn of life experiences that molded that person; not infrequently, such insights allow one to be more tolerant of the other's peculiarities. The further development of the science of management is likely to progress along the lines of understanding in greater psychodynamic depth the assets, liabilities, motivations, and conflicts that shape management styles. Thus, the behavioral science approach to understanding both pathologic and healthy leaders opens a wide field for further development of management science.

Case Illustration

The Judicial Role of the Administrator

A young psychiatrist, who is relied on heavily to bolster the emergency room team, is accused of stealing 12 Dilaudid tablets. When the loss of the tablets is discovered, the administrative nurse on duty calls on security. They start an investigation by quizzing the suspect and then asking for urine and blood tests—

which he refuses. The administrative nurse says, "His pupils were dilated, and he was staring." Further, it is reported that when a staff nurse on duty talked to this particular doctor in the medication room, he stated he was there to get Cogentin for a patient with extrapyramidal syndrome. The staff nurses do submit to blood and urine tests, which are negative.

However, the doctor's performance in the emergency room—where he serves as a casual, as-needed employee—has been satisfactory. He is a highly intelligent and effective worker who says he enjoys the job and wants to stay on, hoping eventually to find a permanent position in the hospital.

All parties were astonished when next morning 12 Dilaudids appeared on the counter of the medication room. No one knew how they got there. To this strange turn of events was added the fact that the administrative nurse's observations about dilated pupils did not withstand critical scrutiny: (1) First, Dilaudid intake is known to cause pupillary constriction, not dilatation; (2) second, the doctor in question was known to "stare" whenever faced with a problem that riveted his attention. The case against the doctor was beginning to collapse. Should the investigations, therefore, be abandoned?

Comment

Of the multiple roles of the administrator, his judicial role is in many ways the most exacting. As he exercises it in appointment, promotions, hiring, and firing, he is deciding issues of life-and-death significance to his employees. He is often in conflict between empathy toward the subject and his loyalties to patient welfare, hospital staff, and hospital goals. Ethics, law, and rules and regulations interplay here in subtle ways. Through such decisions, he establishes his reputation for fairness versus poor judgment and earns, or perhaps loses, respect.

Outcome

In this case, nothing was actually found to incriminate the young doctor. Meanwhile, a petition supporting him as a man of integrity and professional ability, signed by his coworkers, was circulated. The academic head of the emergency service made a personal call pleading for his vindication. Finally, after detailed consultation with administration, it was decided to restore the doctor to his former status, without prejudice.

STRESSES AND STRAINS OF ADMINISTRATION

This section on administrative stresses and strains describes attitudes and feelings of experienced administrators, and gives potential administrators a glimpse into what may lie ahead.

It is no secret that stresses and strains on administrators are numerous and severe; as Truman said, "The buck stops here." In the last analysis, the top administrator has to make final decisions, often with the certain knowledge that some people will be angry and disaffected and will try in various ways to gain redress. Much as he may have consulted experts and tried to foresee the ultimate consequences of his acts, the future is often unclear. A primary complaint, therefore, is, that the administrator's job is a lonely one. One must possess the fortitude and inner strength to make tough decisions, to stand by them, and to accept the consequences, however unpopular they may be. Especially where the job is in the political arena, unpopular decisions may shake the job security of the executive himself. Political appointees are among the most vulnerable of public servants. It is well to know and understand those parties whom one must satisfy to maintain one's tenure; on the other hand, one should not be so dependent on the job that one is afraid to leave it.

Another common complaint is that the physical and mental demands are very great. Unless one is very well prepared for an executive role, overwhelming burdens suddenly descend upon assumption of that role. In our studies of 109 ex-commissioners of mental health[30] and of 18 "sitting" commissioners,[31] my collaborators and I found that sudden elevation from an academic or clinical role to the commissioner's post was often too great an adaptation. The heightened responsibility, increased work load, and demands for quick decision in a system where new information, new relationships, and new values must be quickly integrated can be too much. Acute high vulnerability—and high visibility, too—can be unsettling. Further, there are many watchdogs in the new system who believe they know the rules better than the incumbent, and who want to see to it that things are done "right."

For those transferring from a university/academic setting into a job such as commissioner, the loss of students, research activities, and the relaxed university environment may be regretted. In addition, work overload, excessive demands on time, and the necessity of being up-to-the-minute on loads of new information and always ready to take charge requires each day a high degree of alertness. The job drains one's energies, with consequent fatigue and exhaustion. Under such circumstances, resilience and rapid recuperation from frustrations become necessary qualities for survival. Significantly mentioned also by respondents in the commissioner study are the strains on family ties, which reflexly augment the effects of job stresses.

The constituents to be served in a commissioner's type of job include, first, the governor or other designated appointing body. Since tenure is usually dependent on the goodwill of the appointing authority, his expectations are very important. Then come the legislators, the attorney general, and the support apparatus that surrounds them. Next, the mental health service organization (of which the administrator is the head) must be made effective and efficient, or the administrator loses clout with everyone.

It should be pointed out that a state's mental health organization may be very large, indeed. In Massachusetts, for example, with a population of 5.5 million, the mental health organization (1967–1973) included a total of 17,000 to 18,000 workers, of whom approximately 300 were assigned to the central department. Also, the number of patients served by such an organization may be very large; in Massachusetts (1972), approximately 72,000 patients were served annually. The large size of a state mental health organization and its multiple functions may, indeed, boggle the mind of the novice.

Other constituents that can never be neglected include (a) citizen organizations supporting mental health, the press and other media, and the professional organizations representing different groups of workers (i.e., psychiatry, nursing, psychology, social work, rehabilitation, pastoral counseling, and legal counseling). The goodwill of labor organizations, too, that work aggressively on behalf of both professional and nonprofessional groups is vital to organizational effectiveness, for they possess the powerful tools of job actions and the strike.

Finally, a small but most important constituency—the constituency often overlooked in formal analysis of the executive role—is the executive's own family. I have remarked that the stresses and strains may take a toll on family life. More important than the fact of the executive's frequent absences from the domestic scene is the effect of his public life per se upon his family. For example, if he is criticized publicly in the press or other media, how does this impact upon the morale and occupational/educational life of his wife and children? In their circle of friends and acquaintances, do the family members find themselves defending the public performance of the administrator? Do people try to influence the administrator through pressure on his family? One vital ethical issue here is: How far does the executive allow his job to affect the lives and careers of his family members? This ethical problem has rarely been studied, although its manifestations are often visible in the life of any person who is constantly in the public eye.

As Galbraith[32] has remarked, the more important, central, and powerful the position, the more constraints are imposed upon it. Chief among these are budgetary constraints, but any and all agencies may exert influence. In recent years, budgets have become more and more limiting, leading to curtailments in staff and services and limitations on research and innovation. Under these conditions, disappointment and frustration of service providers and their constituents are inevitable. When budgets expanded, as in the 1960s and early 1970s, the administrator was happily engaged in planning, recruiting, and experimenting with new modalities and services. In periods of funding cutbacks, it is hard to maintain morale, including the morale of the administrator who employs the surgical knife and, therefore, is often seen as the villain.

> The demands are made . . . on all sides, said one executive. "You are blamed for things not under your control. I would brood, lie awake at night thinking about them, the frustrations of my goals."[33]

Another executive, a state commissioner, reacted to his limitations as follows:

> You have 1,000 patients. Should you take care of 100 patients well, and neglect 900, or should you take care of the 1,000 and neglect them all a

little bit? Do you aggressively treat the patients with the best prognosis—
the 100—and horribly neglect the others? That's what I did and I was
never satisfied with it.[34]

Limitations on funds, criticisms from multiple sources—many sensible,
but often impossible to implement—and the political cross fires can cause a
serious erosion of reputation and morale of the top officer. It is impossible to
keep all supplicants happy; thus, in a sense the job is undoable. As an increasing number of individuals or groups become disaffected, hostility projected upward may give rise to a clamor for the administrator's head. In an
essentially political/administrative job, excellence as an executive may not be
sufficient to counteract political embarrassment to the appointing authority.
This means that someone higher up who fears a loss of votes may go so far as
to sacrifice a department head primarily to appease noisy insurgents.

An important feature of a high-level administrative position is concern
about life after the heady but hard job. Is there a market for an ex-commis-
sioner, somewhat battered around the edges and a bit rusty as a clinician or
teacher; or is the commissioner's job a dead end? Fortunately, we have research bearing on this point that answers the question.[35] There *is* life after
commissionership, and some former commissioners even yearn for a return
to the stressful but exciting job they may have left with some regret.

REWARDS

Athough the stresses of an executive position (such as a commissionership) may be great, the rewards are nevertheless substantial. These
rewards include the opportunity to serve large numbers of people in need,
using resources often larger than ever commanded before. This looks good to
many professionals who have spent long hours with only a very few patients.
With this new vista of command comes a greatly enlarged perspective over
the field of mental health, a broadening of concepts and goals, and a fuller
appreciation of the many points of view dominant in the field—points of view
that must be properly blended to ensure effective action.

Anyone hungering for intellectual stimulation and new challenges for
action will immediately find enough to fill every spare minute. The learning
curve ascends rapidly. Personal growth is gratifying, and personal contacts
with new people—many outside the parochial bounds of the mental health
network—are most stimulating. As one executive put it:

There are the prestigious rewards. . . . You're in the papers. You have
dinner with the governor and a justice of the supreme court. You feel you
are a change agent. . . . It is very heady.[36]

One learns much about power—how to wield it subtly and effectively,
without antagonizing people, and with respect for the checks and balances
that always accompany power bestowed. Many watchdogs scrutinize one's
behavior, measuring it against standards of efficiency and integrity. One ap-

preciates as never before the meaning of accountability in the use of public funds. A very important lesson relates to the slow pace of change of large organizations, and the necessity for patience and forbearance before substantial changes can be achieved.

Power brings with it centrality in the arena of action, and heavy involvement in public functions, many of which are honorific. Often, hours away from the office load of work are spent reluctantly, knowing that what is not done during the day must be done at night.

One feature of such jobs that I think rightfully belongs in the category of rewards is the privilege of working with large, complex organizations dedicated to helping the individual client. Mary Parker Follett[37] has made the important point that our very future as a civilization depends on learning how large organizations can best serve the individual man or woman.

For the leader of an organization, the hope is that he will keep the health and welfare of the mentally ill before the public and elevate its importance in the consciousness of the body politic. Another is that the leader will vigorously represent the causes of the poor, minorities, and disenfranchised among the priorities established by the government. And still another is that he will be a guardian of the cherished values of the health profession—that is, the freedom to care for the patient consistent with professional ideals and training, and to teach and do research in the best climate possible.

As an example, in one state, the attorney general decided to control the way research was conducted by requiring that all projects be approved by a state committee appointed by himself. This was at a time when universities were under fire for conducting controlled investigations that allegedly withheld potentially therapeutic drugs from patients. There was also at this time an uproar about carrying out studies on children in the schools, which one investigator proposed to do based on a carefully drawn protocol, approved by the National Institute of Mental Health and generously funded.

After much discussion with the attorney general, pointing out the redundancy of his committee with that already required by federal granting agencies, he withdrew his proposal, but unfortunately not before support for the study of children in the schools ran out due to the procrastinations based on bureaucratic meddling.

REDUCTION OF ADMINISTRATIVE STRESS

Job stress relates to length of service on the job and to turnover rates. In our study of ex-commissioners,[38] we found that the average length of service of commissioners for all the states (in the years 1960–1981)—*excluding* acting commissioners and current sitting commissioners—was 4.3 years. Average length of service *including* acting commissioners (but excluding current commissioners) was 3.5 years. Since it takes many months, even years, for a director to know his job and to exert effective leadership, this record of tenure is not comforting. At the same time, the average length of service of acting commissioners was 0.8 years. Thus, a commissioner hardly gets going when he passes the reins of command to an acting person with much shorter tenure, who because of his acting status conducts to a large extent a holding operation, with its limited ability to meet job demands.

Why did commissioners leave their jobs? The major reasons given were "had enough," "political pressures," and "attractive new offer." Only a few left because of the formal end of an appointment, appointment co-terminus with the governor, or retirement. Clearly, stresses in office made the difference in their tenure.

In view of the above, it is surprising how little attention has been focused on reduction of administrative stress for these important figures who handle billions of the taxpayers' dollars and shoulder responsibility for the lives of many sick people.

How can administrative stress be reduced? I suggest the following:*

1. *Greater emphasis on preparation for the job.* Of 109 commissioners polled,[40] 78 (or 71.5%) did *not* have the American Psychiatric Association certification in mental health administration. That examination is intensive, covering a wide range of subjects, and most candidates study seriously before the ordeal. Is this type of preparation advantageous? Unfortunately, although many examinations have been given, we have no follow-up information on whether those who pass suffer less stress and strain or do a better job than those who flunk.

More important, perhaps, than a paper-and-pencil (or even oral) examination would be the opportunity to learn from observation of executives who have spent years in the saddle, with discussion of their styles of management and ways of handling tensions. In addition, regular consultation and supervision by a successful manager would go far to alleviate stress. Repeated review of problems in a relaxed, objective environment will also promote perspective in situations that evoke disruptive emotions. An astute supervisor would be able to point out where and how the new executive had personally participated in creating the trouble he was in. It is interesting to note here that, in a residency training program, the young psychiatrist receives many hours of supervision in his treatment of an individual patient; but years later, when he takes on a large task running a system responsible for a great many patients, supervision is practically totally neglected.

2. *Brief sabbaticals at selected or prescribed intervals.* Burnout is a hazard when an executive has endured too many stresses over too long a time, or when health is impaired, or when recovery from a routine infection (such as upper respiratory) is unusually slow, or when an added burden from family complications has made him distractible, lowered his morale, or slowed his attention, grasp, and ability to make decisions. Under such conditions, relief

*See Administrative Psychiatry, by M. Greenblatt,[39] especially the section on Reduction of Administrative Stress, p 2453.

from the day-to-day grind is indicated. The executive must have a good deputy in whom he has confidence to take command in his absence, and he must have the privilege of staying out as long as it takes to recover and to recharge his batteries. Such time out will allow for an objective reappraisal of his interest and suitability to carry on. In this task, it is often advisable to consult either an experienced administrator or a wise therapist.

3. *Cross-visiting*.[41,42] In cross-visiting, one executive spends time with an executive in another system whose job is analogous to his own. The very problems faced by an administrator in one system may also be faced by his counterpart in another; yet, surprisingly, what seems almost unsolvable in one situation may be handled with relative ease in another. Innovative programs and projects will be demonstrated in one system that may be applicable, perhaps in modified form, in another. Then there is the sharing of attitudes and affects, the development of valuable friendships, and the cross-consultation and advice that are both learning experiences and morale builders. Cross-visiting reduces the sense of isolation, enhances esteem, and encourages new perspectives on old issues.

4. *Change of role and responsibility.* In the Department of Veterans Affairs, the public health system, and in large businesses with a network of branches, personnel are moved from one unit to another—sometimes at the same level, sometimes upward, and sometimes downward. In the VA, with its 172 hospitals directed from a central department in Washington, D.C., an administrator having trouble in one institution may be moved temporarily to Washington, then moved again to another hospital either at the same or another level. For example, one administrator who got in trouble in an urban hospital that boasted rich teaching and research activities and strong university affiliation was transferred to a distant smaller hospital without academic connections—obviously a downgrading. In these large organizations, such moves may entail uprooting a family and establishing social and educational contacts in a new environment, but that is the practice that the executive employee accepts as a part of his career with such an organization.

A change of role viewed as a promotion acts like a shot in the arm. Although the new position may provide a new set of challenges—and even stresses—many old stresses are left behind with considerable relief. A shift to another environment although the job remains essentially the same may also be invigorating, as again it presents a new scene, different colleagues, and new interpersonal relationships.

What is often difficult to arrange is true interchangeability of roles at the executive level. For example, I considered interchanging superintendents of hospitals with the hope of increasing the learning curves, or just "stirring things up" for superintendents who had become entrenched in their jobs. Some superintendents adapted willingly to the new system: They took on new challenges, became area directors, and also supervised development of community resources in a given catchment area. Others were slow and resistant to change. It was my thought that by interchanging jobs, the resistant director could learn from the accomplishments of a more progressive director, while the latter might teach personnel in the slow hospital how to make the desired changes.

Unfortunately, the necessity to alter the laws of appointment made the plan difficult (but not necessarily unfeasible). I still think it has merit and should be tried.

5. *Organizations and associations of administrators.* In recent years, the following organizations and associations of administrators have come into being:

American Association of Chairmen of Departments of Psychiatry
American Association of Community Mental Health Center Psychiatrists
American Association of Directors of Psychiatric Residency Training
American Association of General Hospital Psychiatrists
American Association of Psychiatric Administrators
American Association of Veterans Affairs Chiefs of Psychiatry
American College of Hospital Administration
American College of Mental Health Administration
Association of Hospital Superintendents

These societies are valuable media for education, exchange of ideas, and renewal of interest and appetite for work. Presentation of research and discussions of changing practices in the field are invaluable assets in keeping abreast of the times.

At the American Psychiatric Association annual meetings, numerous exercises on administration are offered (in the 1989 annual meeting in San Francisco, 2 major lectures, 4 Social Security symposia, and 12 workshops), and at the annual Hospital and Community Psychiatry Institute, as well as at professional meetings of nurses, social workers, occupational therapists, and librarians (not to mention psychiatrists), administrative problems are also discussed.

6. *Academic involvement.* Administrative jobs, even the most demanding, need not take the individual completely away from academe. In Massachusetts, assistant commissioners were accepted into the faculty of the Harvard, Tufts, and Boston University medical schools. Social workers, nurses, and psychologists were also appointed to appropriate academic departments, where they taught students and joined in academic life; an offer of academic contact with one's basic discipline made recruitment easier. Mental health department personnel thus brought state and nationwide perspectives into the classroom, teaching how statewide systems of service were organized to deliver care and treatment to the individual client, and how these systems depended on social/political/economic factors not always explicated fully in the university classroom.

One commissioner of my acquaintance managed to spend a day a week doing research in his electroencephalographic laboratory. A head of a university-affiliated department of psychiatry managed to develop a vigorous ethological laboratory that attracted trainees from several disciplines, some of whom went on to successful research careers. Administration, then, is not counterpoised to academic life, but continues the same—viewing the field from another, sometimes broader perspective. Double appointments that integrate the decision/action component of organizational leadership with the intellectual stimulation of academe can balance the life of executives and reduce stress.

WHAT LIES AHEAD?

A common concern of those who occupy high-level executive positions in the public sector, we learned from the study of former commissioners, was that the job might be a dead end and their value to their profession might be seriously diminished. Reestablishing a practice, or returning to academe, or finding an interesting position in another organization were the primary concerns. In looking forward to finding new employment, our commissioners felt that they might not be helped by their psychiatric society or its district branches, for during their commissionerships, they had received little support from those directions. However, there appeared to be little cause for alarm, as Table 12-1[43] shows.

Of 24 commissioners who wanted jobs in public administration, 22 landed the kind of job they wanted (92%). Similarly good luck obtained for those who wanted to go into private practice, or desired to be public officials (nonadministrative), or wanted to go into private administration. Only those seeking academic jobs were somewhat disappointed—although here, too, 65% succeeded in obtaining academic posts. We can conclude then, that a high executive position is not a dead end, and that the experience gained in such a setting is valued in other settings.

Table 12.1. Jobs Desired and Jobs Obtained by 68 Former Commissioners of State Departments of Mental Health

Type of job	Number who wanted job	Number who obtained job they wanted	
		Number	Percentage
Nonacademic	51	46	90[a]
Public administration	24	22	92
Private practice	10	9	90
Public official	9	8	89
Private administration	8	7	88
Academic	17	11	65[a]
Total	68	57	84

[a]Desired nonacademic jobs were obtained significantly more often than desired academic jobs:$X^2 = 5$, $df = 1$, $p < .05$. From "After commissioner, what?," by M. Greenblatt, K.D. Gaver, and E. Sherwood, *American Journal of Psychiatry, 142*, 752–754, 1985. Copyright 1985, the American Psychiatric Association. Reprinted with permission.

One phenomenon that appeared after the termination of commissionership was a strong sense of loss of power and of centrality in the arena of action, of having fewer supports, and of the apparent necessity to begin all over again. Along with this appeared symptoms of depression. This syndrome we called *decompression,* for it occurred at the point of change from the high-pressure job to one of low pressure, lower status, and low demand (see Chapter 4).

The relationship between decompression and satisfaction in new jobs varied as follows:

1. Those who felt a high degree of decompression after leaving commissionerships found little satisfaction in the new jobs they obtained, and vice versa, those with low manifestations of decompression found a higher degree of satisfaction in jobs they obtained after commissionership.
2. Those with high decompression feelings were more willing to serve again in the commissioner's role than those with low decompression feelings.
3. Those with higher ratings of satisfaction in their new jobs were, in general, less interested in serving again as commissioner than those with lower satisfaction ratings.

We can conclude that there is little foundation for the fear that executive life, for the psychiatrist, is a dead end. Indeed, most found the kind of jobs they wanted. Finally, it appears that administrative experience, although often stressful to be sure, nevertheless adds dimensions of leadership, perspective, challenge, and responsibility not found to the same degree in many other careers.

SUMMARY AND COMMENTS

A strong argument can be made that in any phase of the psychiatrist's career, administrative abilities are needed—whether it be managing a case involving several members of a multidisciplinary team, taking charge of a ward, organizing a teaching program, heading up a day-care program or an outpatient service, or moving up to become head of a facility. Very little is taught in medical school about administration, and in postgraduate education it is often not a formal supervised part of the training program. Many find it a regrettable fact that top leadership of mental health facilities has shifted markedly from psychiatry to nonmedical administrators in recent years.

What does the job of administrator offer the mental health professional? He attains a broader view of the field, hones a new set of skills, and understands social/political/economic realities better in relation to the challenge of improving the lot of a large number of patients.

What do psychiatrists bring to the executive role? A comprehensive view of the patient as a biosocial psychological entity, the Aesculapian authority that goes with the role of doctor, competence in handling crises, understanding of interpersonal dynamics and group processes, and familiarity with hard work and heavy responsibility.

Studies of high-level psychiatric administrators reveal a lack of formal training, but previous practical experience with a diverse number of federal, state, or county jobs. In their earlier lives, they were leaders in school or college, enjoyed running things, and were dissatisfied with individual practice. Many were strongly influenced by mentors coming from the field of administration.

Skills required for leadership may be classified as technical, human, and conceptual; the ability to listen objectively is also a high desideratum. Fortunately, these skills can be learned. Leaders also function in multiple roles, which include managerial/executive roles, paternal or avuncular roles, judicial and social roles, and roles as teachers, scholars, and researchers. A special role is that of spokesman and representative of the institution to the community.

Stresses and strains are indigenous to the job of administrator. It can be a lonely responsibility. Physical and mental demands are great. Many constituencies have to be served, and strains on family life may be acute. Resources may be limited, and one is subject to criticism and sometimes political embarrassment.

To balance these negatives, it must be asserted that rewards can be very gratifying: the opportunity to serve large numbers of clients, broadening of goals and concepts, intellectual stimulation, centrality in the arena of action, use of power, and the privilege of functioning as guardian of the cherished values of the health profession.

Administrative stress can be reduced by better preparation for the job, supervision by an experienced leader, brief sabbaticals, visiting and conferring with other leaders, role interchange with other executives, membership in organizations of administrators, and academic involvement.

Finally, administration is not a dead end. In the study of psychiatric commissioners, it was found that the large majority landed the kind of jobs they wanted after retiring from the commissioner role. Clearly, the experience gained in the commissioner role was valued in other settings.

REFERENCES

1. National Institute of Mental Health: Mental Health Directory. Rockville, Maryland, National Institute of Mental Health, 1971
2. National Association of State Mental Health Program Directors, Washington, D.C.: Data for 1981 received in personal communication.
3. Greenblatt M, Rose SO: Illustrious psychiatric administrators. Amer J Psychiatry 134:626–630, 1977
4. Gaver KD, Norman ML, Greenblatt, M: Life at the state summit: Views and experiences of 18 psychiatric leaders. Hosp & Comm Psychiatry 35:233–238, 1984

5. Greenblatt M, Gaver KD, Sherwood E: After commissioner, what? Amer J Psychiatry 142:752–754, 1985
6. Greenblatt M, Sherwood E: Leadership in mental health, in Pressley LC, Donald, AG (eds), A Symposium on Public Psychiatry in Honor of William S. Hall, M.D. Supplementary Volume to the Psychiatric Forum. Columbia, South Carolina, William S. Hall Psychiatric Institute, 1987, pp 30–37
7. Greenblatt M: Stresses and rewards of administrative life, with some "wise" recommendations, in Liberman RP, Yager J (eds): Stress in Psychiatry (Festschrift volume in honor of Ransom Arthur). (submitted for publication)
8. Gaver KD, Norman, ML, Greenblatt, M: Life at the state summit: Views and experiences of 18 psychiatric leaders. Hosp & Comm Psychiatry 35:233–238, 1984
9. Greenblatt M, Rose SO: Illustrious psychiatric administrators. Amer J Psychiatry 134:626–630, 1977
10. Greenblatt M, Sherwood E, Pasnau, RO: Psychiatric residency, role models, and leadership. Amer J Psychiatry 143:764–767, 1986
11. Perkins DS: From interviews conducted by EGC Collins and P Scott with FJ Lunding, GL Clements, and DS Perkins, in Everyone who makes it has a mentor. Reprinted from Harvard Business Review, July-August 1978, Number 78403, in Harvard Business Review: Paths Toward Personal Progress: Leaders Are Made, Not Born. Cambridge, Mass., President and Fellows of Harvard College, 1983
12. Barton WE: Vanishing American—mental hospital administrators and commissioners. Ment Hosp 13:55–61, 1962
13. Katz RL: Skills of an effective administrator. Reprinted from Harvard Business Review, September-October 1974, Number 74509, in Harvard Business Review: Paths Toward Personal Progress: Leaders Are Made, Not Born. Cambridge, Mass., President and Fellows of Harvard College, 1983
14. Nichols RG, Stevens LA: Listening to people. Reprinted from Harvard Business Review, September-October 1957, Number 57507, in Harvard Business Review: Paths Toward Personal Progress: Leaders Are Made, Not Born. Cambridge, Mass., President and Fellows of Harvard College, 1983
15. Nichols RG, Stevens LA: Listening to people. Reprinted from Harvard Business Review, September-October 1957, Number 57507, in Harvard Business Review: Paths Toward Personal Progress: Leaders Are Made, Not Born. Cambridge, Mass., President and Fellows of Harvard College, 1983
16. Bennis W, Nanus B: Leaders: The Strategies for Taking Charge. New York, Harper & Row, 1985
17. Follett MP: Power, in Metcalf HC, Urwick L (eds): Dynamic Administration: The Collected Papers of Mary Parker Follett. New York, Harper & Bros., 1942
18. Coolidge, C: In statement distributed to agents of New York Life Insurance Co.; according to LE Wikander, Curator, Calvin Coolidge Memorial Room, Forbes Library, Northampton, Mass., in a letter to Abigail Van Buren (Dear Abby), Los Angeles Times, July 22, 1990, p. E4
19. Emerson RW: Self-reliance, in Emerson RW: Essays and English Traits. New York, PF Collier & Son, 1909
20. Kotin J, Sharaf, MR: Management succession and administrative style. Psychiatry 30:237–248, 1967
21. L'Etang H: The Pathology of Leadership. London, Heinemann, 1969. See also L'Etang H: Fit to Lead. London, Heinemann, 1980; L'Etang H: Facing disability. Nursing Times 67:1122–1123, 1971; L'Etang H: Diseases, Decision Makers, and Doctors. Transaction Studies, College of Physicians, Philadelphia 40:30–38, 1972
22. Rogow AA: James Forrestal: A Study of Personality, Politics and Policy. New York, Macmillan, 1963
23. George AL, George JL: Woodrow Wilson and Colonel House. A Personality Study. New York, Dover 1986
24. Wilson TW: A Psychological Study: Sigmund Freud and William C. Bullett. Boston, Houghton Mifflin, 1967
25. Fabricant ND: 13 Famous Patients. Philadelphia, Chilton, 1960
26. Barach AL: Franklin Roosevelt's illness. NY State J Med 2154–2157, 1977
27. Group for the Advancement of Psychiatry, Committee on Governmental Agencies: The VIP with Psychiatric Impairment. New York, Group for the Advancement of Psychiatry, Report No. 83, January 1973

28. Cohen MB, Cohen RA: Personality as a factor in administrative decisions. Psychiatry 14:47–53, 1951
29. Cohen MB, Cohen RA: Personality as a factor in administrative decisions. Psychiatry 14:47–53, 1951
30. Sherwood E, Greenblatt M: Stresses, supports and job satisfactions of psychiatrist executives. Admin in Mental Health 15:47–57, 1987
31. Gaver KD, Norman ML, Greenblatt M: Life at the summit: Views and experiences of 18 psychiatric leaders. Hosp & Comm Psychiatry 35:233–238, 1984
32. Galbraith JK: The Anatomy of Power. Boston, Houghton Mifflin, 1983
33. Greenblatt M, Rose SO: Illustrious psychiatric administrators. Amer J Psychiatry 134:626–630, 1977
34. Greenblatt M, Rose SO: Illustrious psychiatric administrators. Amer J Psychiatry 134:626–630, 1977
35. Greenblatt M, Gaver KD, Sherwood E: After commissioner, what? Amer J Psychiatry 142:752–754, 1985
36. Greenblatt M, Sherwood E: Leadership in mental health, in Pressley LC, Donald, AG (eds): A Symposium on Public Psychiatry in Honor of William S. Hall, M.D. Supplementary Volume to the Psychiatric Forum. Columbia, South Carolina, William S. Hall Psychiatric Institute, 1987, pp 30–37
37. Follett MP: Power, in Metcalf HC, Urwick L (eds): Dynamic Administration: The Collected Papers of Mary Parker Follett. New York, Harper & Bros., 1942
38. Greenblatt M, Sherwood E: Leadership in mental health, in Pressley LC, Donald, AG (eds): A Symposium on Public Psychiatry in Honor of William S. Hall, M.D. Supplementary Volume to the Psychiatric Forum. Columbia, South Carolina, William S. Hall Psychiatric Institute, 1987, pp 30–37
39. See Greenblatt M: Administrative psychiatry, Chapter 51 in Freedman AM, Kaplan HI, Sadock B (eds), Comprehensive Textbook of Psychiatry. Baltimore, Maryland, Williams & Wilkins, 1975, pp 2443–2454, esp. p 2453
40. Greenblatt M, Gaver KD, Norman M: Psychiatric leadership: The paths to the summit: The risks and the rewards. Presented at American College of Mental Health Administration Annual Meeting, October 30–November 1, 1983, St. Petersburg Beach, Florida (unpublished manuscript)
41. Greenblatt M: Administrative psychiatry, Chapter 51 in Freedman AM, Kaplan HI, Sadock B (eds), Comprehensive Textbook of Psychiatry/II. Baltimore, Williams & Wilkins, 1975, pp 2443–2454, esp. p 2453
42. Greenblatt M: Administrative psychiatry, Chapter 51 in Freedman AM, Kaplan HI, Sadock B (eds): Comprehensive Textbook of Psychiatry/II. Baltimore, Williams & Wilkins, 1975, p 2453
43. Greenblatt M, Gaver KD, Sherwood E: After commissioner, what? Amer J Psychiatry 142:752–754, 1985

Index

Abortion, 216
Absenteeism, 32–33, 140–141, 142
Accountability, 29, 73
Accreditation, by Joint Commission on Accreditation of Healthcare Organizations, 5–6, 187, 295–297
  withdrawal of, 288
Acquired immune deficiency syndrome (AIDS), 146, 231–233, 245
Acquired immune deficiency syndrome-related complex (ARC), 146, 232
Administration, diversity of, 2–4
Administrative styles, 3, 345
Administrator, psychiatric, 337–360. *See also* Leader; Leadership
  academic involvement, 355–356
  administrative styles, 3, 345
  advocacy by, 352
  appointment of, 85–86. *See also* Management succession
  burnout, 353–354
  clinical experience, 258
  cross-visiting by, 354
  delegation of work by, 58
  family, 350
  health, 259
  leadership potential, 257–258
  nonpsychiatrist administrators vs., 110–111, 113
  open-door policy of, 156–157
  personality, 3, 346–348
  professional advantages, 338–339

Administrator, psychiatric (*cont.*)
  professional career, 356–357
  professional certification, 260, 353
  professional disadvantages, 338
  professional organizations, 355
  relationship with politicians, 285–286
  research study of, 339–343
  rewards of, 351–352
  role(s), 259
    multiple, 343–345
  role changes, 354–355
  role conflicts and ambiguities, 40
  sabbaticals, 353–354
  skills, 258–259, 340–343
  specialization, 256
  stresses of, 348–351, 358
    reduction of, 352–356, 358
Advertising
  by physicians, 217–218
  by private hospitals, 178
  professional, 182–184
  as revenue-increasing technique, 201–203
Advocacy, of administrators, 352
Agencies, administrators' interaction with, 90
Aggression, 137
AIDS. *See* Acquired immune deficiency syndrome
Aims, organizational, 65
Albert Einstein College of Medicine, 261
Alcohol abuse, incidence, 191
American Association of Chairmen of Departments of Psychiatry, 355